Handbook of Nutrition, Diet and the Eye

Handbook of Nutrition, Diet and the Eye

Editor: Kenya Salley

AMERICAN
MEDICAL PUBLISHERS
www.americanmedicalpublishers.com

AMERICAN
MEDICAL PUBLISHERS
www.americanmedicalpublishers.com

Cataloging-in-Publication Data

Handbook of nutrition, diet and the eye / edited by Kenya Salley.
p. cm.
Includes bibliographical references and index.
ISBN 978-1-63927-686-8
1. Eye--Diseases--Nutritional aspects. 2. Eye--Diseases--Diet therapy.
3. Diet in disease. 4. Nutrition. I. Salley, Kenya.
RE48 .H36 2023
617.7--dc23

American Medical Publishers,
41 Flatbush Avenue,
1st Floor, New York,
NY 11217, USA

ISBN 978-1-63927-686-8 (Hardback)

Contents

Preface VII

Chapter 1 **Resveratrol Based Oral Nutritional Supplement Produces Long-Term Beneficial Effects on Structure and Visual Function in Human Patients** 1
Stuart Richer, Shana Patel, Shivani Sockanathan, Lawrence J. Ulanski II, Luke Miller and Carla Podella

Chapter 2 **Retina, Retinol, Retinal and the Natural History of Vitamin A as a Light Sensor** 18
Ming Zhong, Riki Kawaguchi, Miki Kassai and Hui Sun

Chapter 3 **Dietary Sources of Lutein and Zeaxanthin Carotenoids and their Role in Eye Health** 46
El-Sayed M. Abdel-Aal, Humayoun Akhtar, Khalid Zaheer and Rashida Ali

Chapter 4 **Observation of Human Retinal Remodeling in Octogenarians with a Resveratrol Based Nutritional Supplement** 63
Stuart Richer, William Stiles, Lawrence Ulanski, Donn Carroll and Carla Podella

Chapter 5 **Vitamin A Derivatives as Treatment Options for Retinal Degenerative Diseases** 80
Lindsay Perusek and Tadao Maeda

Chapter 6 **Diminishing Risk for Age-Related Macular Degeneration with Nutrition** 101
Molly Schleicher, Karen Weikel, Caren Garber and Allen Taylor

Chapter 7 **Effects of Lutein and Docosahexaenoic Acid Supplementation on Macular Pigment Optical Density** 153
Alfredo García-Layana, Sergio Recalde, Angel Salinas Alamán and Patricia Fernández Robredo

Chapter 8 **Eye Nutrition in Context: Mechanisms, Implementation and Future Directions** 162
Barbara Demmig-Adams and Robert B. Adams

Chapter 9 **The Relationship between Lutein and Zeaxanthin Status and Body Fat** 181
Emily R. Bovier, Richard D. Lewis and Billy R. Hammond Jr.

Chapter 10 **Retinal Spectral Domain Optical Coherence Tomography in Early Atrophic Age-Related Macular Degeneration (AMD) and a New Metric for Objective Evaluation of the Efficacy of Ocular Nutrition** 189
Stuart Richer, Jane Cho, William Stiles, Marc Levin, James S. Wrobel, Michael Sinai and Carla Thomas

Chapter 11 **The Role of Lutein in Eye-Related Disease** 205
Keyvan Koushan, Raluca Rusovici, Wenhua Li, Lee R. Ferguson and Kakarla V. Chalam

Chapter 12 **Macular Pigment and its Contribution to Vision** 222
Ekaterina Loskutova, John Nolan, Alan Howard and Stephen Beatty

Permissions

List of Contributors

Index

Preface

The eyes are the sensory organs which gather light from the surroundings and transform it into nerve impulses. These signals are sent by the optic nerve to the brain, which interprets them to produce an image and enables sight. Vision and overall eye health can be enhanced by including minerals, vitamins and antioxidants in the diet. Zeaxanthin, lutein, vitamin E, vitamin C and zinc are some of the nutrients that are good for the eyes. These nutrients can help lower the chance of developing significant eye diseases, including cataracts and age-related macular degeneration. Most people can obtain all the nutrients they need for eye health by eating a varied diet that is rich in vegetables, fruits and lean meats. Some of the nutrient rich foods which are good for eye health are nuts, legumes, citrus fruits, carrots, beef, fish, seeds, leafy green vegetables and eggs. This book provides significant information to help develop a good understanding of the relationship between diet, nutrition and the eye. It presents researches and studies performed by experts across the globe. The extensive content of this book provides the readers with a thorough understanding of the subject.

Various studies have approached the subject by analyzing it with a single perspective, but the present book provides diverse methodologies and techniques to address this field. This book contains theories and applications needed for understanding the subject from different perspectives. The aim is to keep the readers informed about the progresses in the field; therefore, the contributions were carefully examined to compile novel researches by specialists from across the globe.

Indeed, the job of the editor is the most crucial and challenging in compiling all chapters into a single book. In the end, I would extend my sincere thanks to the chapter authors for their profound work. I am also thankful for the support provided by my family and colleagues during the compilation of this book.

Editor

1

Resveratrol Based Oral Nutritional Supplement Produces Long-Term Beneficial Effects on Structure and Visual Function in Human Patients

Stuart Richer [1,2,3,*], Shana Patel [3], Shivani Sockanathan [3], Lawrence J. Ulanski II [1,2], Luke Miller [3] and Carla Podella [1]

[1] Eye Clinic 112e, Captain James A Lovell Federal Health Care Center, 3001 Green Bay Rd., North Chicago, IL 60064, USA; E-Mail: larry.ulanski@gmail.com (L.J.U.); cjpstella63@gmail.com (C.P.)

[2] University of Illinois Eye and Ear Infirmary, University of Illinois at Chicago, Chicago, IL 60612, USA; E-Mail: Lulanski@uic.edu

[3] Chicago Medical School, Rosalind Franklin University of Medicine and Science, 3333 Green Bay Rd., North Chicago, IL 60064, USA; E-Mails: shana.patel@my.rfums.org (S.P.); shivani.sockanathan@my.rfums.org (S.S.); luke.miller@my.rfums.org (L.M.)

* Author to whom correspondence should be addressed; E-Mail: stuart.richer1@va.gov

---

Abstract: Background: Longevinex® (L/RV) is a low dose hormetic over-the-counter (OTC) oral resveratrol (RV) based matrix of red wine solids, vitamin D_3 and inositol hexaphosphate (IP6) with established bioavailability, safety, and short-term efficacy against the earliest signs of human atherosclerosis, murine cardiac reperfusion injury, clinical retinal neovascularization, and stem cell survival. We previously reported our short-term findings for dry and wet age-related macular degeneration (AMD) patients. Today we report long term (two to three year) clinical efficacy. Methods: We treated three patients including a patient with an AMD treatment resistant variant (polypoidal retinal vasculature disease). We evaluated two clinical measures of ocular structure (fundus autofluorescent imaging and spectral domain optical coherence extended depth choroidal imaging) and qualitatively appraised changes in macular pigment volume. We further evaluated three clinical measures of visual function (Snellen visual acuity, contrast sensitivity, and glare recovery to a cone photo-stress stimulus). Results: We observed broad bilateral improvements in ocular structure and function over a long time period, opposite to what might be expected due to aging and the natural progression of the patient's pathophysiology. No side effects were observed. Conclusions: These three cases demonstrate that application of epigenetics has long-term efficacy against AMD retinal disease, when the retinal specialist has exhausted other therapeutic modalities.

Keywords: epigenetics; visual structure and function; resveratrol; Longevinex®; age-related macular degeneration; ophthalmology

---

1. Introduction

There is emerging interest in applying epigenetics to the field of ophthalmology, ocular health status, function, and disease(s). Epigenetic modification using small molecular weight nutrients has been discussed in cancer and heart disease, suggesting a potential for cardio-protection against ischemia-reperfusion injuries [1]. However, there remains a dearth of publications applying epigenetics to clinical ophthalmology. There are fewer than a hundred accumulated published articles on PubMed concerning epigenetic regulatory mechanisms and ocular development, health, and diseases.

Epigenetics involves modifications of genetic material that does not impact DNA nucleotide sequences. The complex epigenome results in gene expression and/or gene silencing. While classical genetics concerns itself with inherited mutations (*i.e.*, nucleotide substitutions, omissions), epigenetics involves the variable protein expression that facilitates cellular adaptability, enhancing stem cell survival, and tissue regeneration as manifested through the three specific mechanisms:

(1) DNA methylation, the addition of a methyl group (M) to the DNA base cytosine (C) from folate (B_9) and B_{12}, is most active during embryogenesis and early childhood.

(2) Histone modification include protein spools that control gene expression by winding or unwinding DNA strands around histone bodies by such natural/dietary histone deacetylase (HDAC) inhibitors as sulforaphane in cruciferous vegetables, diallyl disulfide in garlic, nigella sativa in black cumin seed oil, and resveratrol (RV) in red wine.

(3) MicroRNA, short 22 base pair strands of RNA that mesh with messenger RNA, silences a segment of genes during translation. Therefore, microRNAs block the protein-making ability of gene(s). MicroRNA is called the "guiding hand of the human genome" [2].

Significantly, these processes are controlled by environmental cues such as temperature, radiation, oxygen deprivation, food or food deprivation, (the latter doubling the healthspan and lifespan of lab animals as first demonstrated by Clive McCay in the 1930s) [3], as well as provision of small molecular weight molecules in nutrients, such as allicin (garlic) and RV (red wine).

Epigenetic mechanisms have great potential to improve the status and function of ocular tissue. Age-related macular degeneration (AMD) is one of the leading causes of progressive and irreversible vision loss in Western societies. AMD can progress typically from dry (non-exudative) to wet (exudative) form, where the wet form is often visually catastrophic. AMD is distinguished from genetically inherited forms of retinal disease such as Leber's and Stargardt's hereditary retinal dystrophies. This multifactorial aging disorder involves a combination of aging, polygenetic susceptibility genes, and myriad environmental factors, such as smoking and obesity. Epigenetic modifications of the genome modulate this phenotypical variability [4].

RV, a non-flavonoid polyphenol phytoalexin toxin, is produced in response to infection in plants, such as *Vitis vinifera* (a grape) when cultivated in stressful conditions, such as cold or lack of light (*i.e.*, northern altitudes) [5]. This small molecule (molecular weight 228 Daltons) enters all cells, does not need to be nanosized, and acts as a dietary histone deacetylase inhibitor, altering the winding and modulating protective pathways against oxidative stress, DNA damage, excitotoxicity, apoptosis, and inflammation. The activity of RV has been linked to cell-surface receptors, membrane signaling pathways, intracellular signal-transduction machinery, nuclear receptors, gene transcription, and metabolic pathways [6]. RV has germane ophthalmologic biological actions, which include anti-angiogenesis activity and choroidal vasorelaxation [7]. Numerous animal studies have demonstrated that this polyphenol holds promise against numerous age-associated diseases including cancer, diabetes, Alzheimer, and cardiovascular and pulmonary diseases [5].

Short-term anti-neovascular effects of Longevinex (L/RV), a resveratrol-containing supplement, on AMD patients have been published [8], and further mechanistic validation of RVs' suppression of VEGF by human RPE cells has recently been published [9]. We present our clinical experience in the clinic over a multi-year period.

2. Experimental Section

2.1. Selecting an Oral OTC-RV AMD Supplement with Established Bioavailability and Short-Term Efficacy

There is a false concern over RVs' short half-life (minutes) and its lack of bioavailability. Rapid conjugation with glucuronate and sulfate during hepatic detoxification dramatically extending its half-life to 9 h rather than minutes [10]. Generic RV can be photo-isomerized from *trans* to *cis* RV by exposure to ultraviolet radiation. For these reasons we selected a commercially available brand of resveratrol that had been stabilized via microencapsulation and tested and shown to work superiorly to plain resveratrol and has undergone toxicity testing [11]. L/RV, an OTC oral RV-based supplement, contains microencapsulated/microionized RV and a blend of red wine polyphenols, primarily quercetin, along with vitamin D_3, and inositol hexaphosphate (IP6). The process of microencapsulation and miconization of *trans*-RV enhances RV stability to light, heat, and oxygen, while micronization drastically increases blood concentration, lifespan, and epigenetic biological potency.

Studies have shown that quercetin enhances the immediate bioavailability of RV (RV makes more passes through the liver before complete metabolization). Vitamin D_3 controls a variety of genes involved in innate immunity, inflammation, and vascular calcification and has recently emerged as an important nutrient (prohormone) against AMD [12,13]. IP6 (inositol hexaphosphate) from rice bran is nature's divalent mineral binder (*i.e.*, iron and copper) and replaces the need for phlebotomy or chelation, in diseases of iron mismanagement [14]. Multiple polyphenols, in general, and L/RV in particular, exhibit synergistic rather than just additive biological and epigenetic effects [15].

The published synergistic actions of L/RV itself, and/or reference to a component within L/RV, are found at Longevinex® [16], and extend well beyond RV to include:

(1) ↓ Inflammation (COX-2, CRP, TNF)
(2) ↓ HIF-1 and VEGF genes (microRNA 21, 20b, 539)
(3) ↑ Nrf2 endogenous antioxidants (glutathione, SOD, catalase) via the Nrf2 gene.
(4) ↓ Blood clotting (platelet stickiness)
(5) ↑ Vasodilation (nitric oxide)
(6) ↑ Metal chelation (copper)
(7) ↓ Oxidation, peroxidation (mega-dose increases oxidation)
(8) ↓ Cell adhesion (platelets, microbes, tumor)
(9) ↓ Calcification (*i.e.*, Bruch's membrane)
(10) ↓ Bacteria, viruses, fungi
(11) ↑ Kruppel-like factor 4 (KLF4) activities via RV and vitamin D_3, responsible for anti-VEGF therapy failure

Short-term L/RV anti-VEGF type improvements even in octogenarians with ocular pathology, was recently documented at our medical center [8]. L/RV acts as an anti-oxidant to reduce oxidative stress, and our group was also the first to show minimized lipofuscin epoxidation in an octogenarian AMD patient presumably by down-regulation of reactive oxygen species, sparing aging pigment epithelial cells from DNA damage and premature apoptosis, as well as promoting stem cell survival [17].

L/RV activates miRNA genes in murine models nine-fold greater than RV alone [18]. Through such effects, L/RV may outperform anti-VEGF monoclonal antibodies. This can be accomplished because L/RV addresses the known reason why anti-VEGF drugs fail (macrophage polarization via KLF4) and L/RV has superior down-regulation of miRNA 20b expression 1366 times [18] compared to plain RV. The miRNA 20b fragment controls the hypoxia-inducing factor-1 (HIF1) and the VEGF gene, decreasing VEGF to prevent choroidal neovascularization and angiogenesis in as little as one week [8]. This mechanism prevents the conversion from dry to wet AMD.

We have also clinically shown, using spectral domain OCT imaging, that L/RV targets and promotes RPE stem cells to regenerate within the living human eye of another octogenarian (88-year-old) AMD patient, over a 20-week period [19]. Unfortunately, large scale L/RV human clinical trials are lacking. However, a clinical trial in Japan, has demonstrated cardiovascular benefits of L/RV through improvements in endothelial function of adults with metabolic syndrome receiving standard treatment [20].

2.2. Dosage and Clinical Safety Considerations

RV characteristically exhibits a U or J shaped risk curve with hormetic low dose benefits and negative effects at high doses [1]. In rodents it is cardio-protective between 175 and 350 mg human equivalent dose (HED), and cytotoxic at 10-times higher doses between 1750 and 3500 mg HED, and a dose of 3500 mg RV was universally lethal to rat hearts [1]. A Glaxo Smith Kline phase 2 human clinical trial of RV in multiple myeloma patients was suspended in 2010 because several patients developed kidney failure at 5000 mg.

In contradistinction, L/RV has been shown to exhibit a biologically unique L-shaped risk curve and unparalleled margin of safety at high doses up to 2800 mg HED. This margin of safety is clearly superior to RV alone. L/RV passed toxicity testing, meeting the New Dietary Ingredient guidelines described by the FDA [11,21]. This dietary supplement exhibits good safety and the recommended dosage (one capsule per day) and has not produced major side effects among non-anemic subjects over a ten-year period of commercial use [16].

Veteran patients at the James A Lovell Federal Health Care Center, for whom other therapeutic measures had been exhausted (ARED and AREDS II supplements, anti-VEGF treatments, *etc.*), were prescribed one capsule containing low dose nutrients (100 mg *trans* RV) daily and followed clinically. L/RV was compassionately provided when no other options were available beyond the Vision Impairment Service Teams' low vision and blind-rehabilitation services.

2.3. Consent/IRB

An Investigational New Drug (IND) submission is not required to use a marketed product as a part of medical practice for individual patients. However, supervision was requested and approved by the Chief of Staff and IRB (Hines DVA, Chicago, IL, USA).

2.4. Participants

We compiled data from three male AMD patients who were on the L/RV matrix for multi-year periods using an enhanced clinical visual function protocol developed at our medical center [22].

1. Patient 1, a 64-year-old Caucasian glaucoma suspect with photophobia, atrophic AMD (worse right eye), and diabetes with declining vision function right eye, has been on L/RV for 2.5 years and is maintaining visual function.
2. Patient 2, an 89-year-old Caucasian with chronic kidney disease and cataracts, has been on L/RV for 3 years maintaining his visual function requirements to retain his driver's license.
3. Patient 3, a 67-year old Caucasian with bilateral Polypoidal Choroidal Vasculopathy (PCV), a treatment resistant AMD variant, worse right eye. He also has a history of central serous retinopathy above the right optic nerve and a left retinal central foveal photoreceptor integrity line defect and impaired color vision. Improved retinal/choroid structure was observed.

2.5. Methodology

Retina/choroid structure modalities:

1. Retinal Pigment Epithelium (RPE) Fundus Auto Fluorescence (FAF) images were obtained with Optos® 200Tx, (Optos PLC, Dunfermline, UK), a wide-field camera that images the ocular fundus using specialized laser light. It captures a 200-degree field in one image, as compared to standard cameras that image only 50 degrees, allowing for extended evaluation. FAF images were obtained in order to identify lipofuscin granule accumulation in the lysosomal compartment of RPE cells Lipofuscin, is a mixture of autofluorescent pigments that accumulates in the RPE as a byproduct from incomplete degradation of photoreceptor outer segment, and is associated with the disease progression in AMD and retinal disease.

2. Retinal Spectral Domain Optical Coherence Tomographic (SD OCT) images were obtained with an RTVue® instrument (OptoVue, Freemont, CA, USA). These images depict precisely aligned high-resolution *in vivo* histologic sagittal retinal cross sections as well as "extended-depth" choroidal vasculature cross-section images. The OCT highlights retinal alterations in morphology, structure and reflectivity, facilitating baseline and serial clinical evaluation of individual retinal layers. Using "extended depth SD-OCT" the choroid is visible. Choroid thickness decreases with age and even faster in AMD and glaucoma patients, suggestive of diminished choroidal perfusion at least partially responsible for a decline in visual function.
3. Visualized macular pigment volume imaged by ARIS® (Automated Retinal Imaging System) (Visual Pathways, Inc., Prescott, AZ, USA) that also depicts retinal layers by spectral separation. We employ the spectral (visible/IR) separation images for AMD patients because, compared to traditional fundus photographs, there is high sensitivity in identifying intra-retinal pathology (retinal drusen), the critical underlying blood supply underneath the retina (*i.e.*, the choroidal network that becomes less dense in AMD), as well as MPOD typically diminished in AMD. Traditional colored fundus photographs are also derived through wavelength recombination.

Visual function modalities:

1. Visual Acuity (VA—high contrast, high spatial frequency): The clinical best-refracted Snellen acuity was taken in a semi-darkened room using a digital Smart Systems® projection system (M and S Technologies, Skokie, IL, USA).
2. Contrast Sensitivity (CSF—all contrasts, all spatial frequencies): The contrast sensitivity function (CSF), a measure of how an eye sees large objects (low spatial frequencies at 1.5 and 3 cycles/degree) and small objects such as Snellen letters (higher spatial frequencies, *i.e.*, 18 cycles/degree)—*x* axis, at differing contrasts—*y* axis. The area under the curve of the resulting CSF at five spatial frequencies was measured with the validated instrument (Functional Vision Analyzer® (Stereo Optical, Chicago, IL, USA) with best refraction at each visit.
3. Glare Recovery (GR—in seconds): Photo-stress cone glare recovery in seconds to a bright flash that induces retinal-RPE dysfunction was measured with a validated clinical Macular Disease Detection MDD-2® macular adaptometer (Health Research Sciences, Lighthouse Point, FL, USA).

3. Results

Cases 1–3 present patients afflicted with AMD that have taken L/RV over a multi-year period. All other curative measures had been exhausted for these patients, or the patient was either refused intra-vitreal injections, treatment resistant, or classified as non-candidates by conventional retinal ophthalmologic evaluation.

Case 1: A 64-year-old patient with atrophic AMD and diabetes type 2 taking L/RV for 2.5 years. We observed diminishment of retinal lipofuscin, enhanced choroidal thickness (perfusion), qualitatively increased visualized macular pigment volume, CSF, and shortened GR time. Figure 1 depicts decreased RPE FAF over time reflecting lipofuscin resolution in both retinas. Figure 2 shows choroidal thickening, opposite of an expected age-related decline. Figure 3 depicts dramatic improvements in macular pigment volume with no change in carotenoid/omega-3 supplementation. These factors denote improved ocular structure. Figure 4 depicts better CSF and GR over time. Cardiovascular and serum parameters were also reviewed. We observed improvements in HbA1C, body mass index (BMI), blood pressure (BP), pulse, and pulse pressure (Table 1). The following measurements were taken during patient visits before L/RV use (n = 4 from 9/29/10 to 12/9/10) and patient visits after L/RV use (n = 16 from 2/25/11 to 6/12/13); A1C levels decreased by 0.36 mg%; BMI decreased by 1.87; systolic BP decreased by 13.37 mmHg and diastolic BP decreased by 2.69 mmHg; pulse decreased by 9.87 beats/min; pulse pressure decreased by 10.69 mmHg. The patient has been pleased with both his enhanced vision and improved cardiovascular health.

Figure 1. Wide field OPTOS® FAF images of lipofuscin within the neurosensory retina of a 64-year-old male patient with AMD and diabetes type 2. These images are original, untouched, and unaltered. Over time, there is a decrease in autofluorescence in both retinas signifying a decrease in lipofuscin accumulation. Image (*i.e.*, below, center, middle) includes the patient's eyelashes (artifact).

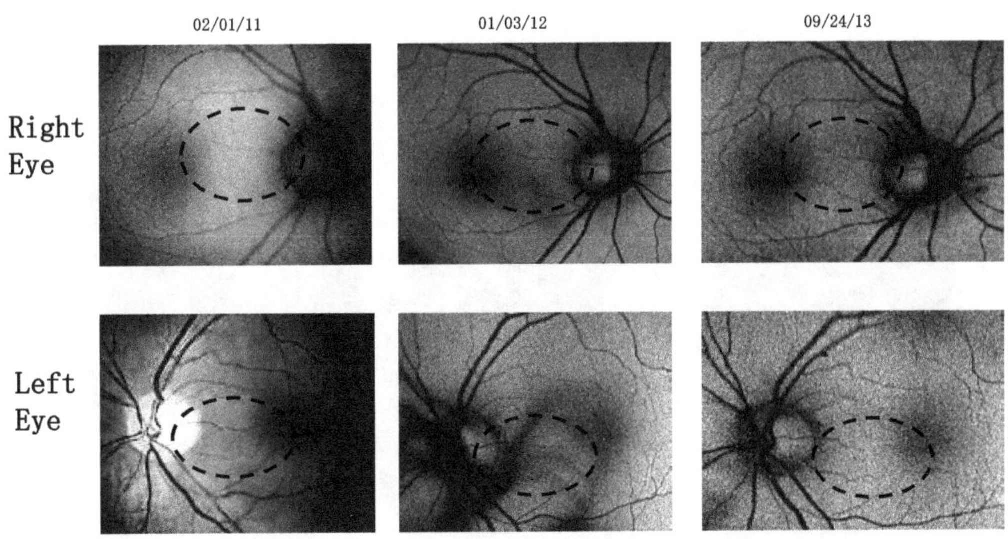

Figure 2. SDOCT "Extended Depth Imaging" of chorodal thickness (microns) of a 64-year-old male patient with AMD and diabetes type 2. Over time, approximately 2.5 years, there is an increase in choroid thickness in both retinas denoting better choroidal perfusion, which is opposite of the expected age-related trend.

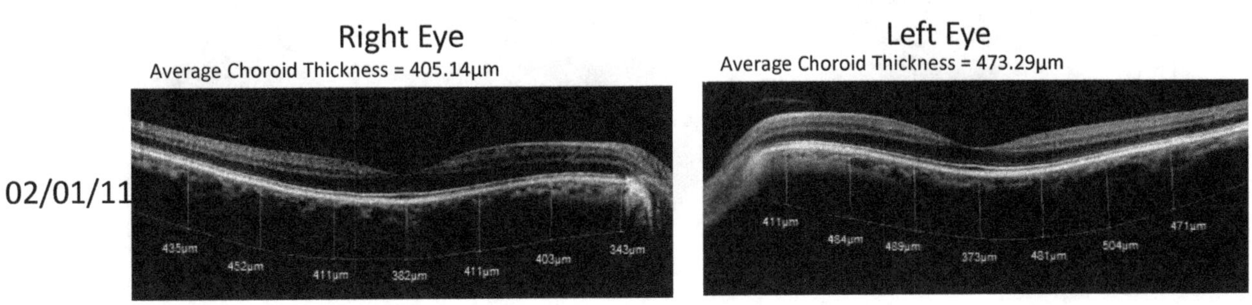

Figure 2. *Cont.*

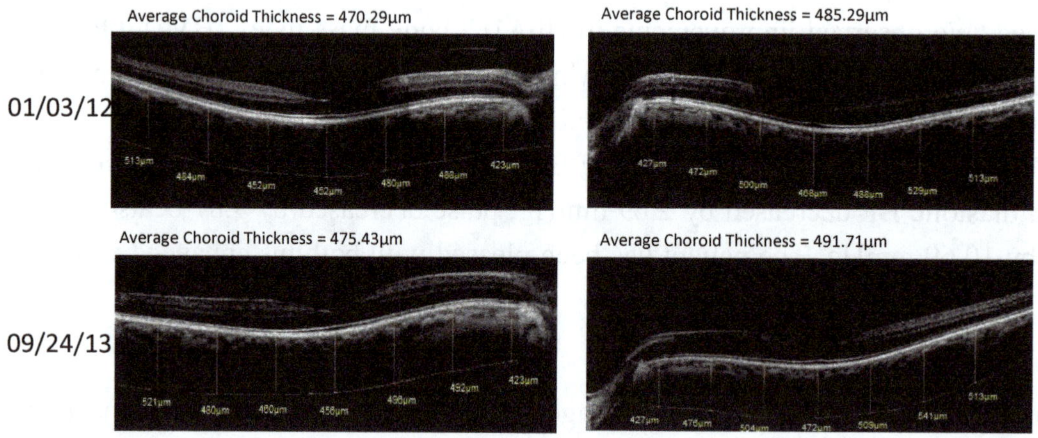

Figure 3. Visualized macular pigment volume of a 64-year-old male patient with AMD and diabetes type 2. With time, approximately 2.5 years, there is bilateral increased macular pigment with no change in reported dietary or supplemental carotenoid/omega-3 intake, an unusual clinical finding.

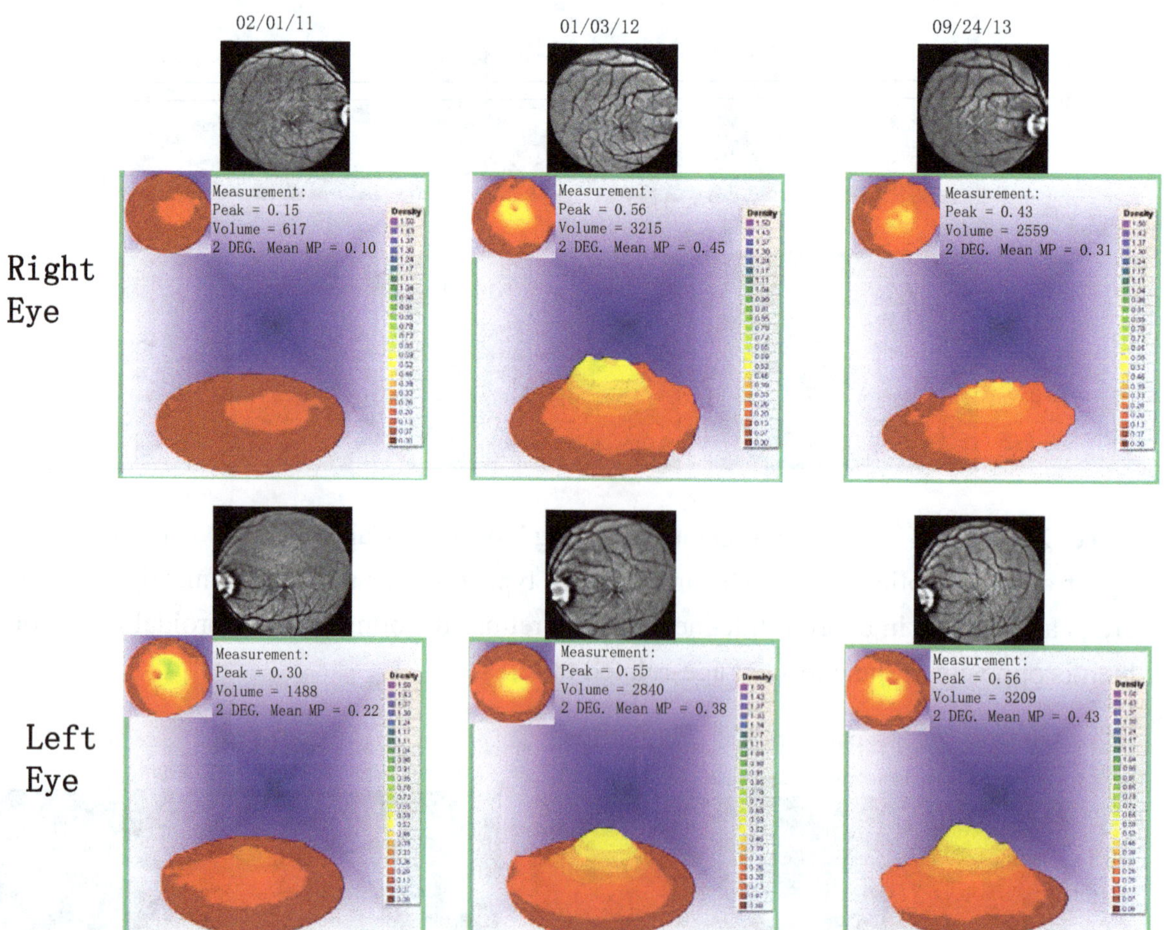

Figure 4. Contrast Sensitivity and Glare Recovery of a 64-year-old male patient with AMD and diabetes type 2. With time, approximately 2.5 years, comprehensive measures of visual function, such as contrast sensitivity, improve in both eyes while glare recovery to a photo stress stimulus improves in his left eye. This is opposite of the expected AMD related decline. Baseline Snellen visual acuity was 20/25 R, 20/20 L and further improved in the right eye to 20/20 by the second visit within one year.

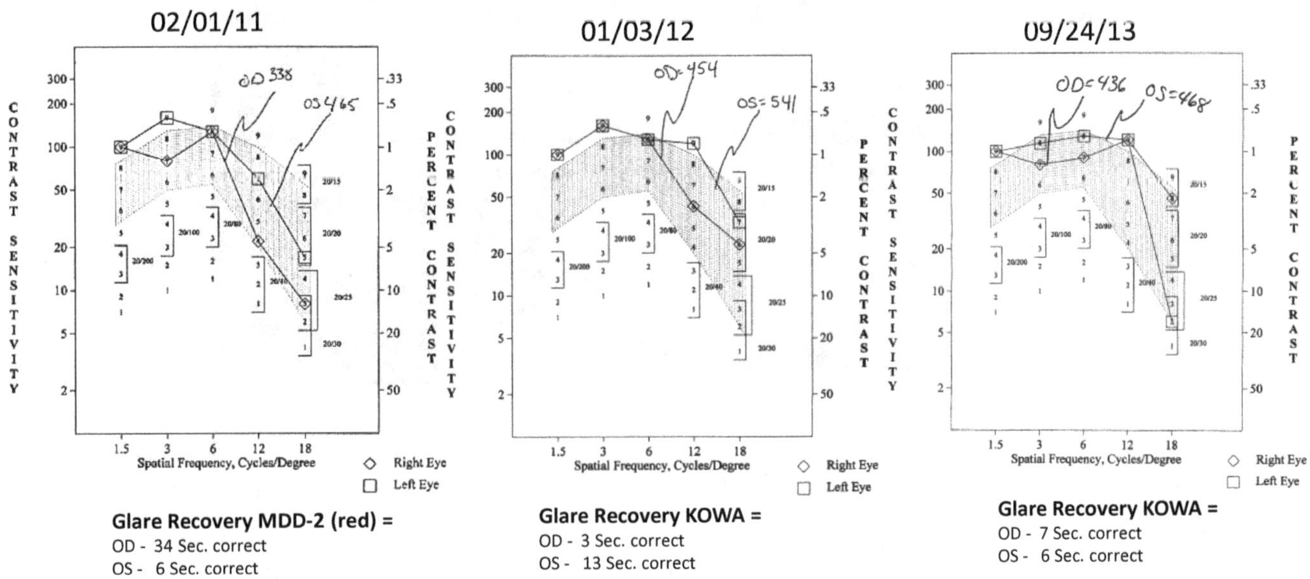

Table 1. Cardiovascular and serum parameters of a 64-year-old male patient with AMD and diabetes type 2. There are broad improvements over time in his HBA1c, BMI (body mass index), systolic, diastolic, pulse and pulse-pressure. Measurements were taken from his medical records months before starting L/RV and months following initiation of epigenetic therapy (see text for details).

Parameter	Average (SD) before Longevinex	Average (SD) While on Longevinex
A1C	6.43 (0.26)	6.07 (0.35)
BMI	35.75 (0.96)	33.88 (0.89)
BP-Systolic	129.50 (4.04)	116.13 (10.19)
BP-Diastolic	76.50 (8.02)	73.81 (6.28)
Pulse	96.50 (9.33)	86.63 (7.23)
Pulse-Pressure	53.00 (7.53)	42.31 (10.52)
RDW	12.42 (1.02)	13.95 (0.49)

Case 2: An 89-year-old Caucasian male with atrophic AMD who has been on L/RV for 2.5 years. We similarly observed a decrease in lipofuscin accumulation (Figure 5), an increase in choroidal thickness (Figure 6), stabilization of visualized macular pigment volume (Figure 7), stabilization of GR right eye, better GR left eye, and better CSF (Figure 8). The patient continues to maintain an unrestricted driver's license, despite his age and expected pathologic decline.

Figure 5. Wide field OPTOS FAF images of lipofuscin within the neurosensory retina of an 89-year-old male patient with AMD. Images of lipofuscin within broad geographic section of the retina is shown to diminish in intensity over time, especially within his left retina.

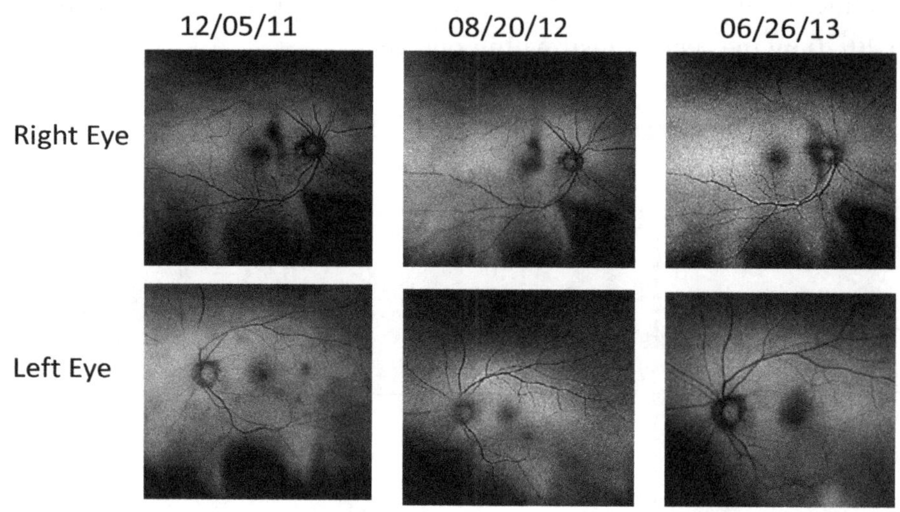

Figure 6. SDOCT "Extended Depth Imaging" of Choroidal Thickness (microns) of an 89-year-old male patient with AMD. With time, approximately 2.5 years, the difference from baseline is +24.4 um of additional right eye choroidal thickening, while the difference from baseline is even greater +34.3 um in the left eye. This represents additional choroidal thickening, well above the 5.0-micron axial resolution of the OptoVue RTVue® SD OCT. Better clinical perfusion of the posterior retina is surmised.

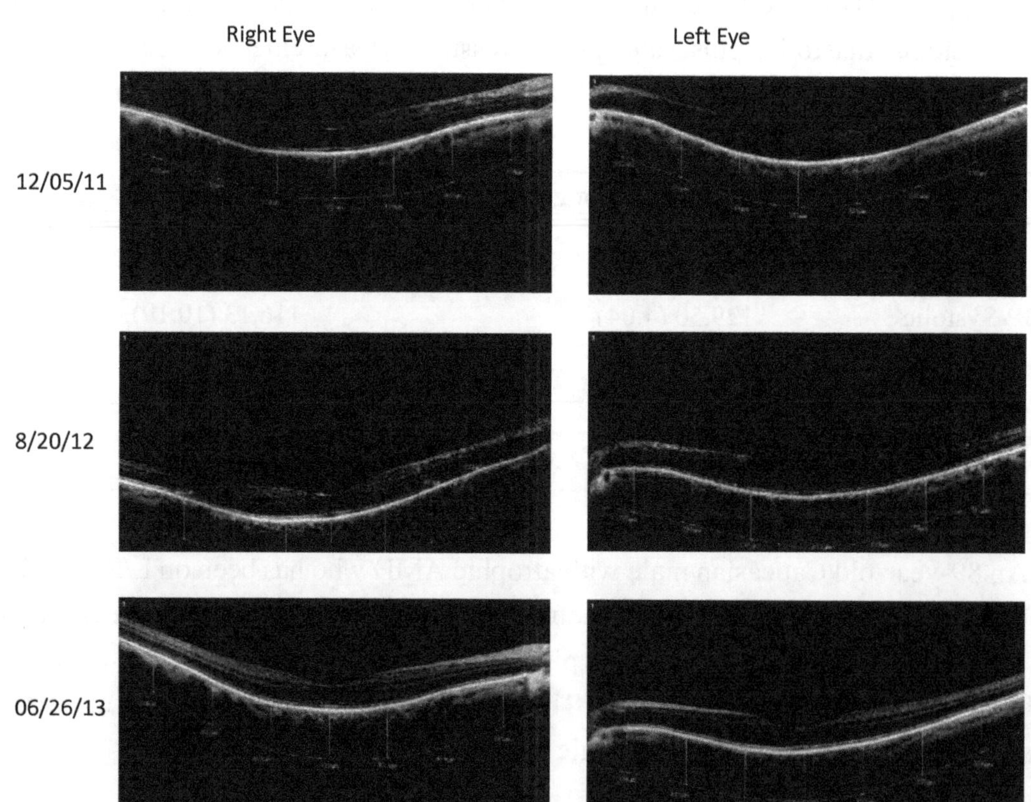

Figure 7. Visualized macular pigment volume of an 89-year-old male patient with AMD. No change in macular pigment over time in both retinas is seen. The patient could not focus on the marker to take 500 nm specular image of left retina on 26 June 2013.

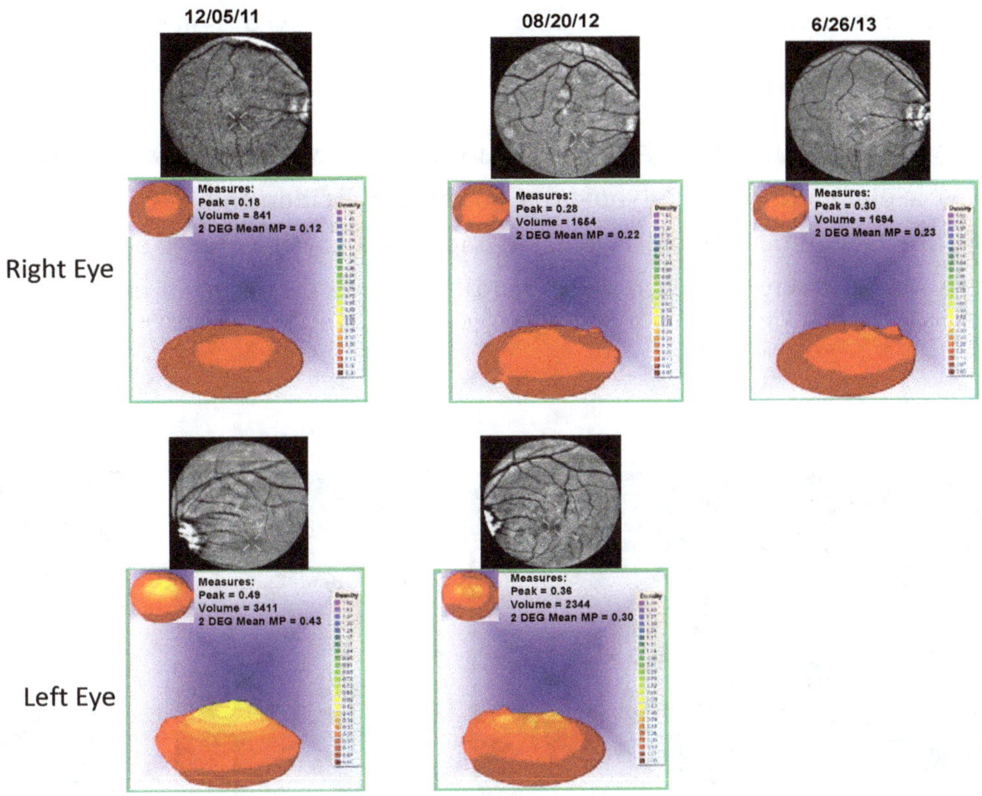

Figure 8. Contrast Sensitivity and Glare Recovery of an 89-year-old male patient with AMD. The contrast sensitivity and glare recovery function right eye are stable, while his left eye has progressive dramatically improved glare recovery (in seconds). Both eyes have an abnormally prolonged glare recovery time that improved but was still abnormal. Expected is 10 to 12 s, in individuals without retinal pathology. This is opposite of the anticipated aging and pathophysiological decline. Baseline Snellen visual acuity was 20/40 in each eye and remained unchanged over 2.5 years allowing the octogenarian to maintain an unrestricted driver's license.

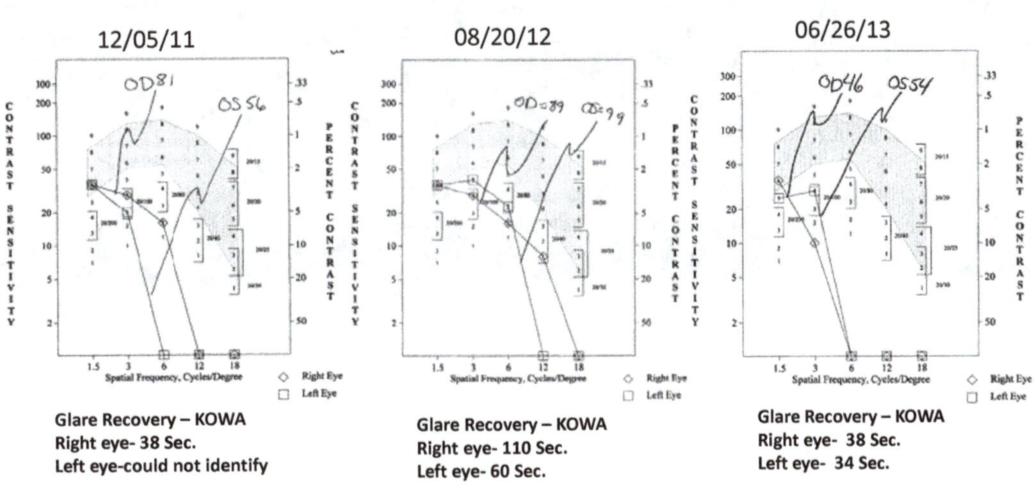

Case 3: A 67-year-old with Polypoidal Choroidal Vasculopathy (PCV), a "treatment resistant" AMD variant who has been on L/RV for almost 2 years. Three measures of ocular structure were enhanced. Retinal autofluorescence diminished (Figure 9), choroid thickened (Figure 10), and macular pigment volume improved (Figure 11). Two measures of visual function, CSF and GR, normalized (Figure 12). Significantly, all five measures were more notable in his more involved right retina.

Figure 9. Wide Field OPTOS® FAF Images of Lipofuscin within the Neurosensory Retina of a 67-year-old male with Polypoidal Choroidal Vasculopathy (PCV), a "treatment resistant" AMD variant. No fluorescein angiography was possible due to a previous allergic reaction to iodine. There is a decrease in auto fluorescence evident in his right retina by Month 22.

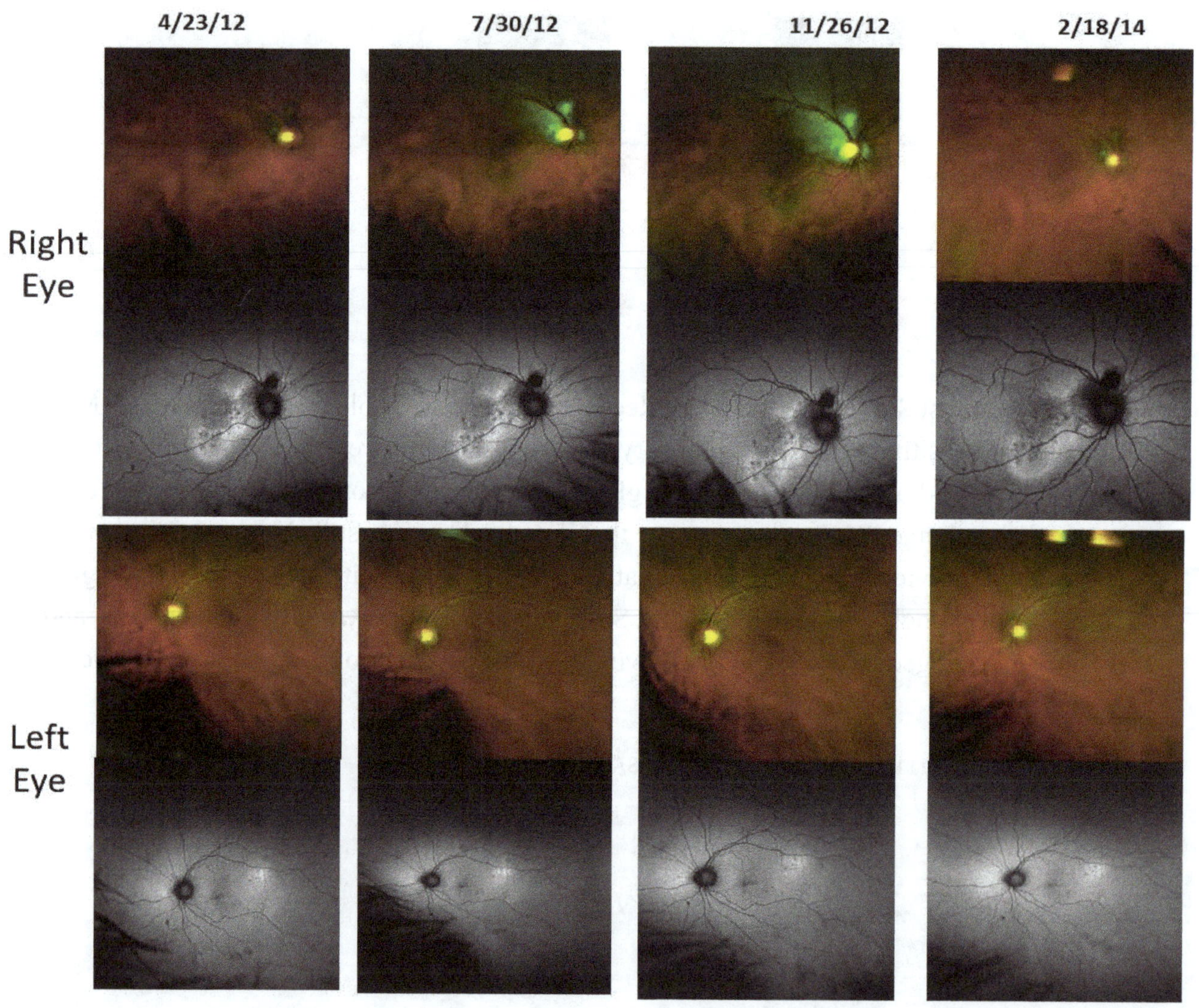

Figure 10. SDOCT "Extended Depth Imaging" of Choroidal Thickness (microns) of a 67-year-old male patient with PCV, an AMD treatment resistant variant. Choroidal thickness (in microns) increased 12% difference right eye and 7% difference left eye by 18 months. This represents additional choroidal thickening, well above the 5.0-micron axial resolution of the OptoVue RTVue® SD OCT. Better clinical perfusion of the posterior retina is presumed.

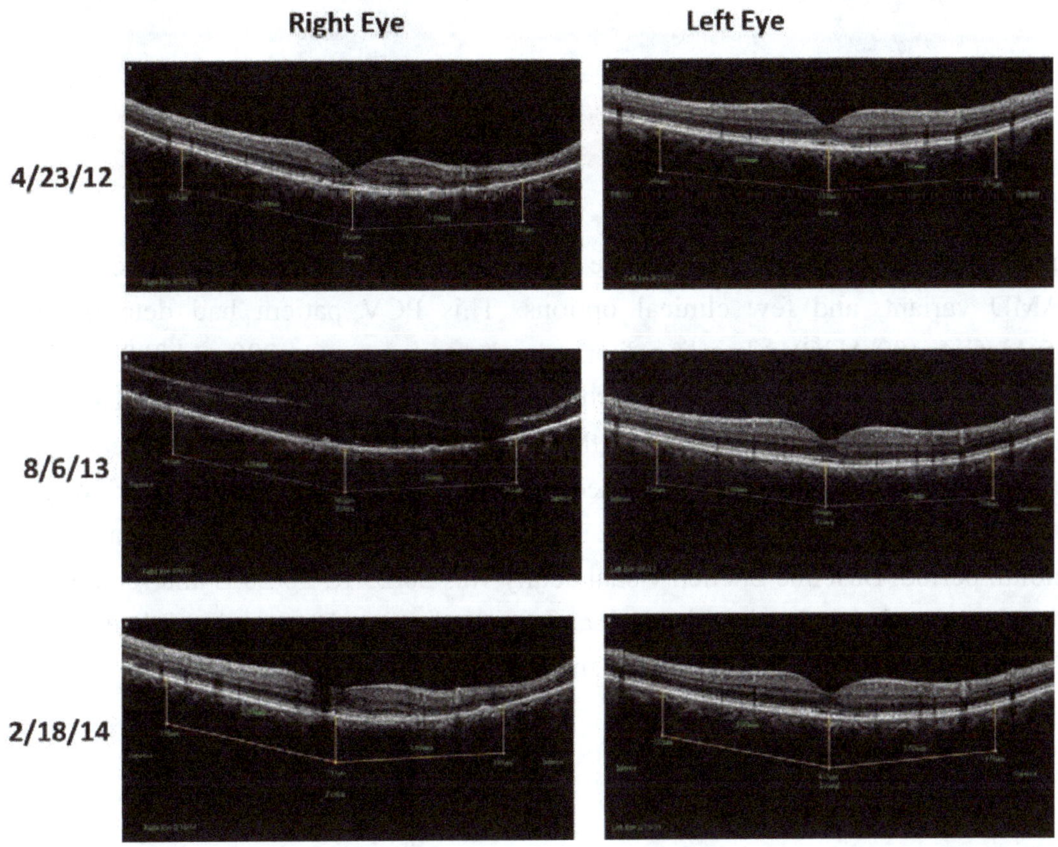

Figure 11. Visualized macular pigment volume, of our 67-year-old male patient with PCV. With time, there is a continual increase in macular pigment volume in the right macula. There was no change in reported dietary or supplemental carotenoid/omega-3 intake. This is an unusual clinical finding, denoting improved cellular health.

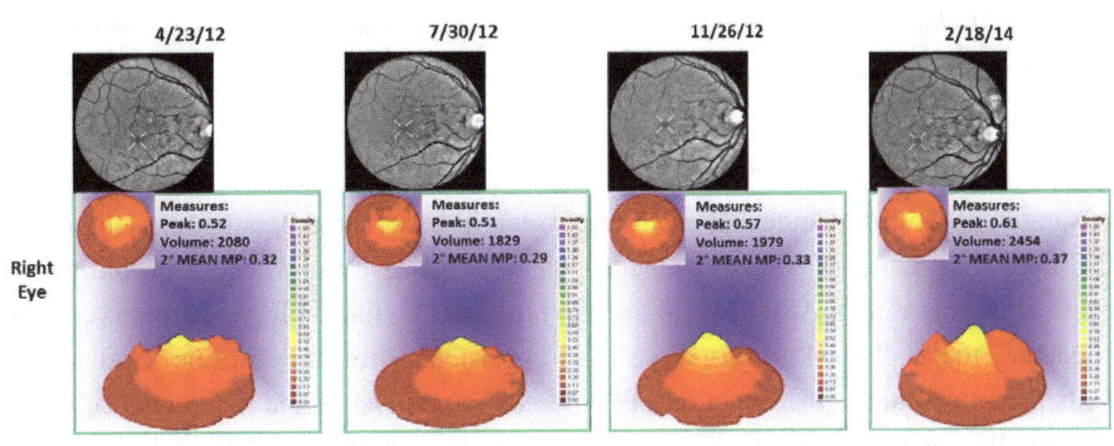

Figure 11. *Cont.*

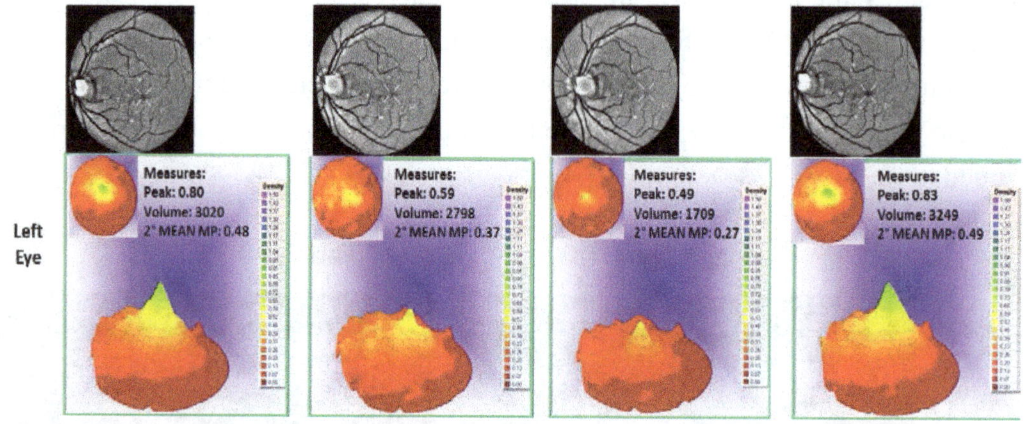

Figure 12. Contrast Sensitivity and Glare Recovery of a 67-year-old male patient with PCV, an AMD variant, and few clinical options. This PCV patient had deteriorated CSF (R 65 AUC, L 109 AUC) at baseline. Normal values are between 200 and 300 AUC. By the second visit, 10 weeks of taking L/RV, the CSF had substantially improved (155 R, 186 L) with continual improvement at the third visit and normalization of each eye by 22 months. The glare recovery quickened dramatically from an abnormal prolonged 30 s right eye and 75 s left eye (normal 10–12 s) at baseline to normal single digit values over the 22-month period. Baseline Snellen visual acuity was 20/25 R, 20/20 L and remained at this level at the second visit. By the third visit at five months, the visual acuity right eye improved to 20/20 and remained unchanged by 22 months.

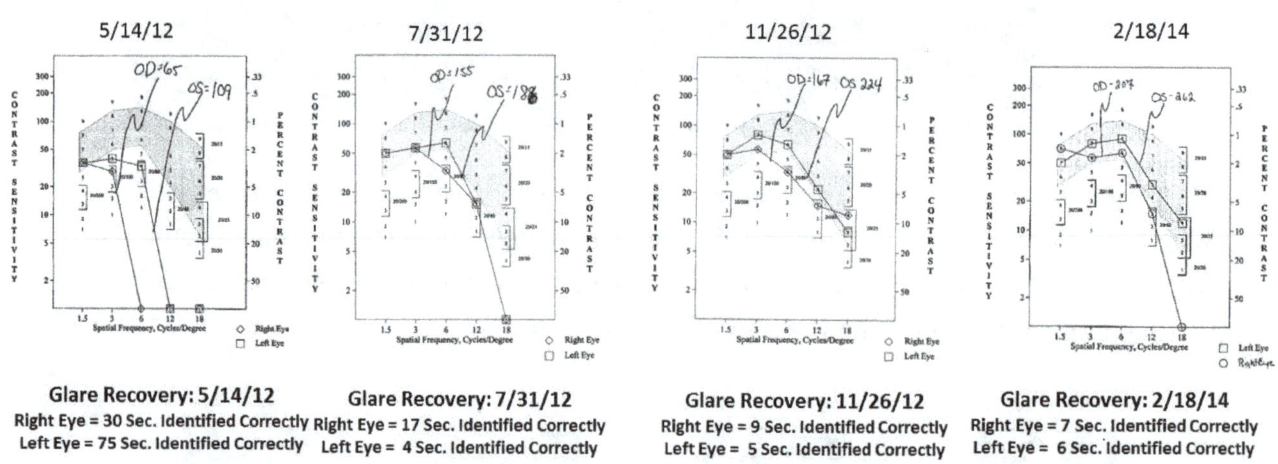

4. Discussion

Diminishment of lipofuscin autofluorescence, as seen in Case 1 and 2, is pathognomonic of healthy retina-RPE-choroidal tissue, as is denser macular pigment (Case 1 and 3). The choroid typically thins with age and at a faster rate in AMD [23,24], yet in our patients, thickening was observed (Cases 1–3). Taken together, these clinical observations are consistent with the murine cardiac reperfusion experiments performed under the direction of Professor Depak Das at the University of Connecticut's Cardiovascular Research Center [25–27], as well as a human clinical trial from Japan demonstrating superior vascular health in patients taking L/RV even for short periods of time [20]. Furthermore, the improved contrast sensitivity and glare recovery we observe are consistent with these improved structural observations.

Foveal health is ultimately affected by drusen deposits that degrade the function and number of cone photoreceptors. Biochemical signs of photoreceptor degeneration, such as decreased expression of synapse-associated proteins and increased expression of stress-response molecules, are seen in AMD patients. The salutary broad and comprehensive effects of L/RV on choroidal thickness, anti-inflammatory markers, regulation of divalent metals, the vitamin D pathway, cellular stress, toxicity genes, up-regulation of Nrf2, and even macular pigment volume appears to ultimately retard degeneration of photoreceptors.

Epigenetics is at the epicenter of modern medicine. It is the study of non-DNA sequence-related heredity that helps explain the relationship between an individual's genetic background, the environment, aging, and disease. In 2013, researchers from a multinational consortium reported results on 19 common susceptibility loci from DNA analyses on nearly 80,000 people, and in aggregate, these loci explain only 10%–30% of the phenotypic variation of AMD [28,29]. The epigenetic state varies among tissues during a lifetime, whereas the DNA sequence remains essentially the same. Dietary recommendations or lack thereof, changes ones DNA and its translation. Clinical reports from our medical center provides us reason to believe that L/RV is beneficial because it reestablishes retinal architecture, decreases lipofuscin accumulation, increases choroidal thickness (perfusion), increases macular pigment volume, improves contrast sensitivity, decreases glare recovery time, and improves visual function—all ostensibly through improved retinal-RPE-choroidal cellular health. These observed clinical benefits in ocular structure and function are seen bilaterally in both eyes with further synergistic effects observed in cardiovascular parameters (*i.e.*, Case 1), consistent with animal data, and the only human clinical trial to date [20,23–25].

5. Conclusions

Randomized placebo controlled ocular-cardiovascular molecular medicine clinical studies are warranted to confirm the proposed dual cardiovascular and ophthalmologic benefits of low-dose epigenetic nutriceutical intervention beyond AREDS II supplementation.

Author Contributions

These medical case reports are based on original clinical work supported by the Optometry/ Ophthalmology sections of Captain James A Lovell Federal Health Care Facility, DVA-Naval Medical Center, North Chicago, IL, USA. The clinical cases were conceived and monitored, the data was analyzed, and the paper was written by Stuart Richer, Shana Patel and Shivani Sockanathan. The collection of data was assisted by Lawrence J. Ulanski II, Luke Miller, and Carla Podella.

References

1. Juhasz, B.; Mukherjee, S.; Das, D.K. Hormetic response of resveratrol against cardioprotection. *Exp. Clin. Cardiol.* **2010**, *15*, 134–138.
2. Dennis, C. Small RNAs: The genome's guiding hand? *Nature* **2002**, *420*, 732, doi:10.1038/420732a.
3. McCay, C.M.; Crowel, M.F.; Maynard, L.A. The effect of retarded growth upon the length of the life span and upon the ultimate body size. *J. Nutr.* **1989**, 5, 155–171.
4. He, S.; Li, X.; Chan, N.; Hinton, D.R. Review: Epigenetic mechanisms in ocular disease. *Mol. Vis.* **2013**, *19*, 665–674.
5. Harikumar, K.B.; Aggarwal, B.B. Resveratrol: A multitargeted agent for age-associated chronic diseases. *Cell Cycle* **2008**, *7*, 1020–1035.
6. Pervaiz, S.; Holme, A.L. Resveratrol: Its biologic targets and functional activity. *Antioxid. Redox. Signal.* **2009**, *11*, 2851–2897.
7. Bola, C.; Bartlett, H.; Eperjesi, F. Resveratrol and the eye: Activity and molecular mechanisms. *Graefes. Arch. Clin. Exp. Ophthalmol.* **2014**, *252*, 699–713.
8. Richer, S.; Stiles, W.; Ulanski, L.; Carroll, D.; Podella, C. Observation of human retinal remodeling in octogenarians with a resveratrol based nutritional supplement. *Nutrients* **2013**, *5*, 1989–2005.
9. Nagineni, C.N.; Raju, R.; Nigineni, K.K.; Kommineni, V.K.; Cherukuri, A.; Kutty, R.K.; Hooks, J.J.; Detrick, B. Reseveratrol suppresses expression of VEGF by human retinal pigment epithelial cells: Potential nutraceutical for age-related macular degeneration. *Aging Dis.* **2014**, *5*, 88–100.
10. Walle, T; Hsieh, F.; DeLegge, M.H.; Oatis, J.E., Jr.; Walle, U.K. High absorption but very low bioavailability of oral resveratrol in humans. *Drug Metab. Dispos.* **2004**, *32*, 1377–1382.
11. Sangeetha, M.K.; Vallabi, D.E.; Sali, V.K.; Thanka, J.; Vasanthi, H.R. Sub-acute toxicity profile of a modified resveratrol supplement. *Food Chem. Toxicol.* **2013**, *59*, 492–500.
12. Roy, S.; Shrinivas, K.; Bagchi, B. A stochastic chemical dynamic approach to correlate autoimmunity and optimal vitamin-D range. *PLoS One* **2014**, *9*, e100635, doi:10.1371/journal.pone.0100635.
13. Itty, S.; Day, S.; Lyles, K.W.; Stinnett, S.S.; Vajzovic, L.M.; Mruthyunjaya, P. Vitamin D deficiency in neovascular *versus* nonneovascular age-related macular degeneration. *Retina* **2014**, *34*, 1779–1786.
14. Weinberg, E.D. Therapeutic potential of iron chelators in diseases associated with iron mismanagement. *J. Pharm. Pharmacol.* **2006**, *58*, 575–584.
15. Kurin, E.; Atanasov, A.G.; Donath, O.; Heiss, E.H.; Dirsch, V.M.; Nagy, M. Synergy study of the inhibitory potential of red wine polyphenols on vascular smooth muscle cell proliferation. *Planta Med.* **2012**, 78, 772–778.
16. Longevinex®. Available online: http://www.longevinex.com/ (accessed on 5 September 2014).
17. Richer, S.; Stiles, W.; Thomas, C. Molecular Medicine in Ophthalmic Care. *Optometry* **2009**, *80*, 695–701.
18. Barger, J.L.; Kayo, T.; Pugh, T.D.; Prolla, T.A. Short-term consumption of a resveratrol-containing nutraceutical mixture mimics gene expression of long-term caloric restriction in mouse heart. *Weindruch R. Exp. Gerontol.* **2008**, *43*, 859–866.

19. Harris, G.; Pratt, S.; Richer, S. Food and nutrients in disease management. In *Strategies for Medical Doctors, Section I. Conditions of the Ears, Eyes, Nose, and Mouth, Age-Related Macular Degeneration*, 2nd ed.; Kohlstadt, I., Ed.; CRC Press: Taylor & Francis Group: Boca Raton, FL, USA, 2013.
20. Fujitaka, K.; Otani, H.; Jo, F.; Jo, H.; Nomura, E.; Iwasaki, M.; Nishikawa, M.; Iwasaka, T.; Das, D.K. Modified resveratrol Longevinex improves endothelial function in adults with metabolic syndrome receiving standard treatment. *Nutr. Res.* **2011**, *12*, 842–847.
21. Longevinex® for Life. Available online: http://www.longevinex.com/articles/longevinex-first-red-wine-anti-aging-capsule-to-pass-sub-acute-toxicity-testing (accessed on 5 May 2014).
22. Richer, S. A protocol for the evaluation and treatment of atrophic age-related macular degeneration. *J. Am. Optom. Assoc.* **1999**, *70*, 13–23.
23. Esmaeelpour, M.; Ansari-Shahrezaei, S.; Glittenberg, C.; Nemetz, S; Kraus, M.F.; Hornegger, J.; Fujimoto, J.G.; Drexler, W.; Binder, S. Choroid, Haller's, and Sattler's layer thickness in intermediate age-related macular degeneration with and without fellow neovascular eyes. *Investig. Ophthalmol. Vis. Sci.* **2014**, *55*, 5074–5080.
24. Sohn, E.H.; Khanna, A.; Tucker, B.A.; Abràmoff, M.D.; Stone, E.M.; Mullins, R.F. Structural and biochemical analyses of choroidal thickness in human donor eyes. *Investig. Ophthalmol. Vis. Sci.* **2014**, *55*, 1352–1360.
25. Mukhopadhyay, P.; Mukherjee, S.; Ahsan, K.; Bagchi, A.; Pacher, P.; Das, D.K. Restoration of altered microRNA expression in the ischemic heart with resveratrol. *PLoS One* **2010**, *5*, e15705, doi:10.1371/journal.pone.0015705.
26. Mukhopadhyay, P.; Das, S.; Ahsan, M.K.; Otani, H.; Das, D.K. Modulation of microRNA 20b with resveratrol and longevinex is linked with their potent anti-angiogenic action in the ischaemic myocardium and synergestic effects of resveratrol and γ-tocotrienol. *J. Cell Mol. Med.* **2012**, *16*, 2504–2517.
27. Juhasz, B.; Das, D.K.; Kertesz, A.; Juhasz, A.; Gesztelyi, R.; Varga, B. Erratum to: Reduction of blood cholesterol and ischemic injury in the hypercholesteromic rabbits with modified resveratrol, longevinex. *Mol. Cell. Biochem.* **2011**, *348*, 205, doi:10.1007/s11010-010-0691-3.
28. SanGiovanni, J.P.; Chew, E.Y. Clinical applications of age-related macular degeneration genetics. *Cold Spring Harb. Perspect. Med.* **2014**, *4*, a017228, doi:10.1101/cshperspect.a017228.
29. Fritsche, L.G.; Chen, W.; Schu, M.; Yaspan, B.L.; Yu, Y.; Thorleifsson, G.; Zack, D.J.; Arakawa, S.; Cipriani, V.; Ripke, S.; *et al.* Seven new loci associated with age-related macular degeneration. *Nat. Genet.* **2013**, *45*, 433–439.

2

Retina, Retinol, Retinal and the Natural History of Vitamin A as a Light Sensor

Ming Zhong, Riki Kawaguchi, Miki Kassai and Hui Sun *

Department of Physiology, Jules Stein Eye Institute, and Howard Hughes Medical Institute, David Geffen School of Medicine, University of California, Los Angeles, CA 90095, USA; E-Mails: mzhong@mednet.ucla.edu (M.Z.); rkawaguchi@mednet.ucla.edu (R.K.); mkassai18@ucla.edu (M.K.)

* Author to whom correspondence should be addressed; E-Mail: hsun@mednet.ucla.edu;

Abstract: Light is both the ultimate energy source for most organisms and a rich information source. Vitamin A-based chromophore was initially used in harvesting light energy, but has become the most widely used light sensor throughout evolution from unicellular to multicellular organisms. Vitamin A-based photoreceptor proteins are called opsins and have been used for billions of years for sensing light for vision or the equivalent of vision. All vitamin A-based light sensors for vision in the animal kingdom are G-protein coupled receptors, while those in unicellular organisms are light-gated channels. This first major switch in evolution was followed by two other major changes: the switch from bistable to monostable pigments for vision and the expansion of vitamin A's biological functions. Vitamin A's new functions such as regulating cell growth and differentiation from embryogenesis to adult are associated with increased toxicity with its random diffusion. In contrast to bistable pigments which can be regenerated by light, monostable pigments depend on complex enzymatic cycles for regeneration after every photoisomerization event. Here we discuss vitamin A functions and transport in the context of the natural history of vitamin A-based light sensors and propose that the expanding functions of vitamin A and the choice of monostable pigments are the likely evolutionary driving forces for precise, efficient, and sustained vitamin A transport.

Keywords: vitamin A; retinoid; opsins; retina; retinol; retinal; STRA6; retinol binding protein

1. Sunlight and Vitamin A

The prevalent light source throughout evolution has been sunlight shining on the surface of the earth. For billions of years, vitamin A biology has been tightly linked to sunlight. Living organisms use sunlight primarily as a source of energy, the source of information for vision, and an indicator of time. Remarkably, vitamin A-based chromophore has evolved as the light sensors for all three usages (Table 1). Archaebacteria use vitamin A-based light-driven pumps to harvest light energy (e.g., by creating the electrochemical gradient of protons to drive ATP synthase). This is an alternative mechanism to chlorophyll-based phototrophy. For adjusting the biological clock, vitamin A-based photoreceptor proteins are used as the light sensors, although flavin-based photoreceptor proteins have also been used for this purpose. However, for vision or the equivalent of vision, the vast majority of species use vitamin A-based chromophore as the light sensor. Vitamin A-based chromophore is the exclusive choice for vision in multicellular organisms.

Even vitamin A's name is tightly linked to vision. The scientific name for vitamin A derivatives is retinoid, which is derived from the word "retina". Retinoids include retinol (the alcohol form), retinal (the aldedyde form, also called retinaldehyde or retinene) and retinoic acid (the acid form). Although vitamin A existed as a chemical before it functioned as a vitamin and retinal existed as a light sensor before there was a retina, we still use these names to refer to these chemicals.

What makes vitamin A so special for vision (the perception of light)? Why was vitamin A repeatedly chosen by evolution as the sensor for sunlight? What determined the region of the electromagnetic spectrum that is visible to the human eye? There are two important factors that provide likely answers for these related questions. First, the conjugation of the aldehyde end of retinal to photoreceptor proteins causes a red shift in its absorbance to the visible range (from the perspective of human vision). Visible light (visible due to vitamin A-based light sensors) generally matches the peak irradiance of sunlight on the earth's surface [1,2]. In contrast, most other light sensors absorb primarily in the UV range (e.g., flavin-based light sensors). Second, the large light-induced conformational change of vitamin A-based chromophore makes it ideal as a ligand for membrane receptors. The large conformational change likely makes it easier for the photoreceptor protein to distinguish the silent state (in the dark) and the activated state (in the light).

1.1. The First Major Switch in the Evolution of Vitamin A-Based Light Sensors

All vitamin A-based photoreceptor proteins are called opsins. All opsins in the animal kingdom that sense light for vision (visual pigments) are G-protein coupled receptors. Visual pigments sense light for daytime and nighttime vision and encode wavelength information of light for color vision [3]. All opsins in the animal kingdom are homologous to visual pigments. In contrast, opsins in unicellular organisms are light-gated channels (for light sensing) or light-driven pumps (for harvesting light energy) [4]. The switch from ion channel and pumps to G-protein coupled receptors is the first major event in the evolution of vitamin A-based light sensors (Table 1). Opsins that are light-gated ion channels or pumps use all-*trans* retinal as the chromophore, while opsins that are G-protein coupled receptors all use 11-*cis* retinal as the chromophore (Table 1 and Figure 1). The vitamin A-based light sensors listed in Table 1 are not meant to be all inclusive because some species contain surprisingly large numbers of opsins, and the functions of some opsins are still not well understood. Using humans and mice as an example, the human retina has long-, medium- and short-wave visual pigments in cone photoreceptor cells [5,6], rhodopsin in rod photoreceptor cells [7–10], melanopsin in ganglion cells [11–17], peropsin in the apical microvilli of the retinal pigment epithelium (RPE) [18] and RGR in the intracellular membranes of the RPE [19–22] (Figure 2). The mouse retina does not express the long-wave cone pigment [23], but has an additional opsin called neuropsin, which is mostly localized to the amacrine and ganglion cell layers [24,25].

Although there is tremendous diversity in the absorption maxima of cone visual pigments, the peak absorbance of rhodopsin, the dim light receptor, in many species is 500 nm. Why not 450 nm or 550 nm? One likely explanation is that the wavelength of the peak irradiance of sunlight on earth surface is 500 nm. Moonlight, the dominant light in natural world at night, is reflected sunlight and thus has same peak irradiance. The peak absorbance of rhodopsin matches this peak irradiance to achieve maximum sensitivity to available light. In contrast, maximum sensitivity is less important for cone visual pigments, which diversify their absorbance maxima for color vision. An extreme example of how available light determines the absorption spectra of visual pigments is the color vision of coelacanth, which lives at a depth about 200 m. To detect color and light in deep ocean where available light spans a very narrow range around 480 nm, coelacanth has only two visual pigments with absorption maxima of 478 nm and 485 nm, respectively [26]. This is in sharp contrast to another extreme example of a fish that has vision both above and below water (*Anableps anableps*). This fish has ten different opsins to adapt to vision both above and below water [27]. Visual pigments can achieve the exact absorption maximum that meets the organism's biological need through several mechanisms of spectral tuning. The common mechanism of spectral tuning is to change the protein environment that surrounds the chromophore [28–35]. Generally, opsin environments that encourage π-electron delocalization of retinal cause a red shift in the absorption maximum. Another mechanism is by changing the structure of the chromophore itself. Although retinal is the universal chromophore for all vitamin A-based light sensors, the exact isomer of retinal can be different between species (Figure 1). For example, aquatic animals are known to shift absorption maxima of visual pigments by using the A1 (11-*cis* retinal) or A2 (11-*cis*-3,4-dehydroretinal) chromophore [36–40]. There are also examples of terrestrial vertebrates using vitamin A2-based visual pigments, which belong to the most red-shifted visual pigments (e.g., absorption maximum of 625 nm) [41]. A2 pigments absorb longer wavelengths of light compared to the A1 version because of the extension of the conjugated chain of the chromophore.

Table 1. Evolution of vitamin A-based light sensors (opsins) from bacteria to humans. The symbol # denotes the sensing of light by visual pigments for the circadian clock and pupillary reflex. Due to the tremendous diversity of opsins and space limitation, this table only depicts opsins that are representative of each kind. Opsin homologs (e.g., RGR in mammals) that function as light-dependent retinoid isomerases are not included.

Kingdom	Species	Photoreceptor Cell or Structure	Physiological Functions	Photoreceptor Proteins	Retinal Chomophore
Animalia	*Homo sapiens* Human	Cones	High luminescence vision and color vision + #	Long-wave cone pigment Medium-wave cone pigment Short-wave cone pigment	11-*cis* retinal
		Rod	Low luminescence vision + #	Rhodopsin	
		Light-sensitive ganglion cell	Light-sensing for the circadian clock and papillary reflex (#)	Melanopsin	
	Mus musculus Mouse	Cones	High luminescence vision and color vision + #	Medium-wave cone pigment UV cone pigment	11-*cis* retinal
		Rod	Low luminescence vision + #	Rhodopsin	
		Light-sensitive ganglion cell	Light-sensing for the circadian clock and papillary reflex (#)	Melanopsin	
	Gallus gallus Chicken	Cones	High luminescence vision and color vision + #	Long-wave cone pigment Medium-wave cone pigment Short-wave cone pigment UV cone pigment	11-*cis* retinal
		Rod	Low luminescence vision + #	Rhodopsin	
		Light-sensitive ganglion cell	Light-sensing for the circadian clock and papillary reflex (#)	Melanopsin	
		pinealocyte	Regulation of pineal circadian cycle	Pinopsin	

Table 1. *Cont.*

Animalia	*Rana catesbeiana* Frog	Rod and cones of adult frog	Vision on land and in water	Visual pigments	11-*cis* retinal
		Photosensitive melanophore	Light-dependent melanosome migration	Melanopsin	
		Rod and cones of tadpole	Vision in water	Visual pigments	11-*cis*-3,4-dehydroretinal
	Watasenia scintillans Squid	Retinal photoreceptors	Vision in water	Visual pigments	11-*cis*-3,4-dehydroretinal 11-*cis*-4-hydroxyretinal 11-*cis* retinal
	Drosophila melanogaster Fly	R1 to R7 photoreceptors	Vision	Visual pigments	11-*cis*-3-hydroxyretinal
Plantae	*Chlamydomonas reinhardtii* Green algea	Eye spot	Phototactic response Photophobic response	Chlamyopsin	All-*trans* retinal
Monera	*Halobacterium halobium* Bacteria	*Halobacterium halobium*	Light-driven chloride pump Light-driven proton pump Phototactic response Photophobic response	Halorhodopsin Bacteriorhodopsin Sensory rhodopsin I Sensory rhodopsin II	All-*trans* retinal

Figure 1. Examples of structural divergence of biologically active retinoids. For simplicity, only representative biologically active endogenous retinoids are shown.

Kingdom	Species	Retinal-Based Light Sensors	Ligands for Nuclear Hormone Receptors
Animalia	*Homo sapiens* *Mus musculus* *Gallus gallus* *Rana catesbeiana*	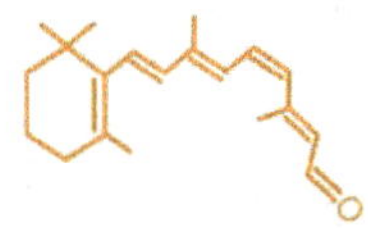 11-cis retinal (A1)	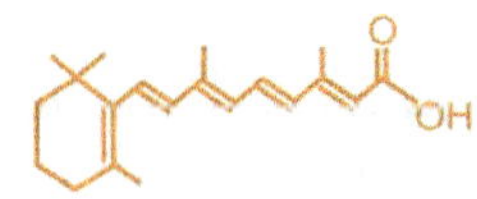 All-trans retinoic acid 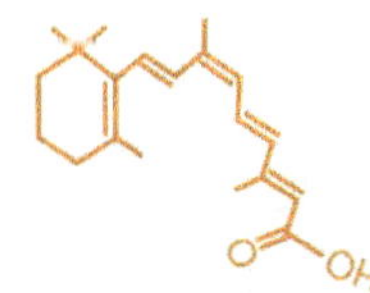 9-cis retinoic acid
		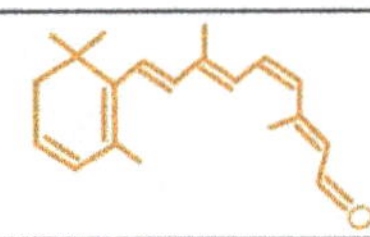 11-cis 3,4-dehydroretinal (A2)	
	Watasenia scintillans	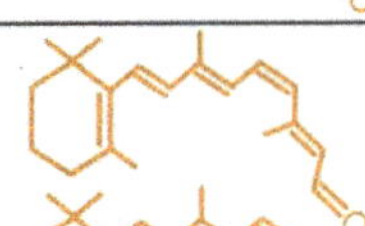 11-cis retinal 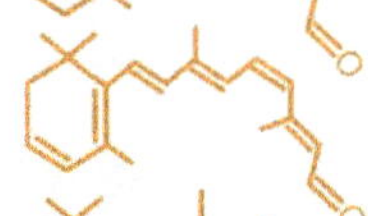 11-cis 3,4-dehydroretinal 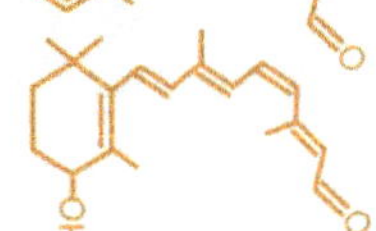 11-cis 4-hydroxyretinal	
	Drosophila melanogaster	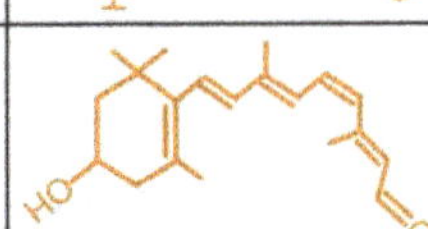 11-cis 3-hydroxyretinal	
Plantae	*Chlamydomonas reinhardtii*	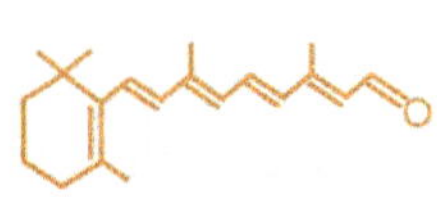 all-trans retinal	
Monera	*Halobacterium halobium*		

Figure 2. Schematic diagram of the localization of various opsins in human and mouse retina and retinal pigment epithelium (RPE). Only cells or cellular structures that express opsins are shown and are color-coded. There are species variations. Human, but not mouse, has the long-wave cone pigment. Neuropsin is expressed in the mouse retina, but not in the human retina.

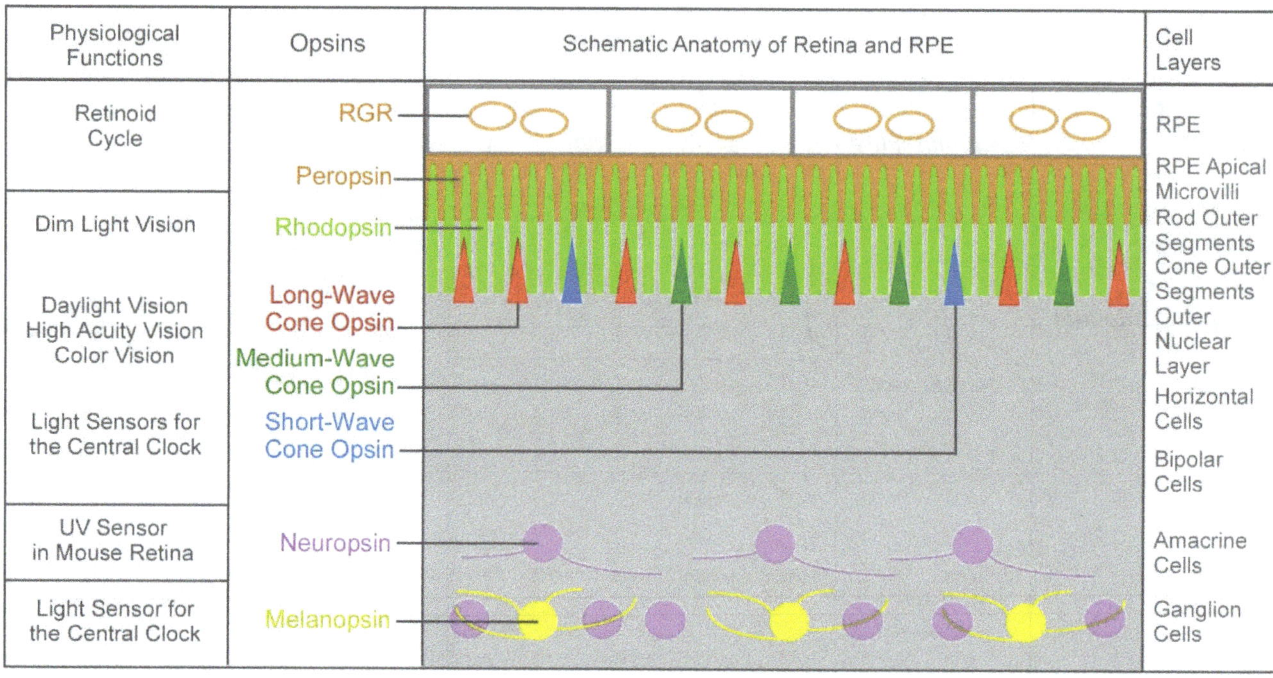

1.2. The Second Major Switch in the Evolution of Vitamin A-Based Light Sensors

The second major change in the evolution of vitamin A-based light sensors is the emergence of monostable pigments (Table 2). All opsins before vertebrate visual pigments (from opsins of unicellular organisms to invertebrate opsins) are bistable pigments, which can be regenerated by light after photobleaching (Table 2). All vertebrate visual pigments are monostable pigments, which release the chromophore after every photoisomerzation event and depend on an enzymatic cycles called the visual cycle to regenerate [42–46]. To compete with bleached rhodopsin for chromophore in daylight, cone visual pigments have their unique regeneration pathway that is different from the visual cycle that regenerates rhodopsin [47–51]. The isomerase in this cone-specific pathway has now been identified [52]. The mechanisms of chromophore release by bleached vertebrate rhodopsin and cone pigments have been studied recently [53,54]. Compared to the regeneration of the bistable pigments by light, the regeneration of monostable pigments requires much more complex mechanisms involving many enzymes and transport proteins (Table 3). The regaining of the 11-*cis* retinal by the monostable pigment after light-induced release is an important factor affecting the dark adaptation of photoreceptor cells [44]. Without the chromophore, the opsin apoprotein itself can activate signal transduction [55,56].

Table 2. Convergent and divergent events in the evolution of vitamin A-based light sensors.

Kingdom	***Monera***	***Plantae***	***Animalia***					
Species	***Halobacterium halobium***	***Chlamydomonas reinhardtii***	***Drosophila melanogaster***	***Watasenia scintillans***	***Rana catesbeiana***	***Gallus gallus***	***Mus musculus***	***Homo sapiens***
Light sensing	Vitamin A-based light sensors for vision or the equivalent of vision							
Opsins	Light-driven pumps or light-gated ion channels		All visual pigments in the animal kingdom are G-protein coupled receptors					
Chromophore	All-*trans* retinal		11-*cis* retinal					
Light-induced isomerization	All-*trans* to 13-*cis*		11-*cis* to all-*trans*					
Photolability	Bistable pigments				Monostable pigments for vision			
Regeneration after photobleaching	Light-dependent				Enzymatic			
Vitamin A functions	Vitamin A's only function is light absorption				Vitamin A has diverse biological functions (e.g., regulating cell growth and differentiation in development and in adult)			
Toxicity of free retinoid	Relatively low				High			
Vitamin A transport	No known mechanism dedicated to long-range vitamin A transport				The emergence of the RBP/STRA6 system for sustained, specific, efficient and controlled delivery			

Vision is known to optimize energy use [57,58]. For chromophore regeneration, vertebrate photoreceptor cells took the seemingly paradoxical evolutionary choice of using the much more energy-inefficient monostable pigments. In contrast, bistable pigments are regenerated by light after photobleaching without any cellular energy. Comparing the energy efficiency of the two mechanisms is analogous to comparing heating a building using fossil fuel versus solar energy. To make it even more "wasteful", we need to constantly consume cellular energy to regenerate bleached rhodopsin in daylight, even when rod photoreceptor cells are completely saturated and do not contribute to visual perception. In contrast, bistable pigments only need enzymatic regeneration when the photoreceptor protein is degraded, not when it is bleached [59]. This regeneration is important during nutritional deficiency.

To convert the released free all-*trans* retinal back to 11-*cis* retinal for monostable pigments, evolution produced many proteins dedicated to the visual cycle. All these proteins are potential causes of blinding diseases. An example is ABCA4 (ABCR) [60,61], whose surprising existence is a testament to the sophistication of the visual cycle. ABCA4 is an ATP-dependent membrane transport protein in photoreceptor disc membranes, and its function is to accelerate the transport of retinal conjugate across photoreceptor disc membranes [62–68]. Loss of ABCA4 function leads to the accumulation of A2E, a toxic bis-retinoid adduct and delayed dark adaptation.

Table 3. Comparison of bistable pigments and monostable pigments.

Advantages / Disadvantages	Bistable pigment	Monostable pigment
Chromophore Release	Chromophore is not released after photoisomerization	Chromophore is released after **every** photoisomerization event
Regeneration Mechanism's Complexity	The pigment can regenerate itself using light	Depends on multiple enzymatic steps and two cell types to regenerate every released chromophore molecule
Consumption of Cellular Energy	Does not depend on cellular energy to regenerate after bleaching and is much more energy efficient	Depends on the cellular energy of two cell types to regenerate every released chromophore molecule
The need of New Vitamin A-Based Chromophore	Vitamin A-based chromophore is only needed during the initial production of the bistable pigment	Constant recycling of retinoid between two cell types during daytime leads to inevitable loss of the chromophore and demands new supply
Sensitivity to Vitamin A Deficiency	Relatively low	High (the eye is the human organ most sensitive to vitamin A deficiency)
Long-Term Toxicity	No toxic retinal is released after light bleaching of the pigment	Toxic retinal is released after every photoisomerization event; free retinal can lead to toxic A2E formation
Frequency of the (Enzymatic) Visual Cycle	Infrequent (A visual cycle is used to recycle chromophore released from degraded opsins)	Highly frequent (A visual cycle is used after every photoisomerization event to regenerate bleached pigment)
"Wasteful" Regeneration	Little or no wasteful regeneration that consumes cellular energy	Constant regeneration of bleached rhodospin in bright daylight when the rod is completely saturated is highly wasteful
Regeneration in the Dark	Depends on light to regenerate; can regenerate in the dark only during the initial formation of the pigment	Due to its ability to be regenerated in complete darkness, it is more sensitive for nighttime vision
Consequence of Photon Absorption	Activation or regeneration	Activation only
Encoding Wavelength Information of Light	Each pigment has two kinds of spectral sensitivity (for bleaching and regeneration)	Each pigment has a distinct spectral sensitivity and is perhaps more precise in encoding wavelength information for color vision

ABCA4 mutations are associated with several blinding diseases in humans, including Stargardt macular dystrophy [69], cone rod dystrophy [70] and retinitis pigmentosa [70,71]. Since ABCA4 functions to accelerate the regeneration of monostable pigments and species that do not have monostable pigments naturally lack ABCA4, human diseases associated with ABCA4 ultimately originated from the choice of monostable pigments during evolution. There may still be other unknown components of the visual cycle. For example, ABCA4 is expressed in the disc membranes of photoreceptor cells where it can play no role in retinal transport between the RPE and photoreceptor cells.

Although vertebrates exclusively use monostable pigments for vision, theydo have endogenous bistable pigments in the inner retina including melanopsin [72–75] and neuropsin [25,76]. Exogenously expressed bistable pigments from unicellular organisms even function well both in the vertebrate retina [77] and the brain (as employed by the technique optogenetics) [78]. Bistable pigments can be repeatedly stimulated by light in vertebrate neurons that have no access to the visual cycle [78]. Why did evolution come up with monostable pigments, which require much more "maintenance"? Despite the many advantages of bistable pigments, there have to be very good reasons for monostable pigments to exist as the universal pigments for vertebrate vision. The first likely reason is survival in the dark. Vision at night can offer tremendous survival advantages for both predators (e.g., to find more prey) and prey (e.g., to avoid predators). Unlike bistable pigments, monostable pigments can regenerate in complete darkness and therefore are likely more suitable for continuous night vision. Bistable pigments can be formed in the dark only in the initial formation of the bistable pigment [79]. Another possible advantage is color vision. Monostable pigments may be more precise in discriminating different wavelengths of light (the basis of color vision) because the response of a bistable pigment to light is confounded by its two absorption maxima (one for activation and one for regeneration). There may be other reasons to justify the choice of this highly energy-consuming and disease-prone regeneration mechanism for visual pigments.

2. Broadening of the Biological Functions of Vitamin A

2.1. Expanding Biological Functions of Vitamin A

If vitamin A is taken in for vision, why not use it for something else? That's exactly what happened in evolution (Figure 1 and Table 2). Vertebrates broaden the use of vitamin A to many other essential biological functions, including its essential roles in embryonic development, maturation of the immune system, maintenance of epithelial integrity, and in the adult brain for learning and memory and neurogenesis [80–87]. This is the third major change in the biology of vitamin A. Most of these new functions are mediated by the acid form of vitamin A (retinoic acid) [88,89]. Since this functional diversification in evolution, vitamin A deficiency would no longer be limited to effects on vision, and vitamin A became an essential nutrient for almost all vertebrate organs.

Vitamin A deficiency affects many vertebrate organs [90,91]. The most well known effects of vitamin A deficiency in humans are night blindness [92] and increased childhood mortality and morbidity [93]. In adults, vitamin A deficiency can lead to profound impairment of hippocampal long-term potentiation and long-term depression [94] and impairment in learning and memory [95]. Vitamin A deficiency can also lead to pathological changes in the lung [96,97], the skin [98], the thyroid [99] and the male and female reproductive systems [90,100]. It was recently discovered that retinol, but not retinoic acid, prevents the differentiation and promotes the feeder-independent culture of embryonic stem cells [101]; retinal inhibits adipogenesis [102]; and retinoic acid regulates protein translation in neurons independent of its roles in regulating gene transcription [103,104]. Given its numerous biological functions, retinoid plays positive or negative roles in a wide-range of human diseases, such as visual disorders [45], cancer [105,106], infectious diseases [82], diabetes [107,108], teratogenicity [109], and skin diseases [110].

2.2. Retinoid Toxicity Associated with the Evolution of Vitamin A Functions

Broadened biological activity of vitamin A is a double-edged sword that also leads to broader toxicity caused by excessive vitamin A or its derivatives (Table 4). Retinoid toxicity can be caused by physical properties of retinoid (e.g., acting like a detergent at sufficient concentrations), chemical reactivity of retinoid (e.g., modification of random proteins by free retinal), or inappropriate biological activities (e.g., retinoic acid activating or suppressing gene expression at the wrong cell type or at the wrong time) (Table 4). Excessive vitamin A uptake can lead to severe toxicity in humans [109,111–113]. Water-miscible, emulsified, and solid forms of retinol are much more toxic than oil-based retinol preparations [114]. Excessive retinoic acid is even more toxic than retinol, consistent with the fact that retinoic acid is more biologically active [115]. Retinoid therapy for human diseases is often associated with side effects such as terotogenicity [109,115,116]. Chronic exposure to clinical doses of 13-*cis* retinoic acid suppresses hippocampal neurogenesis and disrupts hippocampal-dependent memory [117]. In addition, 13-*cis* retinoic acid intake causes night blindness [118].

Retinal is the vitamin A derivative that is most toxic, due to its chemical reactivity. Even when vitamin A is used only for light sensing, retinal can be toxic [119] due to its chemical toxicity in randomly modifying proteins through Schiff base formation. Retinal toxicity becomes more severe for organisms using monostable pigments, which constantly release free retinal in daylight. As a protein that interacts with retinal, ABCA4 in photoreceptor cells is sensitive to retinal-mediated photooxidative damage [120]. A photoreceptor cell culture study revealed that retinal is much more toxic than retinol in mediating photooxidative damage [121]. Photooxidation caused by all-*trans* retinal released from monostable pigments has been observed in single vertebrate photoreceptor cells [122]. Knocking out both ABCA4 and RDH8, two genes that function to reduce retinal toxicity, causes severe retina degeneration [123]. The constant release of free retinal in daylight by the monostable pigments also paves the way for the generation of a toxic chemical derived from retinal called A2E, a unique vitamin A derivative found in vertebrate eyes that has only toxicity but no beneficial function [124–130]. In a sense, A2E ultimately results from the choice of monostable pigments in evolution due to their constant release of free all-*trans* retinal and the demand for 11-*cis* retinal in daylight.

Table 4. Biological functions and toxicities of vitamin A derivatives in vertebrates.

Appropriate Amount		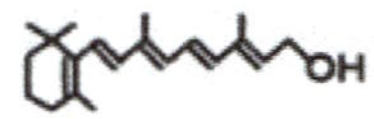	Excessive Amount		
Known Biochemical Basis of Functions	**Examples of Biological Functions**	**Vitamin A Derivatives**	**Example of Toxicity**	**Biochemical Basis of Toxicity**	**Evolutionary Origin of Toxicity**
One the least toxic retinoids; stored by binding to retinol binding proteins	Vitamin A storage and transport	Retinol (Vitamin A alcohol)	Pathological symptoms associated with hypervitaminosis A	Excessive vitamin A intake overwhelms and bypasses dedicated and specific delivery pathway to cause toxicity	Expanding biological roles of vitamin A
One the least toxic retinoids; stored as a lipid	Vitamin A storage and transport	Retinyl Ester (Vitamin A ester)	Excessive retinyl ester in the blood is toxic	Excessive retinyl esters can be converted to biologically active retinoids to cause toxicity	Expanding biological roles of vitamin A
The chromophore for opsins, the photoreceptor proteins for vision and the biological clock	Light absorption for vision and for regulating the biological clock	Retinal (Vitamin A aldehyde)	Excessive accumulation of retinal in retina causes photoreceptor degeneration	Random protein modification through Schiff-base formation; mediates phcto-oxidative damage	Choice of monostable pigments that constantly release free retinal in daylight
Activates nuclear hormone receptors; regulates protein translation	Regulating the growth and differentiation from embryogenesis to adulthood; regulating learning and memory	Retinoic Acid (Vitamin A acid)	Systemic random diffusion of retinoic acid is toxic to many adult organs; also a potent teratogen	The most toxic retinoid due to its activity in activating or suppressing gene expression	Expanding biological roles of vitamin A
		A2E (Retinal Derivative)	The toxic fluorophore that accumulates in the RPE of Stargard disease patients and in aging human eyes	Photo-oxidative damage; Inhibits lysosomal enzymes and retinoid isomerase; activates the complement system	Choice of monostable pigments that constantly release free retinal in daylight

3. The Emergence of a Specific and Stable Vitamin A Transport Mechanism that Coincided with Major Changes in Vitamin A Functions

The tremendous expansion in the biological functions of retinoids, the dependence on vitamin A for survival, and toxicity associated with their random diffusion demand a specific and stable mechanism of vitamin A transport. The concomitant emergence of monostable pigments for vision also demands a specific and stable mechanism of vitamin A transport because the constant release of free retinal by monostable pigments (after every photoisomerization event) and the constant recycling of retinoid between two cell types in daylight inevitably causes loss of vitamin A (absorption of one photon initiates one cycle). Indeed, the diversification of vitamin A functions and the switching of visual pigments from bistable pigments to monostable pigments in evolution coincided with the emergence of a specific and dedicated vitamin A transport mechanism (Figure 3). This mechanism of vitamin A transport is mediated by the plasma retinol binding protein (RBP), a specific and sole carrier of vitamin A in the blood [131–136], and its specific membrane receptor STRA6, which mediates cellular vitamin A uptake [137].

Figure 3. Summary diagram of the key events in the evolution of vitamin A functions that coincide with the emergence of RBP/STRA6-mediated specific vitamin A transport.

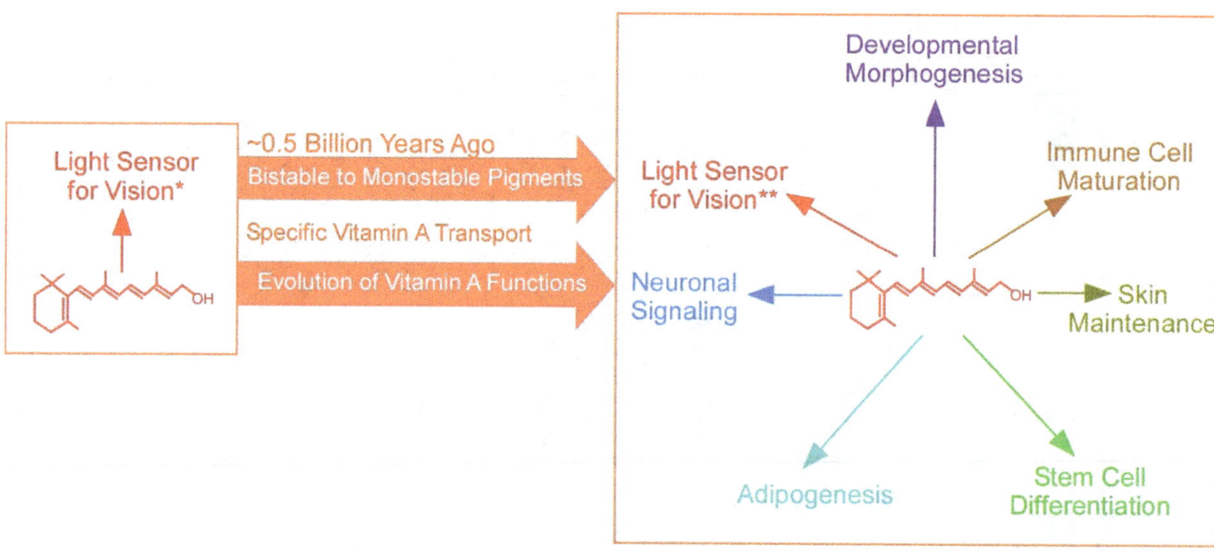

Surprisingly, evolution seems to have produced the RBP receptor STRA6 from scratch because it is not homologous to any membrane receptors or transporters of known function and represents a new type of cell-surface receptor [138]. In contrast, ABCA4, a transporter for vitamin A derivatives, belongs to an ancient family of ATP-dependent transporters. STRA6 employs a membrane transport mechanism distinct from known celluar mechanisms including active transport, channels, and facilitated transport [139,140]. STRA6's vitamin A uptake is coupled to intracellular proteins involved in retinoid storage such as LRAT [137,141,142] or CRBP-I [139], but no single intracellular protein is absolutely required for its vitamin A uptake activity [139,140]. At the biochemical level, STRA6 has diverse catalytic activities such as catalyzing retinol release from holo-RBP [139,140], retinol loading into apo-RBP [139,142], retinol exchange between RBP molecules [140], and retinol transport from holo-RBP to apo-CRBP-I [139]. Depending on extracellular RBP species (the ratio of holo-RBP to apo-RBP) and intracellular proteins (the presence of CRBP-I or LRAT), STRA6 can promote retinol influx, retinol efflux or retinol exchange [140]. How STRA6 achieves its biological activities is not well understood. STRA6 has 9 transmembrane domains, 5 extracellular domains and 5 intracellular domains [143]. Between transmembrane 6 and 7 is an essential RBP binding domain [144].

Studies in human genetics and in animal models have revealed the critical functions of RBP and STRA6. Partial loss of RBP function leads to RPE dystrophy at a young age in humans [145,146]. Complete loss of RBP is embryonic lethal under vitamin A deficient conditions that mimic the natural environment [147]. RBP is required to mobilize liver-stored vitamin A [148]. Complete loss of STRA6 in human causes wide-spread pathogenic phenotypes in many organs [149,150]. Loss of STRA6 causes highly suppressed tissue vitamin A uptake in both zebrafish [142] and mouse [151]. Loss of STRA6 leads to the loss of most stored vitamin A in the eye and subsequent cone photoreceptor degeneration, consistent with previous findings that loss of visual chromophore causes cone photoreceptor degeneration [152–155].

STRA6 knockout causes the loss of 95% of the retinyl ester store in the RPE cells, the key cell type responsible for vitamin A uptake and storage for vision [151]. What is responsible for the STRA6-independent 5%? RBP/STRA6-mediated specific vitamin A transport is not the only mechanism of vitamin A delivery. Vitamin A, like many hydrophobic drugs, has a theoretically much simpler mechanism of transport by random diffusion. However, virtually all vitamin A in vertebrate blood is bound to RBP. The other most dominant mechanism is mediated by retinyl esters in the blood, as revealed by studies of RBP knockout mice [147,156]. Consistently, RPE-specific LRAT knockout also revealed that the RPE can take up retinyl esters without LRAT [157]. The LRAT-independent uptake of retinyl esters by the RPE is more than sufficient to account for the residual retinyl ester in STRA6 knockout mice [151]. This suggests that STRA6 is responsible for virtually all retinol accessible to LRAT in the RPE.

Retinyl ester bound to chylomicron is the primary vehicle that transports dietary vitamin A absorbed by the small intestine to the liver, the primary organ for vitamin A storage [158,159]. There is also strong experimental evidence that a fraction of the retinyl esters can be absorbed by peripheral organs as well [133,159]. This vitamin A transport mechanism is independent of RBP/STRA6. If retinyl ester in the blood can deliver vitamin A, why do we need RBP/STRA6? The many differences between the two mechanisms can answer this question (Table 5). The RBP/STRA6-mediated transport is a sustained and specific mechanism. The high affinity and specificity in RBP's binding to STRA6 can target the vitamin A/RBP complex to specific cells that specialize in vitamin A uptake and storage (e.g., the RPE cell). Although retinyl ester in the blood is capable of partially compensating for the loss of RBP or STRA6 under vitamin A sufficient or excessive conditions, it "borrows" lipid transport pathways, which target a much wider variety of cell types (beyond those specialized in vitamin A uptake and storage) and cannot be relied on during vitamin A deficiency, which is common in natural environments. Studies in both animals [160] and humans [111] revealed that more toxicity is associated with vitamin A delivery independent of RBP. An increase above 10% in retinyl ester in the blood is regarded as a sign of vitamin A overload [111,131].

Table 5. Comparison of vitamin A transport via holo-RBP in the blood *vs.* retinyl esters in the blood.

	RBP-Bound Retinol in Blood	**Retinyl Ester in Blood**
Tissue Origin	Primarily the liver	Primarily the small intestine
Source of Vitamin A	Vitamin A stored in the liver, the primary organ for vitamin A storage	Dietary vitamin A immediately after absorption by the small intestine
Ability to Mobilize Liver-Stored Vitamin A	Yes	No
Dependence on Immediate Diatary Intake	No	Yes
Regulation of its Concentration in the Blood	Yes	No
As a Source of Vitamin A During the Absence of Food	Yes	No
As a Source of Vitamin A in the Absence of Vitamin A in Food	Yes	No
Nature of the Carrier Protein(s) in the Blood	The only known natural ligand of RBP is retinol	Retinyl esters are carried by lipoproteins such as chylomicron remnants, which contain many kinds of lipids
Cellular Uptake Specificity	Cellular retinol uptake by the RBP receptor is not associated with cellular uptake of many other kinds of lipids	Cellular retinyl ester uptake is associated with cellular uptake of many other kinds of lipids
Regulatory Mechanism of Vitamin A Uptake	Unknown	Unknown
As a Cause of Vitamin A Toxicity in Human	No (Healthy people maintain micromolar concentrations in the blood)	Yes (An increase above 10% in retinyl esters in the blood is a sign of vitamin A overload in human)

There exists a STRA6 homolog. The function of this homolog is an intriguing question [161,162]. A recent study found that it is mostly expressed in the liver and the small intestine in mice and can take up vitamin A from holo-RBP similarly to STRA6 [163]. Since transfer of retinol within the liver does not depend on RBP, and liver largely obtains its stored vitamin A from chylomicron remnants [159], this receptor may help certain liver cells to obtain vitamin A from holo-RBP in the circulation. The small intestine absorbs vitamin A or its precursors from food and secretes retinyl esters bound to chylomicrons to be delivered to the liver for storage [158,159]. Because there is no retinol/RBP complex in the intestinal lumen, this receptor likely helps small intestine cells not directly accessible to vitamin A from food to obtain vitamin A from the circulation.

4. The Eye and Vitamin A

The earliest structure remotely related to an eye is the eyespot, a light sensing structure in the green alga *Chlamydomonas*. Although the human eye is vastly more complex than the eyespot, and the structures are separated by billions of years of evolutionary time, both serve a similar biological function in perceiving light, and both depend on vitamin A (Figure 4). Despite the growing dependence of other organs on vitamin A in evolution, the eye is still the organ most dependent on vitamin A. For human, the eye is the organ most sensitive to vitamin A deficiency, the loss of RBP, or the loss of STRA6 (Table 6). Given both the essential functions and toxicity of retinoids, how the eye regulates its vitamin A uptake to obtain a sufficient but not excessive amount is still poorly understood.

Figure 4. Comparison of two retinal-based light sensing structures: the eyespot in Chlamydomonas reinhardtii and the human eye. The human eye depends on vitamin A not only for light sensing for vision and the biological clock, but also for embryonic development and for the maintenance of the cornea. Cells or structures that depend on vitamin A are labeled in red.

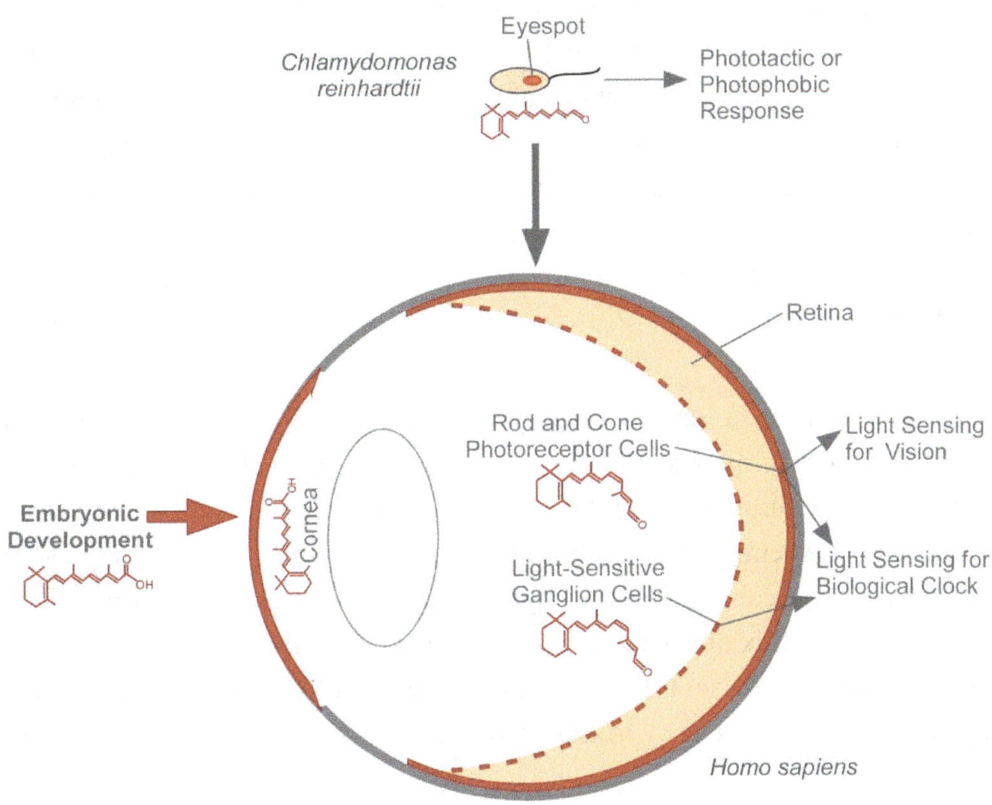

Table 6. In both mice and humans, the eye is the organ most sensitive to vitamin A deficiency, loss of RBP, or loss of STRA6.

	The Most Sensitive Organ in Mouse	The Most Sensitive Organ in Human	The Most Severe Systemic Phenotype
Vitamin A deficiency	The Eye	The Eye	Embryonic Lethality
Loss of RBP	The Eye	The Eye	Embryonic Lethality
Loss of STRA6	The Eye	The Eye	Embryonic Lethality

Nutritional blindness due to vitamin A deficiency is still a leading cause of blindness in the world. Vitamin A deficiency can deprive the photoreceptor cells of the visual chromophore [164]. In addition, vitamin A deficiency causes the disorganization of rod photoreceptor outer segments, degeneration of cone photoreceptor cells, and the loss of LRAT expression in the RPE [165]. If rod and cone photoreceptor cells that sense light for vision depend on vitamin A, what about sensing light for the biological clock, which needs to be frequently readjusted by light? An early study using a mammalian model showed that the spectral sensitivity of the photoreceptors that mediate light's entrainment of the biological clock is indicative of a vitamin A-based light sensor that peaks at 500 nm [166]. Although there was a debate on whether it might be flavin-based, recent studies confirmed that it is vitamin A based and revealed that visual pigments in rod and cone and melanopsin in light-sensitive ganglion cells all contribute to this light sensing function.

Vitamin A, a chemical originally used only for light sensing, is now also an essential molecule for eye development. Retinoic acid, the acid form of vitamin A, plays critical roles in retina and eye development [167–172]. The human eye does not develop without STRA6, the RBP receptor that mediates vitamin A uptake [149,150,173]. STRA6's influence on eye development may not be limited to its expression within the eye itself. One of the organs that expresses the highest level of STRA6 is the placenta, the maternal-fetal barrier which supplies essential nutrients for fetal development. STRA6 can also influence eye development by supplying retinoid to developing embryos in general.

In addition to sensing light for vision and circadian rhythm and eye development, vitamin A also plays crucial roles in maintaining a healthy cornea [174,175]. Without vitamin A, the cornea develops ulceration. Corneal dryness due to vitamin A deficiency is another common cause of human blindness. This role of vitamin A is likely related to one of vitamin A's general functions in epithelial maintenance and stem cell differentiation. How the cornea absorbs vitamin A physiologically is still poorly understood.

Although human vision in a sense perfectly serves our daily needs, we are living with the consequences of the choice of monostable pigments in evolution. If this choice helped our ancestors survive at night, it came at surprisingly high costs. It is astonishing to realize that "every" photon we see depends on a complex enzymatic cycle that consumes cellular energy and releases free toxic retinoid. As we see using our cones in natural daylight or artificial light, a staggering amount of energy is consumed, and a constant flux of toxic free retinoid is cycling between cells to regenerate rhodopsin, which plays no role in daylight vision. In a sense, a whole range of human diseases, from our vision's high sensitivity to vitamin A deficiency to Stargardt macular dystrophy, are the price we pay for this evolutionary choice.

5. Conclusion

For most of evolutionary history starting about 3 billion years ago, vitamin A has functioned as a light sensor. Vitamin A-based light sensors span a wide range of absorption maxima from UV to near infrared. This range matches the peak irradiance of sunlight on earth's surface, the dominant light source in evolution that determines the "visible" light for fish in deep sea or human beings. The major changes during the evolution of vitamin A-based light sensors are the switch from light-gated ion channels to light-activated G-protein coupled receptors and the switch from bistable pigments to monostable pigments for vision. Vitamin A's biological functions have also been tremendously expanded to include its crucial roles in regulating cell growth and differentiation from embryogenesis to adulthood. The likely driving forces for the evolution of a sustained, efficient and precise system of vitamin A transport are the high demand for vitamin A by vision (due to monostable pigments that constantly release the chromophore in daylight), the high toxicity associated with excess vitamin A, and the need to survive vitamin A deficiency, which is common in the natural environments. Because an imbalance in vitamin A homeostasis is associated with diverse human diseases including blindness and birth defects, a better understanding of how vitamin A is transported to the right cell type in the appropriate amount will help to devise new strategies to treat many human diseases caused by insufficient or excessive tissue retinoid levels or to use retinoids as therapeutic agents.

Acknowledgment

Supported by National Institutes of Health grant R01EY018144. H.S. is an Early Career Scientist of the Howard Hughes Medical Institute.

References

1. Brine, D.T.; Iqbal, M. Diffuse and global solar spectral irradiance under cloudless skies. *Sol. Energy* **1983**, *30*, 447–453.
2. Lean, J. Evolution of the sun's spectral irradiance since the maunder minimum. *Geophys. Res. Lett.* **2000**, *27*, 2425–2428.
3. Nathans, J. The evolution and physiology of human color vision: Insights from molecular genetic studies of visual pigments. *Neuron* **1999**, *24*, 299–312.
4. Spudich, J.L.; Yang, C.S.; Jung, K.H.; Spudich, E.N. Retinylidene proteins: Structures and functions from archaea to humans. *Annu. Rev. Cell Dev. Biol.* **2000**, *16*, 365–392.
5. Nathans, J.; Piantanida, T.P.; Eddy, R.L.; Shows, T.B.; Hogness, D.S. Molecular genetics of inherited variation in human color vision. *Science* **1986**, *232*, 203–210.
6. Nathans, J.; Thomas, D.; Hogness, D.S. Molecular genetics of human color vision: The genes encoding blue, green, and red pigments. *Science* **1986**, *232*, 193–202.
7. Nathans, J. Rhodopsin: Structure, function, and genetics. *Biochemistry* **1992**, *31*, 4923–4931.
8. Khorana, H.G. Rhodopsin, photoreceptor of the rod cell. An emerging pattern for structure and function. *J. Biol. Chem.* **1992**, *267*, 1–4.
9. Hubbell, W.L.; Altenbach, C.; Hubbell, C.M.; Khorana, H.G. Rhodopsin structure, dynamics, and activation: A perspective from crystallography, site-directed spin labeling, sulfhydryl reactivity, and disulfide cross-linking. *Adv. Protein Chem.* **2003**, *63*, 243–290.
10. Palczewski, K. G protein-coupled receptor rhodopsin. *Annu. Rev. Biochem.* **2006**, *75*, 743–767.
11. Provencio, I.; Rodriguez, I.R.; Jiang, G.; Hayes, W.P.; Moreira, E.F.; Rollag, M.D. A novel human opsin in the inner retina. *J. Neurosci.* **2000**, *20*, 600–605.
12. Hattar, S.; Liao, H.W.; Takao, M.; Berson, D.M.; Yau, K.W. Melanopsin-containing retinal ganglion cells: Architecture, projections, and intrinsic photosensitivity. *Science* **2002**, *295*, 1065–1070.
13. Panda, S.; Provencio, I.; Tu, D.C.; Pires, S.S.; Rollag, M.D.; Castrucci, A.M.; Pletcher, M.T.; Sato, T.K.; Wiltshire, T.; Andahazy, M.; *et al.* Melanopsin is required for non-image-forming photic responses in blind mice. *Science* **2003**, *301*, 525–527.

14. Dacey, D.M.; Liao, H.W.; Peterson, B.B.; Robinson, F.R.; Smith, V.C.; Pokorny, J.; Yau, K.W.; Gamlin, P.D. Melanopsin-expressing ganglion cells in primate retina signal colour and irradiance and project to the lgn. *Nature* **2005**, *433*, 749–754.
15. Melyan, Z.; Tarttelin, E.E.; Bellingham, J.; Lucas, R.J.; Hankins, M.W. Addition of human melanopsin renders mammalian cells photoresponsive. *Nature* **2005**, *433*, 741–745.
16. Do, M.T.; Kang, S.H.; Xue, T.; Zhong, H.; Liao, H.W.; Bergles, D.E.; Yau, K.W. Photon capture and signalling by melanopsin retinal ganglion cells. *Nature* **2009**, *457*, 281–287.
17. Guler, A.D.; Ecker, J.L.; Lall, G.S.; Haq, S.; Altimus, C.M.; Liao, H.W.; Barnard, A.R.; Cahill, H.; Badea, T.C.; Zhao, H.; *et al.* Melanopsin cells are the principal conduits for rod-cone input to non-image-forming vision. *Nature* **2008**, *453*, 102–105.
18. Sun, H.; Gilbert, D.J.; Copeland, N.G.; Jenkins, N.A.; Nathans, J. Peropsin, a novel visual pigment-like protein located in the apical microvilli of the retinal pigment epithelium. *Proc. Natl. Acad. Sci. USA* **1997**, *94*, 9893–9898.
19. Shen, D.; Jiang, M.; Hao, W.; Tao, L.; Salazar, M.; Fong, H.K. A human opsin-related gene that encodes a retinaldehyde-binding protein. *Biochemistry* **1994**, *33*, 13117–13125.
20. Morimura, H.; Saindelle-Ribeaudeau, F.; Berson, E.L.; Dryja, T.P. Mutations in RGR, encoding a light-sensitive opsin homologue, in patients with retinitis pigmentosa. *Nat. Genet.* **1999**, *23*, 393–394.
21. Wenzel, A.; Oberhauser, V.; Pugh, E.N., Jr.; Lamb, T.D.; Grimm, C.; Samardzija, M.; Fahl, E.; Seeliger, M.W.; Reme, C.E.; von Lintig, J. The retinal G protein-coupled receptor (RGR) enhances isomerohydrolase activity independent of light. *J. Biol. Chem.* **2005**, *280*, 29874–29884.
22. Radu, R.A.; Hu, J.; Peng, J.; Bok, D.; Mata, N.L.; Travis, G.H. Retinal pigment epithelium-retinal G protein receptor-opsin mediates light-dependent translocation of all-*trans*-retinyl esters for synthesis of visual chromophore in retinal pigment epithelial cells. *J. Biol. Chem.* **2008**, *283*, 19730–19738.
23. Applebury, M.L.; Antoch, M.P.; Baxter, L.C.; Chun, L.L.; Falk, J.D.; Farhangfar, F.; Kage, K.; Krzystolik, M.G.; Lyass, L.A.; Robbins, J.T. The murine cone photoreceptor: A single cone type expresses both s and m opsins with retinal spatial patterning. *Neuron* **2000**, *27*, 513–523.
24. Tarttelin, E.E.; Bellingham, J.; Hankins, M.W.; Foster, R.G.; Lucas, R.J. Neuropsin (Opn5): A novel opsin identified in mammalian neural tissue. *FEBS Lett.* **2003**, *554*, 410–416.
25. Kojima, D.; Mori, S.; Torii, M.; Wada, A.; Morishita, R.; Fukada, Y. UV-sensitive photoreceptor protein OPN5 in humans and mice. *PLoS One* **2011**, *6*, e26388.
26. Yokoyama, S.; Zhang, H.; Radlwimmer, F.B.; Blow, N.S. Adaptive evolution of color vision of the Comoran coelacanth (*Latimeria chalumnae*). *Proc. Natl. Acad. Sci. USA* **1999**, *96*, 6279–6284.
27. Owens, G.L.; Windsor, D.J.; Mui, J.; Taylor, J.S. A fish eye out of water: Ten visual opsins in the four-eyed fish, anableps anableps. *PLoS One* **2009**, *4*, e5970.
28. Merbs, S.L.; Nathans, J. Role of hydroxyl-bearing amino acids in differentially tuning the absorption spectra of the human red and green cone pigments. *Photochem. Photobiol.* **1993**, *58*, 706–710.
29. Sun, H.; Macke, J.P.; Nathans, J. Mechanisms of spectral tuning in the mouse green cone pigment. *Proc. Natl. Acad. Sci. USA* **1997**, *94*, 8860–8865.

30. Fasick, J.I.; Lee, N.; Oprian, D.D. Spectral tuning in the human blue cone pigment. *Biochemistry* **1999**, *38*, 11593–11596.
31. Kochendoerfer, G.G.; Lin, S.W.; Sakmar, T.P.; Mathies, R.A. How color visual pigments are tuned. *Trends Biochem. Sci.* **1999**, *24*, 300–305.
32. Lin, S.W.; Sakmar, T.P. Colour tuning mechanisms of visual pigments. *Novartis Found. Symp.* **1999**, *224*, 124–135; discussion 135–141, 181–190.
33. Fasick, J.I.; Applebury, M.L.; Oprian, D.D. Spectral tuning in the mammalian short-wavelength sensitive cone pigments. *Biochemistry* **2002**, *41*, 6860–6865.
34. Kusnetzow, A.K.; Dukkipati, A.; Babu, K.R.; Ramos, L.; Knox, B.E.; Birge, R.R. Vertebrate ultraviolet visual pigments: Protonation of the retinylidene schiff base and a counterion switch during photoactivation. *Proc. Natl. Acad. Sci. USA* **2004**, *101*, 941–946.
35. Yokoyama, S. Evolution of dim-light and color vision pigments. *Annu. Rev. Genomics Hum. Genet.* **2008**, *9*, 259–282.
36. Tsin, A.T.; Beatty, D.D.; Bridges, C.D.; Alvarez, R. Selective utilization of vitamins A1 and A2 by goldfish photoreceptors. *Investig. Ophthalmol. Vis. Sci.* **1983**, *24*, 1324–1327.
37. Ma, J.X.; Kono, M.; Xu, L.; Das, J.; Ryan, J.C.; Hazard, E.S., III; Oprian, D.D.; Crouch, R.K. Salamander UV cone pigment: Sequence, expression, and spectral properties. *Vis. Neurosci.* **2001**, *18*, 393–399.
38. Temple, S.E.; Plate, E.M.; Ramsden, S.; Haimberger, T.J.; Roth, W.M.; Hawryshyn, C.W. Seasonal cycle in vitamin A1/A2-based visual pigment composition during the life history of coho salmon (*Oncorhynchus kisutch*). *J. Comp. Physiol. A Neuroethol. Sens. Neural Behav. Physiol.* **2006**, *192*, 301–313.
39. Ala-Laurila, P.; Donner, K.; Crouch, R.K.; Cornwall, M.C. Chromophore switch from 11-*cis*-dehydroretinal (A2) to 11-*cis*-retinal (aA1) decreases dark noise in salamander red rods. *J. Physiol.* **2007**, *585*, 57–74.
40. Saarinen, P.; Pahlberg, J.; Herczeg, G.; Viljanen, M.; Karjalainen, M.; Shikano, T.; Merila, J.; Donner, K. Spectral tuning by selective chromophore uptake in rods and cones of eight populations of nine-spined stickleback (*Pungitius pungitius*). *J. Exp. Biol.* **2012**, *215*, 2760–2773.
41. Provencio, I.; Loew, E.R.; Foster, R.G. Vitamin A2-based visual pigments in fully terrestrial vertebrates. *Vis. Res.* **1992**, *32*, 2201–2208.
42. Dowling, J.E. Chemistry of visual adaptation in the rat. *Nature* **1960**, *188*, 114–118.
43. Crouch, R.K.; Chader, G.J.; Wiggert, B.; Pepperberg, D.R. Retinoids and the visual process. *Photochem. Photobiol.* **1996**, *64*, 613–621.
44. Lamb, T.D.; Pugh, E.N., Jr. Dark adaptation and the retinoid cycle of vision. *Prog. Retin. Eye Res.* **2004**, *23*, 307–380.
45. Travis, G.H.; Golczak, M.; Moise, A.R.; Palczewski, K. Diseases caused by defects in the visual cycle: Retinoids as potential therapeutic agents. *Annu. Rev. Pharmacol. Toxicol.* **2007**, *47*, 469–512.
46. Von Lintig, J.; Kiser, P.D.; Golczak, M.; Palczewski, K. The biochemical and structural basis for *trans*-to-*cis* isomerization of retinoids in the chemistry of vision. *Trends Biochem. Sci.* **2010**, *35*, 400–410.

47. Mata, N.L.; Radu, R.A.; Clemmons, R.C.; Travis, G.H. Isomerization and oxidation of vitamin A in cone-dominant retinas: A novel pathway for visual-pigment regeneration in daylight. *Neuron* **2002**, *36*, 69–80.
48. Fleisch, V.C.; Schonthaler, H.B.; von Lintig, J.; Neuhauss, S.C. Subfunctionalization of a retinoid-binding protein provides evidence for two parallel visual cycles in the cone-dominant zebrafish retina. *J. Neurosci.* **2008**, *28*, 8208–8216.
49. Wang, J.S.; Estevez, M.E.; Cornwall, M.C.; Kefalov, V.J. Intra-retinal visual cycle required for rapid and complete cone dark adaptation. *Nat. Neurosci.* **2009**, *12*, 295–302.
50. Travis, G.H.; Kaylor, J.; Yuan, Q. Analysis of the retinoid isomerase activities in the retinal pigment epithelium and retina. *Methods Mol. Biol.* **2010**, *652*, 329–339.
51. Wang, J.S.; Kefalov, V.J. The cone-specific visual cycle. *Prog. Retin. Eye Res.* **2011**, *30*, 115–128.
52. Kaylor, J.J.; Yuan, Q.; Cook, J.; Sarfare, S.; Makshanoff, J.; Miu, A.; Kim, A.; Kim, P.; Habib, S.; Roybal, C.N.; *et al.* Identification of DES1 as a vitamin A isomerase in muller glial cells of the retina. *Nat. Chem. Biol.* **2012**, doi:10.1038/nchembio.1114.
53. Jastrzebska, B.; Palczewski, K.; Golczak, M. Role of bulk water in the hydrolysis of rhodopsin's chromophore. *J. Biol. Chem.* **2011**, *286*, 18930–18937.
54. Chen, M.H.; Kuemmel, C.; Birge, R.R.; Knox, B.E. Rapid release of retinal from a cone visual pigment following photoactivation. *Biochemistry* **2012**, *51*, 4117–4125.
55. Woodruff, M.L.; Wang, Z.; Chung, H.Y.; Redmond, T.M.; Fain, G.L.; Lem, J. Spontaneous activity of opsin apoprotein is a cause of Leber congenital amaurosis. *Nat. Genet.* **2003**, *35*, 158–164.
56. Kefalov, V.J.; Estevez, M.E.; Kono, M.; Goletz, P.W.; Crouch, R.K.; Cornwall, M.C.; Yau, K.W. Breaking the covalent bond—A pigment property that contributes to desensitization in cones. *Neuron* **2005**, *46*, 879–890.
57. Okawa, H.; Sampath, A.P.; Laughlin, S.B.; Fain, G.L. ATP consumption by mammalian rod photoreceptors in darkness and in light. *Curr. Biol.* **2008**, *18*, 1917–1921.
58. Emran, F.; Rihel, J.; Adolph, A.R.; Dowling, J.E. Zebrafish larvae lose vision at night. *Proc. Natl. Acad. Sci. USA* **2010**, *107*, 6034–6039.
59. Wang, X.; Wang, T.; Jiao, Y.; von Lintig, J.; Montell, C. Requirement for an enzymatic visual cycle in drosophila. *Curr. Biol.* **2010**, *20*, 93–102.
60. Molday, R.S.; Zhong, M.; Quazi, F. The role of the photoreceptor abc transporter ABCA4 in lipid transport and stargardt macular degeneration. *Biochim. Biophys. Acta* **2009**, *1791*, 573–583.
61. Tsybovsky, Y.; Molday, R.S.; Palczewski, K. The ATP-binding cassette transporter ABCA4: Structural and functional properties and role in retinal disease. *Adv. Exp. Med. Biol.* **2010**, *703*, 105–125.
62. Weng, J.; Mata, N.L.; Azarian, S.M.; Tzekov, R.T.; Birch, D.G.; Travis, G.H. Insights into the function of rim protein in photoreceptors and etiology of Stargardt's disease from the phenotype in ABCR knockout mice. *Cell* **1999**, *98*, 13–23.
63. Sun, H.; Molday, R.S.; Nathans, J. Retinal stimulates ATP hydrolysis by purified and reconstituted ABCR, the photoreceptor-specific ATP-binding cassette transporter responsible for Stargardt disease. *J. Biol. Chem.* **1999**, *274*, 8269–8281.

64. Mata, N.L.; Weng, J.; Travis, G.H. Biosynthesis of a major lipofuscin fluorophore in mice and humans with ABCR-mediated retinal and macular degeneration. *Proc. Natl. Acad. Sci. USA* **2000**, *97*, 7154–7159.
65. Sun, H.; Nathans, J. Mechanistic studies of ABCR, the ABC transporter in photoreceptor outer segments responsible for autosomal recessive Stargardt disease. *J. Bioenergy Biomembr.* **2001**, *33*, 523–530.
66. Zhong, M.; Molday, R.S. Binding of retinoids to ABCA4, the photoreceptor ABC transporter associated with Stargardt macular degeneration. *Methods Mol. Biol.* **2010**, *652*, 163–176.
67. Boyer, N.P.; Higbee, D.; Currin, M.B.; Blakeley, L.R.; Chen, C.; Ablonczy, Z.; Crouch, R.K.; Koutalos, Y. Lipofuscin and *N*-retinylidene-*N*-retinylethanolamine (A2E) accumulate in retinal pigment epithelium in absence of light exposure: Their origin is 11-*cis*-retinal. *J. Biol. Chem.* **2012**, *287*, 22276–22286.
68. Quazi, F.; Lenevich, S.; Molday, R.S. ABCA4 is an *N*-retinylidene-phosphatidylethanolamine and phosphatidylethanolamine importer. *Nat. Commun.* **2012**, *3*, 925.
69. Allikmets, R.; Singh, N.; Sun, H.; Shroyer, N.F.; Hutchinson, A.; Chidambaram, A.; Gerrard, B.; Baird, L.; Stauffer, D.; Peiffer, A.; *et al.* A photoreceptor cell-specific ATP-binding transporter gene (ABCR) is mutated in recessive Stargardt macular dystrophy. *Nat. Genet.* **1997**, *15*, 236–246.
70. Cremers, F.P.; van de Pol, D.J.; van Driel, M.; den Hollander, A.I.; van Haren, F.J.; Knoers, N.V.; Tijmes, N.; Bergen, A.A.; Rohrschneider, K.; Blankenagel, A.; *et al.* Autosomal recessive retinitis pigmentosa and cone-rod dystrophy caused by splice site mutations in the Stargardt's disease gene ABCR. *Hum. Mol. Genet.* **1998**, *7*, 355–362.
71. Martinez-Mir, A.; Paloma, E.; Allikmets, R.; Ayuso, C.; del Rio, T.; Dean, M.; Vilageliu, L.; Gonzalez-Duarte, R.; Balcells, S. Retinitis pigmentosa caused by a homozygous mutation in the stargardt disease gene ABCR. *Nat. Genet.* **1998**, *18*, 11–12.
72. Fu, Y.; Zhong, H.; Wang, M.H.; Luo, D.G.; Liao, H.W.; Maeda, H.; Hattar, S.; Frishman, L.J.; Yau, K.W. Intrinsically photosensitive retinal ganglion cells detect light with a vitamin A-based photopigment, melanopsin. *Proc. Natl. Acad. Sci. USA* **2005**, *102*, 10339–10344.
73. Panda, S.; Nayak, S.K.; Campo, B.; Walker, J.R.; Hogenesch, J.B.; Jegla, T. Illumination of the melanopsin signaling pathway. *Science* **2005**, *307*, 600–604.
74. Walker, M.T.; Brown, R.L.; Cronin, T.W.; Robinson, P.R. Photochemistry of retinal chromophore in mouse melanopsin. *Proc. Natl. Acad. Sci. USA* **2008**, *105*, 8861–8865.
75. Sexton, T.J.; Golczak, M.; Palczewski, K.; van Gelder, R.N. Melanopsin is highly resistant to light and chemical bleaching *in vivo*. *J. Biol. Chem.* **2012**, *287*, 20888–20897.
76. Yamashita, T.; Ohuchi, H.; Tomonari, S.; Ikeda, K.; Sakai, K.; Shichida, Y. Opn5 is a UV-sensitive bistable pigment that couples with Gi subtype of G protein. *Proc. Natl. Acad. Sci. USA* **2010**, *107*, 22084–22089.
77. Bi, A.; Cui, J.; Ma, Y.P.; Olshevskaya, E.; Pu, M.; Dizhoor, A.M.; Pan, Z.H. Ectopic expression of a microbial-type rhodopsin restores visual responses in mice with photoreceptor degeneration. *Neuron* **2006**, *50*, 23–33.
78. Zhang, F.; Wang, L.P.; Brauner, M.; Liewald, J.F.; Kay, K.; Watzke, N.; Wood, P.G.; Bamberg, E.; Nagel, G.; Gottschalk, A.; *et al.* Multimodal fast optical interrogation of neural circuitry. *Nature* **2007**, *446*, 633–639.

79. Oberhauser, V.; Voolstra, O.; Bangert, A.; von Lintig, J.; Vogt, K. NinaB combines carotenoid oxygenase and retinoid isomerase activity in a single polypeptide. *Proc. Natl. Acad. Sci. USA* **2008**, *105*, 19000–19005.
80. Ross, A.C.; Gardner, E.M. The function of vitamin A in cellular growth and differentiation, and its roles during pregnancy and lactation. *Adv. Exp. Med. Biol.* **1994**, *352*, 187–200.
81. Napoli, J.L. Biochemical pathways of retinoid transport, metabolism, and signal transduction. *Clin. Immunol. Immunopathol.* **1996**, *80*, S52–S62.
82. Stephensen, C.B. Vitamin A, infection, and immune function. *Annu. Rev. Nutr.* **2001**, *21*, 167–192.
83. Drager, U.C. Retinoic acid signaling in the functioning brain. *Sci. STKE* **2006**, *2006*, pe10.
84. Maden, M. Retinoic acid in the development, regeneration and maintenance of the nervous system. *Nat. Rev. Neurosci.* **2007**, *8*, 755–765.
85. Duester, G. Retinoic acid synthesis and signaling during early organogenesis. *Cell* **2008**, *134*, 921–931.
86. Niederreither, K.; Dolle, P. Retinoic acid in development: Towards an integrated view. *Nat. Rev. Genet.* **2008**, *9*, 541–553.
87. Takahashi, J.; Palmer, T.D.; Gage, F.H. Retinoic acid and neurotrophins collaborate to regulate neurogenesis in adult-derived neural stem cell cultures. *J. Neurobiol.* **1999**, *38*, 65–81.
88. Evans, R.M. The molecular basis of signaling by vitamin A and its metabolites. *Harvey Lect.* **1994**, *90*, 105–117.
89. Mark, M.; Ghyselinck, N.B.; Chambon, P. Function of retinoid nuclear receptors: Lessons from genetic and pharmacological dissections of the retinoic acid signaling pathway during mouse embryogenesis. *Annu. Rev. Pharmacol. Toxicol.* **2006**, *46*, 451–480.
90. Wolbach, S.R.; Howe, P.R. Tissue change following deprivation of fat-soluble A vitamin. *J. Exp. Med.* **1925**, *42*, 753–777.
91. West, K.P., Jr. Vitamin A deficiency: Its epidemiology and relation to child mortality and morbidity. In *Vitamin A in Health and Disease*; Blomhoff, R., Ed.; Marcel Dekker, Inc.: New York, NY, USA, 1994.
92. Dowling, J.E. Night blindness. *Sci. Am.* **1966**, *215*, 78–84.
93. Sommer, A. Vitamin A: Its effect on childhood sight and life. *Nutr. Rev.* **1994**, *52*, S60–S66.
94. Misner, D.L.; Jacobs, S.; Shimizu, Y.; de Urquiza, A.M.; Solomin, L.; Perlmann, T.; de Luca, L.M.; Stevens, C.F.; Evans, R.M. Vitamin A deprivation results in reversible loss of hippocampal long-term synaptic plasticity. *Proc. Natl. Acad. Sci. USA* **2001**, *98*, 11714–11719.
95. Cocco, S.; Diaz, G.; Stancampiano, R.; Diana, A.; Carta, M.; Curreli, R.; Sarais, L.; Fadda, F. Vitamin A deficiency produces spatial learning and memory impairment in rats. *Neuroscience* **2002**, *115*, 475–482.
96. Biesalski, H.K. The significance of vitamin A for the development and function of the lung. *Forum Nutr.* **2003**, *56*, 37–40.
97. Ross, A.C. On the sources of retinoic acid in the lung: Understanding the local conversion of retinol to retinoic acid. *Am. J. Physiol. Lung Cell. Mol. Physiol.* **2004**, *286*, L247–L248.
98. Vahlquist, A. Role of retinoids in normal and diseased skin. In *Vitamin A in Health and Disease*; Blomhoff, R., Ed.; Marcel Dekker, Inc.: New York, NY, USA, 1994; pp. 365–424.

99. Morley, J.E.; Damassa, D.A.; Gordon, J.; Pekary, A.E.; Hershman, J.M. Thyroid function and vitamin A deficiency. *Life Sci.* **1978**, *22*, 1901–1905.

100. Livera, G.; Rouiller-Fabre, V.; Pairault, C.; Levacher, C.; Habert, R. Regulation and perturbation of testicular functions by vitamin A. *Reproduction* **2002**, *124*, 173–180.

101. Chen, L.; Khillan, J.S. Promotion of feeder-independent self-renewal of embryonic stem cells by retinol (vitamin A). *Stem Cells* **2008**, *26*, 1858–1864.

102. Ziouzenkova, O.; Orasanu, G.; Sharlach, M.; Akiyama, T.E.; Berger, J.P.; Viereck, J.; Hamilton, J.A.; Tang, G.; Dolnikowski, G.G.; Vogel, S.; *et al.* Retinaldehyde represses adipogenesis and diet-induced obesity. *Nat. Med.* **2007**, *13*, 695–702.

103. Chen, N.; Onisko, B.; Napoli, J.L. The nuclear transcription factor RARα associates with neuronal RNA granules and suppresses translation. *J. Biol. Chem.* **2008**, *283*, 20841–20847.

104. Aoto, J.; Nam, C.I.; Poon, M.M.; Ting, P.; Chen, L. Synaptic signaling by all-*trans* retinoic acid in homeostatic synaptic plasticity. *Neuron* **2008**, *60*, 308–320.

105. Chytil, F.; Ong, D.E. Mediation of retinoic acid-induced growth and anti-tumour activity. *Nature* **1976**, *260*, 49–51.

106. Love, J.M.; Gudas, L.J. Vitamin A, differentiation and cancer. *Curr. Opin. Cell Biol.* **1994**, *6*, 825–831.

107. Yang, Q.; Graham, T.E.; Mody, N.; Preitner, F.; Peroni, O.D.; Zabolotny, J.M.; Kotani, K.; Quadro, L.; Kahn, B.B. Serum retinol binding protein 4 contributes to insulin resistance in obesity and type 2 diabetes. *Nature* **2005**, *436*, 356–362.

108. Basu, T.K.; Basualdo, C. Vitamin A homeostasis and diabetes mellitus. *Nutrition* **1997**, *13*, 804–806.

109. Nau, H.; Chahoud, I.; Dencker, L.; Lammer, E.J.; Scott, W.J. Teratogenicity of vitamin A and retinoids. In *Vitamin A in Health and Disease*; Blomhoff, R., Ed.; Marcel Dekker, Inc.: New York, NY, USA, 1994; pp. 615–664.

110. Orfanos, C.E.; Zouboulis, C.C.; Almond-Roesler, B.; Geilen, C.C. Current use and future potential role of retinoids in dermatology. *Drugs* **1997**, *53*, 358–388.

111. Smith, F.R.; Goodman, D.S. Vitamin A transport in human vitamin A toxicity. *N. Engl. J. Med.* **1976**, *294*, 805–808.

112. Collins, M.D.; Mao, G.E. Teratology of retinoids. *Annu. Rev. Pharmacol. Toxicol.* **1999**, *39*, 399–430.

113. Penniston, K.L.; Tanumihardjo, S.A. The acute and chronic toxic effects of vitamin A. *Am. J. Clin. Nutr.* **2006**, *83*, 191–201.

114. Myhre, A.M.; Carlsen, M.H.; Bohn, S.K.; Wold, H.L.; Laake, P.; Blomhoff, R. Water-miscible, emulsified, and solid forms of retinol supplements are more toxic than oil-based preparations. *Am. J. Clin. Nutr.* **2003**, *78*, 1152–1159.

115. Adams, J. Structure-activity and dose-response relationships in the neural and behavioral teratogenesis of retinoids. *Neurotoxicol. Teratol.* **1993**, *15*, 193–202.

116. Nau, H. Teratogenicity of isotretinoin revisited: Species variation and the role of all-*trans*-retinoic acid. *J. Am. Acad. Dermatol.* **2001**, *45*, S183–S187.

117. Crandall, J.; Sakai, Y.; Zhang, J.; Koul, O.; Mineur, Y.; Crusio, W.E.; McCaffery, P. 13-*cis*-retinoic acid suppresses hippocampal cell division and hippocampal-dependent learning in mice. *Proc. Natl. Acad. Sci. USA* **2004**, *101*, 5111–5116.
118. Sieving, P.A.; Chaudhry, P.; Kondo, M.; Provenzano, M.; Wu, D.; Carlson, T.J.; Bush, R.A.; Thompson, D.A. Inhibition of the visual cycle *in vivo* by 13-*cis* retinoic acid protects from light damage and provides a mechanism for night blindness in isotretinoin therapy. *Proc. Natl. Acad. Sci. USA* **2001**, *98*, 1835–1840.
119. Voolstra, O.; Oberhauser, V.; Sumser, E.; Meyer, N.E.; Maguire, M.E.; Huber, A.; von Lintig, J. NinaB is essential for drosophila vision but induces retinal degeneration in opsin-deficient photoreceptors. *J. Biol. Chem.* **2010**, *285*, 2130–2139.
120. Sun, H.; Nathans, J. ABCR, the ATP-binding cassette transporter responsible for Stargardt macular dystrophy, is an efficient target of all-*trans*-retinal-mediated photooxidative damage *in vitro*. Implications for retinal disease. *J. Biol. Chem.* **2001**, *276*, 11766–11774.
121. Kanan, Y.; Moiseyev, G.; Agarwal, N.; Ma, J.X.; Al-Ubaidi, M.R. Light induces programmed cell death by activating multiple independent proteases in a cone photoreceptor cell line. *Investig. Ophthalmol. Vis. Sci.* **2007**, *48*, 40–51.
122. Masutomi, K.; Chen, C.; Nakatani, K.; Koutalos, Y. All-*trans* retinal mediates light-induced oxidation in single living rod photoreceptors (dagger). *Photochem. Photobiol.* **2012**, *88*, 1356–1361.
123. Maeda, A.; Maeda, T.; Golczak, M.; Palczewski, K. Retinopathy in mice induced by disrupted all-*trans*-retinal clearance. *J. Biol. Chem.* **2008**, *283*, 26684–26693.
124. Sparrow, J.R.; Cai, B.; Jang, Y.P.; Zhou, J.; Nakanishi, K. A2E, a fluorophore of RPE lipofuscin, can destabilize membrane. *Adv. Exp. Med. Biol.* **2006**, *572*, 63–68.
125. Sparrow, J.R.; Boulton, M. RPE lipofuscin and its role in retinal pathobiology. *Exp. Eye Res.* **2005**, *80*, 595–606.
126. De, S.; Sakmar, T.P. Interaction of A2E with model membranes. Implications to the pathogenesis of age-related macular degeneration. *J. Gen. Physiol.* **2002**, *120*, 147–157.
127. Vives-Bauza, C.; Anand, M.; Shirazi, A.K.; Magrane, J.; Gao, J.; Vollmer-Snarr, H.R.; Manfredi, G.; Finnemann, S.C. The age lipid A2E and mitochondrial dysfunction synergistically impair phagocytosis by retinal pigment epithelial cells. *J. Biol. Chem.* **2008**, *283*, 24770–24780.
128. Zhou, J.; Kim, S.R.; Westlund, B.S.; Sparrow, J.R. Complement activation by bisretinoid constituents of RPE lipofuscin. *Investig. Ophthalmol. Vis. Sci.* **2009**, *50*, 1392–1399.
129. Moiseyev, G.; Nikolaeva, O.; Chen, Y.; Farjo, K.; Takahashi, Y.; Ma, J.X. Inhibition of the visual cycle by A2E through direct interaction with RPE65 and implications in stargardt disease. *Proc. Natl. Acad. Sci. USA* **2010**, *107*, 17551–17556.
130. Radu, R.A.; Hu, J.; Yuan, Q.; Welch, D.L.; Makshanoff, J.; Lloyd, M.; McMullen, S.; Travis, G.H.; Bok, D. Complement system dysregulation and inflammation in the retinal pigment epithelium of a mouse model for Stargardt macular degeneration. *J. Biol. Chem.* **2011**, *286*, 18593–18601.
131. Goodman, D.S. Plasma retinol-binding protein. In *The Retinoids*; Sporn, M.B., Boberts, A.B., Goodman, D.S., Eds.; Academic Press, Inc.: Orlando, FL, USA, 1984; Volume 2, pp. 41–88.

132. Rask, L.; Anundi, H.; Bohme, J.; Eriksson, U.; Fredriksson, A.; Nilsson, S.F.; Ronne, H.; Vahlquist, A.; Peterson, P.A. The retinol-binding protein. *Scand. J. Clin. Lab. Investig. Suppl.* **1980**, *154*, 45–61.

133. Blomhoff, R.; Green, M.H.; Berg, T.; Norum, K.R. Transport and storage of vitamin A. *Science* **1990**, *250*, 399–404.

134. Quadro, L.; Hamberger, L.; Colantuoni, V.; Gottesman, M.E.; Blaner, W.S. Understanding the physiological role of retinol-binding protein in vitamin A metabolism using transgenic and knockout mouse models. *Mol. Aspects Med.* **2003**, *24*, 421–430.

135. Zanotti, G.; Berni, R. Plasma retinol-binding protein: Structure and interactions with retinol, retinoids, and transthyretin. *Vitam. Horm.* **2004**, *69*, 271–295.

136. Newcomer, M.E.; Ong, D.E. Plasma retinol binding protein: Structure and function of the prototypic lipocalin. *Biochim. Biophys. Acta* **2000**, *1482*, 57–64.

137. Kawaguchi, R.; Yu, J.; Honda, J.; Hu, J.; Whitelegge, J.; Ping, P.; Wiita, P.; Bok, D.; Sun, H. A membrane receptor for retinol binding protein mediates cellular uptake of vitamin A. *Science* **2007**, *315*, 820–825.

138. Sun, H.; Kawaguchi, R. The membrane receptor for plasma retinol-binding protein, a new type of cell-surface receptor. *Int. Rev. Cell Mol. Biol.* **2011**, *288*, 1–41.

139. Kawaguchi, R.; Yu, J.; Ter-Stepanian, M.; Zhong, M.; Cheng, G.; Yuan, Q.; Jin, M.; Travis, G.H.; Ong, D.; Sun, H. Receptor-mediated cellular uptake mechanism that couples to intracellular storage. *ACS Chem. Biol.* **2011**, *6*, 1041–1051.

140. Kawaguchi, R.; Zhong, M.; Kassai, M.; Ter-Stepanian, M.; Sun, H. STRA6-catalyzed vitamin A influx, efflux and exchange. *J. Membr. Biol.* **2012**, *245*, 731–745.

141. Golczak, M.; Maeda, A.; Bereta, G.; Maeda, T.; Kiser, P.D.; Hunzelmann, S.; von Lintig, J.; Blaner, W.S.; Palczewski, K. Metabolic basis of visual cycle inhibition by retinoid and nonretinoid compounds in the vertebrate retina. *J. Biol. Chem.* **2008**, *283*, 9543–9554.

142. Isken, A.; Golczak, M.; Oberhauser, V.; Hunzelmann, S.; Driever, W.; Imanishi, Y.; Palczewski, K.; von Lintig, J. RBP4 disrupts vitamin A uptake homeostasis in a STRA6-deficient animal model for Matthew-Wood syndrome. *Cell Metab.* **2008**, *7*, 258–268.

143. Kawaguchi, R.; Yu, J.; Wiita, P.; Ter-Stepanian, M.; Sun, H. Mapping the membrane topology and extracellular ligand binding domains of the retinol binding protein receptor. *Biochemistry* **2008**, *47*, 5387–5395.

144. Kawaguchi, R.; Yu, J.; Wiita, P.; Honda, J.; Sun, H. An essential ligand-binding domain in the membrane receptor for retinol-binding protein revealed by large-scale mutagenesis and a human polymorphism. *J. Biol. Chem.* **2008**, *283*, 15160–15168.

145. Seeliger, M.W.; Biesalski, H.K.; Wissinger, B.; Gollnick, H.; Gielen, S.; Frank, J.; Beck, S.; Zrenner, E. Phenotype in retinol deficiency due to a hereditary defect in retinol binding protein synthesis. *Investig. Ophthalmol. Vis. Sci.* **1999**, *40*, 3–11.

146. Folli, C.; Viglione, S.; Busconi, M.; Berni, R. Biochemical basis for retinol deficiency induced by the I41N and G75D mutations in human plasma retinol-binding protein. *Biochem. Biophys. Res. Commun.* **2005**, *336*, 1017–1022.

147. Quadro, L.; Hamberger, L.; Gottesman, M.E.; Wang, F.; Colantuoni, V.; Blaner, W.S.; Mendelsohn, C.L. Pathways of vitamin A delivery to the embryo: Insights from a new tunable model of embryonic vitamin A deficiency. *Endocrinology* **2005**, *146*, 4479–4490.

148. Quadro, L.; Blaner, W.S.; Salchow, D.J.; Vogel, S.; Piantedosi, R.; Gouras, P.; Freeman, S.; Cosma, M.P.; Colantuoni, V.; Gottesman, M.E. Impaired retinal function and vitamin A availability in mice lacking retinol-binding protein. *EMBO J.* **1999**, *18*, 4633–4644.

149. Pasutto, F.; Sticht, H.; Hammersen, G.; Gillessen-Kaesbach, G.; Fitzpatrick, D.R.; Nurnberg, G.; Brasch, F.; Schirmer-Zimmermann, H.; Tolmie, J.L.; Chitayat, D.; *et al.* Mutations in STRA6 cause a broad spectrum of malformations including anophthalmia, congenital heart defects, diaphragmatic hernia, alveolar capillary dysplasia, lung hypoplasia, and mental retardation. *Am. J. Hum. Genet.* **2007**, *80*, 550–560.

150. Golzio, C.; Martinovic-Bouriel, J.; Thomas, S.; Mougou-Zrelli, S.; Grattagliano-Bessieres, B.; Bonniere, M.; Delahaye, S.; Munnich, A.; Encha-Razavi, F.; Lyonnet, S.; *et al.* Matthew-Wood syndrome is caused by truncating mutations in the retinol-binding protein receptor gene STRA6. *Am. J. Hum. Genet.* **2007**, *80*, 1179–1187.

151. Ruiz, A.; Mark, M.; Jacobs, H.; Klopfenstein, M.; Hu, J.; Lloyd, M.; Habib, S.; Tosha, C.; Radu, R.A.; Ghyselinck, N.B.; *et al.* Retinoid content, visual responses and ocular morphology are compromised in the retinas of mice lacking the retinol-binding protein receptor, STRA6. *Investig. Ophthalmol. Vis. Sci.* **2012**, *53*, 3027–3039.

152. Znoiko, S.L.; Rohrer, B.; Lu, K.; Lohr, H.R.; Crouch, R.K.; Ma, J.X. Downregulation of cone-specific gene expression and degeneration of cone photoreceptors in the *Rpe65*$^{-/-}$ mouse at early ages. *Investig. Ophthalmol. Vis. Sci.* **2005**, *46*, 1473–1479.

153. Rohrer, B.; Lohr, H.R.; Humphries, P.; Redmond, T.M.; Seeliger, M.W.; Crouch, R.K. Cone opsin mislocalization in *Rpe65*$^{-/-}$ mice: A defect that can be corrected by 11-*cis* retinal. *Investig. Ophthalmol. Vis. Sci.* **2005**, *46*, 3876–3882.

154. Rohrer, B.; Crouch, R. Rod and cone pigment regeneration in *Rpe65*$^{-/-}$ mice. *Adv. Exp. Med. Biol.* **2006**, *572*, 101–107.

155. Zhang, H.; Fan, J.; Li, S.; Karan, S.; Rohrer, B.; Palczewski, K.; Frederick, J.M.; Crouch, R.K.; Baehr, W. Trafficking of membrane-associated proteins to cone photoreceptor outer segments requires the chromophore 11-*cis*-retinal. *J. Neurosci.* **2008**, *28*, 4008–4014.

156. Quadro, L.; Hamberger, L.; Gottesman, M.E.; Colantuoni, V.; Ramakrishnan, R.; Blaner, W.S. Transplacental delivery of retinoid: The role of retinol-binding protein and lipoprotein retinyl ester. *Am. J. Physiol. Endocrinol. Metab.* **2004**, *286*, E844–E851.

157. Ruiz, A.; Ghyselinck, N.B.; Mata, N.; Nusinowitz, S.; Lloyd, M.; Dennefeld, C.; Chambon, P.; Bok, D. Somatic ablation of the *Lrat* gene in the mouse retinal pigment epithelium drastically reduces its retinoid storage. *Investig. Ophthalmol. Vis. Sci.* **2007**, *48*, 5377–5387.

158. Harrison, E.H. Mechanisms of digestion and absorption of dietary vitamin A. *Annu. Rev. Nutr.* **2005**, *25*, 87–103.

159. D'Ambrosio, D.N.; Clugston, R.D.; Blaner, W.S. Vitamin A metabolism: An update. *Nutrients* **2011**, *3*, 63–103.

160. Mallia, A.K.; Smith, J.E.; Goodman, D.W. Metabolism of retinol-binding protein and vitamin A during hypervitaminosis A in the rat. *J. Lipid Res.* **1975**, *16*, 180–188.

161. Wyatt, N.; Ponting, C.; Dorin, J.; Fitzpatrick, D.; Hill, R. STRA6.2: A novel member of the STRA6 gene family. *Mech. Dev.* **2009**, *126*, S259.
162. Sun, H. Membrane receptors and transporters involved in the function and transport of vitamin A and its derivatives. *Biochim. Biophys. Acta* **2012**, *1821*, 99–112.
163. Alapatt, P.; Guo, F.; Komanetsky, S.M.; Wang, S.; Cai, J.; Sargsyan, A.; Díaz, E.R.; Bacon, B.T.; Aryal, P.; Graham, T.E. Liver retinol transporter and receptor for serum retinol binding protein (RBP4). *J. Biol. Chem.* **2012**, doi:10.1074/jbc.M112.369132.
164. Dowling, J.E.; Wald, G. Vitamin A deficiency and night blindness. *Proc. Natl. Acad. Sci. USA* **1958**, *44*, 648–661.
165. Hu, Y.; Chen, Y.; Moiseyev, G.; Takahashi, Y.; Mott, R.; Ma, J.X. Comparison of ocular pathologies in vitamin A-deficient mice and RPE65 gene knockout mice. *Investig. Ophthalmol. Vis. Sci.* **2011**, *52*, 5507–5514.
166. Takahashi, J.S.; DeCoursey, P.J.; Bauman, L.; Menaker, M. Spectral sensitivity of a novel photoreceptive system mediating entrainment of mammalian circadian rhythms. *Nature* **1984**, *308*, 186–188.
167. Dowling, J.E.; Wald, G. The biological function of vitamin A acid. *Proc. Natl. Acad. Sci. USA* **1960**, *46*, 587–608.
168. Marsh-Armstrong, N.; McCaffery, P.; Gilbert, W.; Dowling, J.E.; Drager, U.C. Retinoic acid is necessary for development of the ventral retina in zebrafish. *Proc. Natl. Acad. Sci. USA* **1994**, *91*, 7286–7290.
169. Hyatt, G.A.; Schmitt, E.A.; Fadool, J.M.; Dowling, J.E. Retinoic acid alters photoreceptor development *in vivo*. *Proc. Natl. Acad. Sci. USA* **1996**, *93*, 13298–13303.
170. Kelley, M.W.; Turner, J.K.; Reh, T.A. Retinoic acid promotes differentiation of photoreceptors *in vitro*. *Development* **1994**, *120*, 2091–2102.
171. Hyatt, G.A.; Dowling, J.E. Retinoic acid. A key molecule for eye and photoreceptor development. *Investig. Ophthalmol. Vis. Sci.* **1997**, *38*, 1471–1475.
172. Duester, G. Keeping an eye on retinoic acid signaling during eye development. *Chem. Biol. Interact.* **2009**, *178*, 178–181.
173. Casey, J.; Kawaguchi, R.; McGettigan, P.; Sun, H.; Morrissey, M.; Nielsen, J.; Conroy, J.; Regan, R.; Tormey, P.; Ni Chroinin, M.; *et al.* First implication of STRA6 mutations in isolated anophthalmia, microphthalmia and coloboma: Adding a new dimension to the STRA6 phenotype. *Hum. Mutat.* **2011**, *32*, 1417–1426.
174. Rask, L.; Geijer, C.; Bill, A.; Peterson, P.A. Vitamin A supply of the cornea. *Exp. Eye Res.* **1980**, *31*, 201–211.
175. Tielsch, J.M.; Sommer, A. The epidemiology of vitamin A deficiency and xerophthalmia. *Annu. Rev. Nutr.* **1984**, *4*, 183–205.

3

Dietary Sources of Lutein and Zeaxanthin Carotenoids and their Role in Eye Health

El-Sayed M. Abdel-Aal [1,*], Humayoun Akhtar [1], Khalid Zaheer [2] and Rashida Ali [3,4]

1 Guelph Food Research Centre, Agriculture and Agri-Food Canada, Guelph, ON N1G 5C9, Canada; E-Mail: humayoun.akhtar@agr.gc.ca
2 Consultant, Toronto, ON M3M 2E9, Canada; E-Mail: kzaheer2000@gmail.com
3 Department of Food Science and Technology, ICCBS, University of Karachi, Karachi 75270, Pakistan; E-Mail: rashida338@gmail.com
4 English Biscuit Manufacturers Pvt. Ltd., Korangi Industrial Area, Karachi 74900, Pakistan

* Author to whom correspondence should be addressed; E-Mail: elsayed.abdelaal@agr.gc.ca;

Abstract: The eye is a major sensory organ that requires special care for a healthy and productive lifestyle. Numerous studies have identified lutein and zeaxanthin to be essential components for eye health. Lutein and zeaxanthin are carotenoid pigments that impart yellow or orange color to various common foods such as cantaloupe, pasta, corn, carrots, orange/yellow peppers, fish, salmon and eggs. Their role in human health, in particular the health of the eye, is well established from epidemiological, clinical and interventional studies. They constitute the main pigments found in the yellow spot of the human retina which protect the macula from damage by blue light, improve visual acuity and scavenge harmful reactive oxygen species. They have also been linked with reduced risk of age-related macular degeneration (AMD) and cataracts. Research over the past decade has focused on the development of carotenoid-rich foods to boost their intake especially in the elderly population. The aim of this article is to review recent scientific evidences supporting the benefits of lutein and zexanthin in preventing the onset of two major age-related eye diseases with diets rich in these carotenoids. The review also lists major dietary sources of lutein and zeaxanthin and refers to newly developed foods, daily intake, bioavailability and physiological effects in relation to eye health. Examples of the newly developed high-lutein functional foods are also underlined.

Keywords: lutein and zeaxanthin carotenoids; dietary sources; eye health; high-lutein foods; bioavailability

---

1. Introduction

Nutrition plays a vital role in human health with no exception to the eye. Healthy eyes provide good vision, which is essential for an enjoyable and productive lifestyle. There is a growing global concern about eye health related issues. To address these issues the World Health Organization (WHO) report on visual impairment in 2010 identifies the principal causes of visual impairment as follows: uncorrected refractive errors (43%), cataracts (33%), glaucoma (2%), age-related macular degeneration (AMD) (1%), diabetic retinopathy (1%) and about 18% are of undetermined nature [1]. The report also lists the three major causes of blindness as cataract (51%), glaucoma (8%), AMD (5%), diabetic retinopathy (1%) and undetermined causes (21%). Cataract is the principal cause of blindness among people over 40 years of age predominantly in developing countries due to improper nutrition (e.g., lack of carotenoids in diet), infectious diseases [2]. AMD, on the other hand, is the leading cause of legal blindness with limited treatment options in people over 65 years of age in industrial countries, and costs many billions of dollars worldwide [2]. There are two types of AMD—dry (atrophic) and wet (neovascular or exudative). In most cases AMD starts as "Dry", which then progresses slowly in approximately 20% cases to "Wet" stage. There is no known treatment for dry AMD. The wet AMD is responsible for almost 90% of the severe cases of blindness [3]. The prevalence of AMD is estimated to be a one-third increase in UK [4] and a 50% increase in USA by 2020 [5]. A similar estimate is also reported for Australia [6]. Both diseases are expected to sharply increase in the elderly population within the next 10–15 years. The Vision 2020, a global initiative for the elimination of avoidable blindness in partnership between WHO and International Agency for the Prevention of Blindness [IAPB] projects blindness due to cataracts alone in elderly to reach 40 million globally by 2025 [7]. It is clear that AMD and cataract incidences will continue to rise substantially in the coming years causing a great impact on health care. This requires global collective efforts to develop strategies for the prevention of the two most important common age-related diseases with appropriate diets/supplements. Several high-lutein functional foods that would be useful in developing such preventive strategies are discussed in the current article.

Oxidative stress, aging and smoking are known to cause cataract and AMD [8,9]. A typical US diet contains 1–3 mg/day of lutein and zeaxanthin, while ~6 mg/day have been related to decrease risk of AMD [8]. Lutein and zeaxanthin have been associated with reduced risk of cataract development and AMD [10]. A longitudinal study has shown that plasma zeaxanthin reduces the risk of cataract [11]. Hence lutein and zeaxanthin, both potent antioxidants, are very important to retard the onset of both cataract and AMD [12]. Additional sources of lutein and zeaxanthin either in the food form or dietary supplements would enhance their intake on regular basis. There are also reports that do not support the protective role of dietary lutein and zeaxanthin against cataracts [13] and AMD [14]. Recently an article that traces the modern history of lutein and zeaxanthin in health and diseases of retina identified four areas for further investigation: (i) ultra-structural localization of xanthophyll affected proteins in the retina, (ii) genetic analysis-genotyping efforts, (iii) model system for the metabolism of lutein and zeaxanthin and (iv) integrated system based approaches to trace the fate of lutein and zeaxanthin, its precursor(s) and metabolites [15].

This review article mainly focuses on lutein and zeaxanthin carotenoids in terms of their sources of common and newly developed foods, daily intake, bioavailability and physiological effects in relation to eye health. Examples of the newly developed high-lutein functional foods are underlined as well.

2. Lutein and Zeaxanthin Carotenoids

2.1. Chemistry

Lutein and zeaxanthin are relatively polar carotenoid pigments found at high levels in parsley, spinach, kale, egg yolk and lutein-fortified foods. They have demonstrated several beneficial health effects due to their ability to act as scavengers for reactive oxygen species and to bind with physiological proteins in humans [16]. In general, carotenoids are tetra-terpenoid having 40 carbon skeleton made up of 8 isoprene units and comprise of two classes, namely carotenes (purely unsaturated hydrocarbons) and carotenoids with oxygen atoms which are referred to as oxygenated carotenoids or xanthophyll carotenoids. The macular carotenoids are dietary lutein and zeaxanthin, and their conversion isomer *meso*-zeaxanthin, which are non-provitamin A carotenoids, (*i.e.*, it cannot be converted into vitamin A). Important members of oxygenated carotenoids are lutein, zeaxanthin, β-cryptoxanthin, capsanthin, astaxanthin, and fucoxanthin. Figure 1 lists the chemical structure of the macular pigments found in the retina. It is estimated that about 90% of the total carotenoids in North American diets consist of lycopene, β-carotene, α-carotene, lutein, β-cryptoxanthin and zeaxanthin [17]. In nature more than 600 carotenoids have been isolated and characterized, yet only about 40 carotenoids have been detected in human milk, serum and tissues. Percentage of main carotenoids inhuman serum is lutein (20%), lycopene (20%), β-carotene (10%); β-cryptoxanthin (8%), α-carotene (6%) and zeaxanthin (3%) [18,19]. Lutein and zeaxanthin are the main dietary carotenoids found in human retina [20] and they protect the macula from damage by blue light, improve visual acuity and scavenge harmful reactive oxygen. Lutein and zeaxanthin along with their common metabolite *meso*-zeaxanthin, commonly referred to as macular pigments (MP) [21]. The ratio between lutein, zeaxanthin and *meso*-zeaxanthin changes as the eccentricity moves away from fovea [21–23]. Although lutein and zeaxanthin were also detected in prenatal eyes, they did not form visible yellow spot. No age-related (between the ages of 3 and 95 years) differences were observed in the quantity of lutein and zeaxanthin [21]. But, the ratio of lutein to zeaxanthin differed between infants and adults. In infants, lutein predominates over zeaxanthin in fovea, and the opposite is true after 3 years of age [21,24]. Structurally the difference between lutein and zeaxanthin is in the type of ionone ring, lutein contains a β-ionone ring and a ε-ionone ring, whereas zeaxanthin has two β-ionone rings. Lutein and zeaxanthin are isomers, but not stereoisomers, which differ in the location of a double bond unsaturation in the end ring (Figure 1). Lutein can exist in possible eight stereoisomeric forms because of three chiral centers, but in nature it exists mainly in Z (*cis*)-form (*R*,*R*,*R*). Zeaxanthin, on the other hand, has two chiral centers but, because of symmetry exists only in 3-stereoisomeric forms (*R*,*R*), (*S*,*S*) and (*R*,*S*-*meso*) (Figure 1).

Figure 1. Chemical structures of macula pigments in retina.

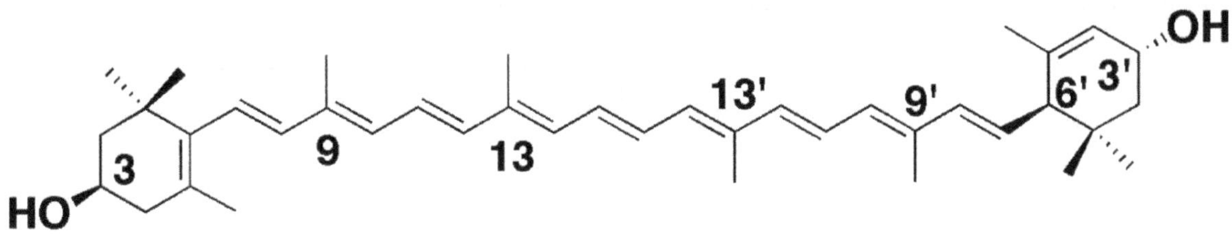

[(3*R*,3′*R*,6′*R*)-Lutein]

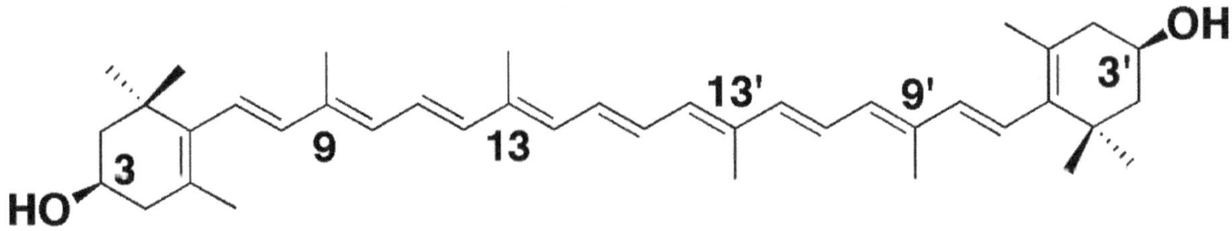

[(3*R*,3′*R*)-Zeaxanthin]

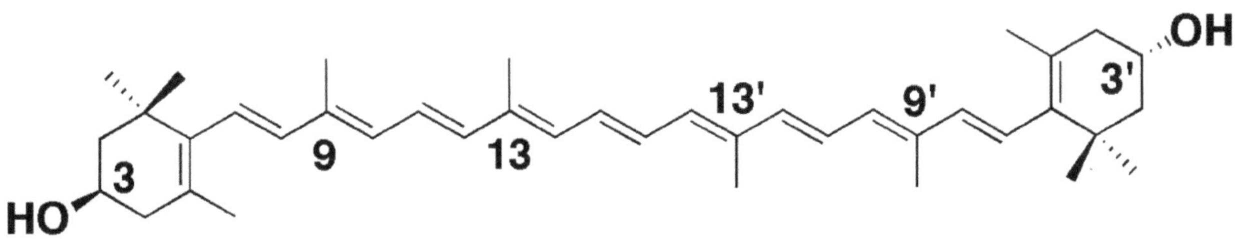

[(3*R*,3′*S*; *meso*)-Zeaxanthin]

2.2. Dietary Sources

Lutein and zeaxanthin are the most common xanthophylls in green leafy vegetables (e.g., kale, spinach, broccoli, peas and lettuce) and egg yolks [25] (Table 1). They are also found at relatively high levels in einkorn, Khorasan and durum wheat and corn and their food products [26–29] (Table 1). The ratio of lutein and zeaxanthin in green vegetables has been reported to range between 12 to 63, highest being in kale, while in yellow-orange fruits and vegetable this ratio ranges between 0.1 and 1.4 [30]. They also quantified small amounts of lutein and zeaxanthin in breads prepared from modern wheat varieties, Pioneer and Catoctin, while breads prepared from green-harvested wheat, Freekeh, an ancient grain, contained considerably large amounts of lutein and zeaxanthin compared to the North American breads. Lutein to zeaxanthin ratio followed the order Pioneer > Catochtin > Freekeh [30]. Chicken egg yolk is deemed a better source of lutein and zeaxanthin compared to fruits and vegetables because of its increased bioavailability due to the high fat content in eggs [31,32]. The concentrations of lutein and zeaxanthin in chicken egg yolk are 292 ± 117 μg/yolk and 213 ± 85 μg/yolk (average weight of yolk is about 17–19 g), respectively and are likely dependent on the type of feed, found mainly in on-esterified form with minute amounts of lycopene and β-carotene [33]. It is not surprising that egg noodle had almost 6 times more xanthophyll carotenoids than lasagne [30]. Astaxanthin and fucoxanthin are abundant in green and brown algae, respectively, which are eaten by fish. Capsanthin is found mainly in pepper. β-Cryptoxanthin is a pro-vitamin A and found in many fruits and vegetables, but mainly in corn, oranges, peaches, papaya, watermelon, and egg yolk [34,35].

Table 1. Selected commonly consumed foods as high sources of xanthophylls (μg/g fresh weight except for corn tortilla and chips μg/g dry matter) [25].

Food	Lutein	Zeaxanthin
Vegetables		
Basil [a]	70.5	in
Parsley [a]	64.0–106.5	in
Spinach [a]	59.3–79.0	in
Kale [a]	48.0–114.7	-
Leek [a]	36.8	in
Pea [a]	19.1	in
Lettuce [a]	10.0–47.8	-
Green pepper [a]	8.8	-
Broccoli [a]	7.1–33.0	in
Carrot [a]	2.5–5.1	in
Red pepper [a]	2.5–85.1	5.9–13.5
Eggs		
Egg yolk [a]	3.84–13.2	-
Nuts		
Pistachio [a]	7.7–49.0	-
Baked foods		
High lutein bread [b]	36.7	3.3
High lutein cookie [b]	21.3	2.9
High lutein muffin [b]	26.1	3.7
Corn tortilla [c]	72.5	105.3
Corn chips [c]	61.1	92.5
Grains		
Corn [d]	21.9	10.3
Einkorn wheat [d]	7.4	0.9
Khorasan wheat [d]	5.5	0.7
Durum wheat [d]	5.4	0.5

Data obtained from: a, [26]; b, [27]; c, [28]; d, [29]; in = included with lutein.

In general carotenoids are very minor constituents in cereal grains except for einkorn and durum wheat and corn that contain relatively high levels of carotenoids or yellow pigments [27,29,36]. The common carotenoids in cereal grains are α and β-carotene, β-cryptoxanthin, lutein and zeaxanthin with lutein being the dominant carotenoid compound. In common wheat flour (low in carotenoids), the bran/gem fraction had 4-fold more lutein, 12-fold more zeaxanthin, and 2-fold more β-cryptoxanthin than the endosperm fractions [37]. Higher amounts of lutein were found in durum, Kamut and Khorasan (5.4–5.8 μg/g) compared with common bread and pastry wheat (2.0–2.1 μg/g). Einkorn, on the other hand, had the highest concentration of all-*trans*-lutein, which is influenced by environmental growing conditions [29] and processing [27]. Corn also contains exceptionally high levels of non-provitamin A carotenoids primarily lutein and zeaxanthin [29,38].

2.3. Bioavailability

In order to exert and deliver their physiological effects carotenoids must be absorbed and transported into the blood stream. In general, carotenoids are lipophilic or hydrophobic which are soluble in fat and insoluble in aqueous media, the medium of human digestive system. Because of the hydroxyl groups, lutein and zeaxanthin are polar compounds compared with the hydrocarbon carotenoids (α-, β-carotene, and lycopene). Thus, a good understanding of carotenoid release, absorption, transportation and accumulation in eye is essential to evaluate the benefits.

The major factors that influence the absorption of carotenoids including lutein and zeaxanthin from food include (i) nature of the food matrix, e.g., in natural format, cooked or supplement, (ii) amount and nature of the dietary fat, which aids in the solubilisation of released carotenoids, (iii) phospholipids, (iv) dietary fiber, (v) nature of carotenoids [39–41]. The absorption of carotenoid released from food include several steps (i) dispersion in the gastric emulsion to be incorporated into lipid droplets, (ii) followed by transfer to mixed micelles involving bile salts, biliary phospholipids, dietary lipids and others. Solubilized carotenoids are then absorbed by the intestinal cell for transportation into blood system. These steps may include simple diffusion, uptake by micelles and receptor mediated and other transporter, as schematically presented by Nagao and colleagues [42,43]. The highest concentration of carotenoids in micelles (*i.e.*, solubilisation), corresponds to greater absorption and transportation into plasma. In general, bioavailability of carotenoids is affected by a number of factors including food matrix, processing conditions and fat content [39,44], while the rate of bio-accessibility of carotenoids is greatly impacted by food matrix and processing. It was observed that the in vitro rate of lutein, zeaxanthin and β-cryptoxanthin transfer almost 100% from fruits (orange, kiwi, grapefruit and sweet potato) compared to between 19% and 38% from spinach and broccoli, respectively [45]. The release of carotenoids from a food matrix followed by absorption is the determining factors for delivering the anticipated health benefits. Since carotenoids are found in a food matrix, they could be released prior to consumption by processing and heat treatment [46]. In other words, the intestinal absorption and metabolic transformation determine the efficacies of carotenoids including transportation and accumulation of macula pigments (MP) in retina that leads to protection of retina, possible prevention and/or slowing the progress of blindness.

Dietary lutein and zeaxanthin and the metabolite *meso*-zeaxanthin are concentrated (~25% of the total carotenoids) in the macula region of healthy eye as a yellow spot, but considerably less in deceased eyes [47–49]. *meso*-Zeaxanthin a non-dietary carotenoid is not found in serum, but only in retina. It has been suggested that lutein and zeaxanthin are transported into retina in the same ratio as in plasma, and then transferred to macula where lutein is preferentially converted into *meso*-zeaxanthin [47–51]. These observations strongly suggest the importance of lutein, zeaxanthin and *meso*-zeaxanthin in the management of good eye health [51–53]. Several studies have shown that incidences of AMD can be reduced by consuming diets with high levels of lutein and zeaxanthin and supplementation by increasing their concentration in serum and parallel increase in macular pigment optical density (MPOD) [54–58]. For example, lutein supplementation over a 140-day period increased serum lutein level [55]. Similarly, consuming increased spinach and kale in diet for a 4-week period increased the MPOD by 4%–5%. Recently, a systematic review and meta-analysis of several longitudinal studies have concluded that lutein and zeaxanthin affect positively in the case of late

AMD but not early AMD [59]. The early or dry AMD was defined by the presence of drusen pigment abnormalities in retina pigment epithelium (RPE) or both whereas the late or wet AMD includes neovascular AMD and geographic atrophy by the presence of choroidal neovascularization, detachment of RPE or geographic atrophy [59].

Concentration and nature of various carotenoids in eye (macula and retina) were established in early 1990. In the fovea, the carotenoid concentration approaches 1 mM, and the ratio of lutein to zeaxanthin to *meso*-zeaxanthin is 1:1:1 [47]. The concentration of macular carotenoids declines over 100-fold just a few millimeters from the foveal center, and the composition ratio approaches 3:1:0 in the peripheral retina (around 21 mm) *i.e.*, lutein concentration is considerably higher with no zeaxanthin in peripheral retina [47,50,60]. The exclusiveness (>80% of total carotenoids) of lutein and zeaxanthin in retina from among 40 carotenoids found in serum is unique and intriguing since the presence of about 20%–25% of total carotenoids in human plasma cannot account for by routine transportation systems [61,62]. In general, carotenoids are transported mainly by low-density lipoprotein (LDL, 55%), followed by high-density lipoprotein (HDL, 33%) and very low density lipoprotein (VLDL, 10% to 19%) and others [63]. However, lutein and zeaxanthin are distributed equally in LDL and HDL, with more infinity towards HDL [64]. These data suggest that lipoprotein profile of serum would play important role in transport and concentration of lutein and zeaxanthin in retina and MPOD. A study reported negative relationship between serum triglycerides and MP, and no relations between MPOD and HDL and LDL [65]. The authors also observed lower than the normal serum lutein and zeaxanthin levels. On the other hand, another study found positive relationships between serum lutein and zeaxanthin with total cholesterol and HDL, inversely related to triacylglycerols, but none with LDL [58]. A most recent cross-sectional study observed that serum lutein and zeaxanthin and lipoprotein concentrations are significantly related [66]. The study concludes that changing lipoprotein concentrations may impact retinal lutein and zeaxanthin levels. Evidences for HDL primary role in the transport of lutein and zeaxanthin were provided when it was reported that feeding high lutein diet to the Wisconsin Hypoalpha Mutant Chicken deficient in HDL increased lutein concentration significantly in various tissues/organ except in retina [67]. Egg, a rich source of lutein and zeaxanthin, is an integral part of the American diet, but with continued concerns for increasing serum lipids and lipoproteins concentrations. A randomized cross-over design study involving 33 men and women consuming 1 egg per day for 5 weeks reported increased serum lutein (26%), and zeaxanthin (38%), but serum concentrations of total cholesterol, LDL cholesterol, HDL cholesterol and triacylglycerols were not affected [68]. Most recently it was reported that daily intake of 3 eggs for 12 weeks increased the lutein and zeaxanthin by 21% and 48%, respectively in 20 adults [69]. Thus, egg yolk could be an important dietary source to improve lutein and zeaxanthin status for the prevention of cataracts and AMD in adults. Similarly, a separate study with simultaneous administration of large amounts of lutein, zeaxanthin and β-carotene affected their concentrations in plasma, tissues and retina [70]. The retinal concentration of lutein and zeaxanthin increased 128% and 116% respectively, when fed diet with high lutein (27.2 mg/kg) and zeaxanthin (15.3 mg/kg) for 28 days compared to the control diet with lutein (5.2 mg/kg) and zeaxanthin (1.7 mg/kg). Further, it was observed that supplementation of β-carotene increased its value in plasma very little, and none in the other tissues and retina. However, high supplementation of β-carotene in conjunction with high lutein and zeaxanthin diet decreased lutein and zeaxanthin concentration in plasma, tissue and retina [70]. The mechanism is not well understood. A recent explanatory study using a formulation consisting of all the three MP carotenoids (7.3 mg *meso*-zeaxanthin, 3.7 mg lutein and 0.8 mg zeaxanthin) over an 8 week period significantly increased the serum concentration of these carotenoids as well as the MPOD [71].

It is more likely that transportation and accumulation of lutein and zeaxanthin involve preferential and efficacious complex-binding with other circulating proteins. Such xanthophyll-lipoprotein complex(s) are then circulated in blood stream. It is interesting to note that blue colouration in lobster shell has been shown to be due to the complex-binding of carotenoid (astaxanthin) with a protein referred to as crustacyanin [72]. It would, therefore, be reasonable to explore similar complex-binding protein(s) in humans and other vertebrates that may be responsible for transportation of lutein and zeaxanthin to the macula. Bhosale and co-workers [73] reported that Pi isoform of glutathione transferase protein (GSTPi) in the human macula has a greater interaction with zeaxanthin and *meso*-zeaxanthin compared with lutein which has a weaker interaction. Subsequently, these researchers also purified and identified a lutein-binding protein in the macula of human eye labeled as StARD3 (Steroidogmic regulatory domain), also known as MNL64 [74,75]. Another team investigated the mechanism for preferential uptake of xanthophylls by retina pigment epithelial (RPE) cells. They reported that RPE cells preferentially take up xanthophylls than other carotenes by SR-BI dependent-dependent process(s) to preferentially accumulate in the macula of retina [76]. Overall, absorption and transportation of carotenoids in foods are complex multi-step processes.

2.4. Eye Health

Considerable research has been undertaken on global level to generate new knowledge to understand the causes, and define steps/processes to slow the onset of cataract and AMD through diets. Evidences show that lutein and zeaxanthin are important dietary carotenoids in preventing and reducing cataracts and AMD. A multi-center eye disease case-control study involving five ophthalmology centers in the US showed that a higher dietary intake of carotenoids, specifically lutein and zeaxanthin is associated with reduced AMD risk [8]. Thus, our efforts will be limited to reviewing the existing literature on the role of dietary carotenoids in reducing the incidences of cataract and AMD. In general, the ageing processes cause biochemical, physiological and physical changes that are directly or indirectly responsible for the onset of many diseases including cataract and AMD. The pathogeneses of both cataract and AMD formation are not fully established. However, over the years research has identified major contributing factors for both diseases. Ageing (greater than 50 years of age) seems to be the major cause in both cases. In addition, other factors include exposure to ultraviolet light (up to around 380 nm) and blue light (400–500 nm high energy), oxidative stress due to access of oxygen radical species, environmental factors, and high polyunsaturated fatty acids responsible for AMD [77]. High incidences of cataract have been linked to poverty and poor nutrition, and strict vegetarian diets lacking in antioxidants [78,79].

High macular pigment density (MPD), macular pigment optical density (MPOD) and macular pigment (MP) have been associated with reduced AMD. There are studies that have linked ethnicity to the development of AMD because of differences in the MPD, MPOD and MP distribution in retina among various races. For example, Wolf-Schnurrbusch and co-workers [80] recorded significantly higher MPD in African subjects compared to White non-Hispanic subjects (0.59 ± 0.14 DU *versus*

0.36 ± 0.13 DU). This provides scientific explanations for previously observed higher incidences of AMD in white non-Hispanic compared to African populations in East Baltimore, USA. Further, a reverse trend was observed for cataracts, *i.e.*, its incidence is 4 times higher in Blacks than White non-Hispanic subjects [81]. These observations have been supported by several other studies that have linked lutein and zeaxanthin concentrations to the reduction of cataracts in North Indian population [82], in older American women [83] and in Australian population [84]. Recent studies also reported the prevalence of major eye diseases and showed that high plasma concentrations of lutein and zeaxanthin reduced the risk of age-related cataract in the elderly Finnish population by about 41% [85,86]. Studies involving older Europeans from Norway, Estonia, United Kingdom, France, Italy, Greece and Spain have reported high AMD prevalence (4% to 12%) depending on age [87]. However, studies from China, India and Korea show a prevalence rate of around 4% [88–90]. The Beijing study [88] involved 4439 subjects over 40 years of age residing in rural and urban areas and the Korean studies had 10,449 subjects over 40 years [90]. These studies suggest less prevalence of AMD in Asians than Caucasians. In addition, several epidemiological studies have found a close relationship between dietary carotenoids, more specifically the amount of lutein and zeaxanthin, and the incidences of AMD [91–93].

3. High-Lutein Functional Foods

As mentioned earlier a number of wheat species such as einkorn (ancient wheat) and durum (pasta wheat) and corn hold a potential for developing high-lutein staple foods. These cereals were identified as promising ingredients for the development of high-lutein functional foods based on their relatively higher levels of lutein compared with other wheat species such as spelt, soft and hard wheat [94,95]. Lutein content ranges from 5.4 to 7.4 μg/g in high-lutein wheat species and about 21.9 μg/g in corn. Lutein and zeaxanthin are the major carotenoids in corn milled fractions and account for about 70% of the total carotenoids [96]. This makes corn a promising blending flour ingredient in the development of high-lutein functional foods.

Three wholegrain functional foods with high level of lutein (about 1 mg per 30 g serving) were developed and evaluated in terms of lutein stability during baking process [27], lutein digestibility in vitro using fasted and fed model [44], phenolic antioxidants [97], and antioxidant properties [98]. The wholegrain bakery products include high-lutein flat bread, high-lutein cookie and high-lutein muffin. Lutein was found to drop significantly during baking process (28% to 64% loss) due to oxidation and isomerization. A number of *cis*-isomers were found in the three products with 13- and 13′-*cis*-lutein being the dominant *cis*-isomers. Due to the significant losses of lutein a fortification approach was used to boost lutein in the functional food products and to compensate for the losses of lutein occurred during processing and/or storage. Other approaches could also be used such as protection of lutein during processing or developing wheat and corn verities with higher lutein content than the existing ones. Despite the significant losses of lutein during processing, the developed fortified baked products still contain reasonable concentrations (up to 1 mg/serving) of lutein and would hold a promise as high-lutein staple functional foods. Bioavailability of lutein in the wholegrain bread, cookie and muffin was also investigated using fasted and fed digestion model in which food products were subjected to an *in vitro* simulation of human salivary, gastric and duodenal digestion, and then followed by Caco-2 monolayer absorption [44]. The fed model resulted in much higher estimates of bioavailability of lutein and the higher fat products (cookie and muffin) resulted in higher overall bioavailability. Antioxidant capacity of the products varied among the baked products subject to product type, type of bioactive components (e.g., unbound *versus* bound phenolic compounds) and antioxidant assay [98]. In the ORAC assay similar antioxidant capacities were obtained for unbound phenol extracts either from fortified or unfortified high-lutein products, while significant differences were observed for bound phenol extracts. Significant differences were also found between unbound and bound phenol extracts in their ability to scavenge ABTS radical cation. In the DPPH assay lutein-fortified products had scavenging capacities significantly higher than that of the unfortified ones. In general, the bound phenolic extracts contribute significantly higher than the unbound phenol extracts to the antioxidant capacity. Only the DPPH test showed the contribution of lutein to the antioxidant capacity. The baking process was found to increase free phenolic acids in the three products, while bound phenolic acids was decreased in bread and slightly changed in cookie and muffin products [97]. Though the effect of baking appeared to be dependent on type of baked product, type of phenolic, recipe and baking conditions, the wholegrain products should be considered good sources of phenolic antioxidants.

Corn products are also rich in carotenoids primarily lutein and zeaxanthin and would be potential candidates for making cereal-based functional foods if high carotenoids varieties are chosen for processing. Lutein, zeaxanthin and other carotenoids in processed corn including canned corn, corn meal, corn flour and corn flake were found to vary between the products and between brands of the same product, but variations between lots of the same brand was small [28]. Among five corn types including white, yellow, high-carotenoid, blue and red corns, lutein content was highest in yellow corn (406 μg/100 g) and lowest in blue and white corns (5.2 and 5.7 μg/100 g, respectively) [99]. Lime-cooking significantly decreased lutein content in yellow, red and high-carotenoid corns. Further processing into tortillas and tortilla chips did not significantly affect lutein content except for yellow corn chips. The contents of lutein and zeaxanthin in corn tortilla and chips made from high-carotenoid variety are presented in Table 1.

4. Conclusions

Increasing age is the dominating factor for the onset of cataracts and AMD because of physiological and biochemical changes due to old age. Global researchers have identified lack of lutein and zeaxanthin as dietary causes in cataract and AMD related blindness. To date large scale prevalence studies provide serious data that conclude ethnicity may be the other major factors. But, age, diet and ethnicity are not the only factors for cataract and AMD. Hence prevention programs should not be solely based on these factors. Other factors such as living (geographic location) and working environment, socio-economic standing and hitherto unidentified factors should also be investigated. More research looking into the development of high-xanthophyll functional foods is essential in order to develop dietary strategies for the management of cataract and AMD in particular for elderly people.

References

1. World Health Organization. Global data on visual impairments, 2012. Available online: http://www.WHO.int/blindness/GLOBALDATAFINALforweb.pdf (accessed on 17 October 2012).
2. Gottlieb, J.L. Age-related macular degeneration. *JAMA* **2002**, *288*, 2233–2236.
3. Mogk, L. The differences between wet and dry age-related macular degeneration, 2013. Available online: http://www.visionaware.org/section.aspx?FolderID=6&SectionID=134&DocumentID=5972 (accessed on 7 March 2013).
4. Owen, C.G.; Tarrar, Z.; Wormald, R.; Cook, D.G.; Fletcher, A.E.; Rudnicka, A.R. The estimated prevalence and incidence of late stage age-related macular degradation in the UK. *Br. J. Ophthalmol.* **2012**, *96*, 752–756.
5. Friedman, D.S.; O'Colmain, B.J.; Munoz, B. Prevalence of age-related macular degeneration in the United States. *Arch. Ophthalmol.* **2004**, *122*, 564–572.
6. Taylor, H.; Guymer, R.; Keefe, J. *The Impact of Age-Related Macular Degeneration*; Limited, A.E.P., Ed.; University of Melbourne: Melbourne, Australia, 2006; pp. 1–72.
7. IAPB (The International Agency for the Prevention of Blindness). Vision 2020—The Right to Sight. Available online: http://www.iapb.org (accessed on 3 April 2013).
8. Seddon, J.M.; Ajani, U.A.; Sperduto, R.D.; Hiller, R.; Blair, N.; Burton, T.C.; Farber, M.D.; Gragoudas, E.S.; Haller, J.; Mille, D.T.; *et al.* Dietary carotenoids, vitamin A,C and E, and advanced age-related macular degeneration. Eye Disease Case-Control Study Group. *JAMA* **1994**, *272*, 1413–1420.
9. Richer, S.; Stiles, W.; Statkute, L.; Pulido, J.; Frankowski, J.; Rudy, D.; Pei, K.; Tsipursky, M.; Nyland, J. Double-masked, placebo-controlled, randomized trial of lutein and antioxidant supplementation in the intervention of atrophic age-related macular degeneration: The Veterans LAST study (Lutein Antioxidant Supplementation Trial). *Optometry* **2004**, *75*, 216–230.
10. Basu, H.N.; Del Vacchio, A.; Flider, F.; Orthoefer, F.T. Nutritional and potential disease prevention properties of carotenoids. *J. Am. Oil Chem. Soc.* **2001**, *78*, 665–675.
11. Delcourt, C.; Carriere, I.; Delage, M.; Barberger-Gateau, P.; Schalch, W. Plasma lutein and zeaxanthin and other carotenoids as modifiable risk factors for age-related maculopathy and cataract: The POLA Study. *Invest. Ophthalmol. Vis. Sci.* **2006**, *47*, 2329–2335.
12. Tan, J.S.L.; Wang, J.J.; Flood, V.; Rochtina, E.; Smith, W.; Mitchell, P. Dietary antioxidants and the long-term incidences of age-related macular degeneration—The Blue Mountains Eye Study. *Ophthalmology* **2008**, *115*, 334–341.
13. Lyle, B.J.; Mares-Perlman, J.A.; Klein, B.E.; Klein, R.; Patta, M.; Bowen, P.E.; Greger, J.L. Serum carotenoids and tocopherols and incidence of age-related nuclear cataract. *Am. J. Clin. Nutr*. **1999**, *69*, 272–277.
14. Cho, E.; Hankinson, S.E.; Rosner, B.; Willet, W.C.; Colditz, G.A Prospective study of lutein/zeaxanthin intake and risk of age-related macular degeneration. *Am. J. Clin. Nutr*. **2008**, *87*, 1837–1843.
15. SanGiovanni, J.P.; Neuringer, M. The putative role of lutein and zeaxanthin as protective agents against age-related macular degeneration: promise of macular genetics for guiding mechanism and translational research in the field. *Am. J. Clin. Nutr*. **2012**, *96*, 1223S–1233S.

16. Snodderly, D.M. Evidence for protection against age-related macular degeneration by carotenoids and antioxidant vitamins. *Am. J. Nutr.* **1995**, *62*, 1448s–1461s.
17. Rao, A.V.; Rao, L.G. Carotenoids and human health. *Pharmacol. Res.* **2007**, *55*, 207–216.
18. Khachik, F.; Beecher, G.R.; Goli, M.B. Separation and identification of carotenoids and their oxidation products in the extrcats of human plasma. *Anal. Chem.* **1992**, *64*, 2111–2122.
19. Khachik, F.; Spangler, C.J.; Smith, J.C., Jr.; Canfield, L.M.; Steck, A.; Pfander, H. Identification, quantification, and relative concentration of carotenoids and their metabolites in human milk and serum. *Anal. Chem.* **1997**, *69*, 1873–1881.
20. Krinsky, N.I.; Landrum, J.I.; Bone, R.A. Biological mechanisms of the protective role of lutein and zeaxanthin in the eye. *Ann. Rev. Nutr.* **2003**, *23*, 171–201.
21. Bone, R.A.; Landrum, J.T.; Fernandez, L.; Tarsis, S.L. Analysis of macular pigment by HPLC: Retinal distribution and age study. *Invest. Ophthalmol. Vis. Sci.* **1988**, *28*, 843–849.
22. Handelmam, G.J.; Dratz, E.A.; Reay, C.C.; van Kuijk, J.G. Carotenoids in the human macula and whole retina. *Invest. Ophthalmol. Vis. Sci.* **1988**, *29*, 850–855.
23. Landrum, J.T.; Bone, R.A. Lutein, zeaxanthin, and the macular pigment. *Arch. Biochem. Biophys.* **2001**, *385*, 28–40.
24. Moukarzel, A.A.; Bejjani, R.A.; Fares, F.N. Xanthophylls and eye health in infants and adults. *J. Med. Liban.* **2009**, *57*, 261–267.
25. Perry, A.; Rasmussen, H.; Johnson, E.J. Xanthophyll (lutein, zeaxanthin) content of fruits, vegetables and corn and egg products. *J. Food Comp. Anal.* **2009**, *22*, 9–15.
26. Maiani, G.; Periago Caston, M.J.; Catasta, G.; Toti, E.; Cambrodon, I.G.; Bysted, A.; Granado-Lorencio, F.; Olmedilla-Alonso, B.; Knuthsen, P.; Valoti, M.; *et al.* Carotenoids: Actual knowledge on food sources, intakes, stability and bioavailability and their protective role in humans. *Mol. Nutr. Food Res.* **2009**, *53*, S194–S218.
27. Abdel-Aal, E.-S.M.; Young, J.C.; Akhtar, H.; Rabalski, I. Stability of lutein in wholegrain bakery products naturally high in lutein or fortified with free lutein. *J. Agric. Food Chem.* **2010**, *58*, 10109–10117.
28. De La Parra, C.; Saldivar, S.O.S.; Lui, R.H. Effect of processing on the phytochemical profiles and antioxidant activity of corn for production of masa, tortillas and tortilla chips. *J. Agric. Food Chem.* **2007**, *55*, 4177–4183.
29. Abdel-Aal, E.-S.M.; Young, J.C.; Rabalski, I.; Frégeau-Reid, J.; Hucl, P. Identification and quantification of seed carotenoids in selected wheat species. *J. Agric. Food Chem.* **2007**, *55*, 787–794.
30. Humphries, J.M.; Khachik, F. Distribution of lutein, zeaxanthin, and related geometrical isomers in fruits, vegetable, wheat, and pasta products. *J. Agric. Food Chem.* **2003**, *51*, 1322–1327.
31. Mangels, A.R.; Holden, J.M.; Beecher, G.R.; Forman, M.R.; Lanza, E. Carotenoid contents of fruits and vegetables—an evaluation of analytical data. *J. Am. Diet. Assoc.* **1993**, *93*, 284–296.
32. Schaeffer, T.L.; Tyczkowski, J.R.; Parkhurst, C.R.; Hamilton, P.B. Carotenoid composition of serum and egg yolk of hens fed diets varying in carotenoid composition. *Poultry Sci.* **1988**, *67*, 608–614.

33. Handleman, G.H.; Nightingale, Z.D.; Lichtenstein, A.H.; Schaefer, E.J.; Blumberg, J.P. Lutein and zeaxnathin concentrations in plasm after dietary supplementation with egg yolk. *Am. J. Clin. Nutr.* **1999**, *70*, 247–251.
34. Chandrika, U.G.; Jansz, E.R.; Wickranasinghe, S.M.D.N.; Warnasuriya, N.D. Carotenoids in yellow and red-fleshed papaya (*Carcia papaya* L). *J. Sci. Food Agric.* **2003**, *83*, 1279–1282.
35. United States Department of Agriculture. Nutritional data laboratory home page. USDA Nutritional database for standard reference release 22, 2009. Available online: http://www.ars.usda.gov/Services/docs.htm?docid=20960 (accessed on 24 November 2012).
36. Abdel-Aal, E.-S.M.; Young, J.C.; Wood, P.J.; Rabalski, I.; Hucl, P.; Fregeau-Reid, J. Einkorn: A potential candidate for developing high lutein wheat. *Cereal Chem.* **2002**, *79*, 455–457.
37. Adom, K.K.; Sorrells, M.E.; Liu, R.H. Phytochemicals and antioxidant activity of milled fractions of different wheat varieties. *J. Agric. Food Chem.* **2005**, *53*, 2297–2306.
38. Moros, E.E.; Darnoko, D.; Cheryan, M.; Perkins, E.G.; Jerrell, J. Analysis of xanthophylls in corn by HPLC. *J. Agric. Food Chem.* **2002**, *50*, 5787–5790.
39. Van Het Hof, K.H.; Weststrate, J.A.; Hautvast, J.G. Dietary factors that affect the bioavailability of carotenoids. *Nutr. Res.* **1999**, *130*, 503–506.
40. Castenmiller, J.J.; West, C.E. Bioavailability and bioconversion of carotenoids. *Annu. Rev. Nutr.* **1998**, *18*, 19–38.
41. Bohn, T. Bioavailability of non-provitamin A carotenoids. *Curr. Nutr. Food Sci.* **2008**, *4*, 240–258.
42. Yonekura, L.; Nagao, A. Intestinal absorption of dietary carotenoids. *Mol. Nutr. Food Res.* **2007**, *51*, 107–115.
43. Nagao, A. Absorption and metabolism of dietary carotenoids. *BioFactors* **2011**, *37*, 83–87.
44. Read, A. Influence of digestion model, product type and enrichment level on *in vitro* bioavailability of lutein from high lutein functional bakery products. M.Sc. Thesis, University of Guelph, Guelph, Canada, 2011.
45. O'Connell, O.F.; Ryan, L.; O'Brien, N.B. Xanthophyll carotenoids are more bioaccessible from fruits than dark green vegetables. *Nutr. Res.* **2007**, *27*, 258–264.
46. Thurnham, D.I. Macular zeaxanthins and lutein- a review of dietary sources and bioavailability and some relationships with macular optical density and age-related disease. *Nutr. Res. Rev.* **2007**, *20*, 163–179.
47. Bone, R.A.; Landrum, J.T.; Friedes, L.M.; Gomez, C.M.; Kilburn, M.D.; Menendez, E.; Vidal, I.; Wang, W. Distribution of lutein and zeaxanthin stereoisomers in the human retina. *Exp. Eye Res.* **1997**, *64*, 211–218.
48. Bone, R.A.; Landrum, J.T.; Dixon, Z.; Chen, Y.; Llerena, C.M. Lutein and zeaxanthin in the eyes, serum and diet of human subjects. *Exp. Eye Res.* **2000**, *71*, 239–245.
49. Whitehead, A.J.; Mares, J.A.; Danis, R.P. Macular pigment: A review of current knowledge. *Arch. Ophthalmol.* **2006**, *124*, 1038–1045.
50. Bone, R.A.; Landrum, J.T.; Hime, G.W.; Cains, A.; Zamor, J. Stereochemistry of the human macular carotenoids. *Invest. Ophthalmol. Vis. Sci.* **1993**, *34*, 2033–2040.

51. Mozaffarieh, M.; Sacu, S.; Wedrich, A. The role of the carotenoids lutein and zeaxanthin, in protecting against age-related macular degeneration: A review based on controversial evidence. *Nutr. J.* **2003**, *2*, 20.
52. Bone, R.A.; Landrum, J.T.; Beatty, S.; Nolan, J. Targeting AMD with a critical carotenoid. *Rev. Ophthalmol.* **2011**, *7*, 91–94.
53. Albert, G.; Hoeller, U.; Schierle, J.; Neuringer, M.; Johnson, E.; Schaich, W. Metabolism of lutein and zeaxanthin in Rhesus monkey: Identification of (3*R*,6′*R*)-, and (3*R*,6′*S*)-3′-hydro-lutein as common metabolites and comparison of humans. *Comp. Biochem. Physisol. B Biochem. Mol. Biol.* **2008**, *15*, 70–78.
54. Hammond, B.R.; Johnson, E.J.; Russell, R.M.; Krinsky, N.I.; Yeum, K.J.; Edwards, R.B.; Snodderly, D.; Russell, R.M. Dietary modification of human macular pigment density. *Invest. Ophthalmol. Vis. Sci.* **1997**, *38*, 1795–1801.
55. Berendschot, T.T.M.; Goldbohn, R.A.; Klopping, W.A.A.; van der Kraats, J.; van Norel, J.; van Norren, D. Influence of lutein supplementation on macular pigment assessed with two objective techniques. *Invest. Ophthalmol. Vis. Sci.* **2000**, *41*, 3322–3326.
56. Johnson, E.J.; Hammond, B.R.; Yeum, K.-J.; Qin, J.; Wang, X.D.; Castaneda, C.; Snodderly, D.; Russell, R.M. Relation among serum and tissue concentrations of lutein and zeaxanthin and macular pigment density. *Am. J. Clin. Nutr.* **2000**, *71*, 1555–1562.
57. Landrum, J.T.; Bone, R.A.; Joa, H.; Kilburn, M.D.; Moore, L.L.; Sprague, K.E. A one-year study on the macular pigment—the effect of 140 days of a lutein supplementation. *Exp. Eye Res.* **1997**, *65*, 57–62.
58. Loane, E.; Nolan, J.M.; Beatty, S. The respective relationships between lipoprotein profile, macular pigment optical density, and serum concentrations of lutein and zeaxanthin. *Invest. Ophthalmol. Vis. Sci.* **2010**, *51*, 5897–5905.
59. Ma, L.; Dou, H.-L.; Wu, Y.-Q.; Huang, Y.-M.; Huang, Y.-B.; Zou, Z.-Y.; Lin, X.-M. Lutein and zeaxanthin intake and the risk of age-related macular degeneration: A systematic review and meta-analysis. *Br. J. Nutr.* **2012**, *107*, 350–359.
60. Khachik, F.; de Moura, F.F.; Zhao, D.Y.; Aebischer, C.P.; Bernstein, P.S. Transformations of selected carotenoids in plasma, liver, and ocular tissues of humans and in nonprimate animal models. *Invest. Ophthalmol. Vis. Sci.* **2002**, *43*, 3383–3392.
61. Handelman, G.J.; Snodderly, D.M.; Adler, A.J.; Russett, M.D.; Dratz, E.A. Measurement of carotenoids in human and monkey reina. *Methods Enzymol.* **1992**, *213*, 220–230.
62. Handelman, G.J.; Shen, B.; Kinsky, N.L. High resolution analysis of carotenoids in human plasma by high performance liquid chromatography. *Methods Enzymol.* **1992**, *213*, 336–356.
63. Clevendice, B.A.; Bieri, J.G. Association of carotenoids with human plasma lipoproteins. *Methods Enzymol.* **1993**, *214*, 33–46.
64. Goulinet, S.; Chapman, M.J. Plasma LDL and HDL subspecies are heterogeneous in particle content of tocopherols and oxygenated and hydrocarbon carotenoids. Relevance to oxidative resistance and atherogenesis. *Arterioscler. Thromb. Vasc. Biol.* **1997**, *17*, 786–796.
65. Broekmans, W.M.R.; Berendschot, T.T.J.M.; Klopping-Ketelaars, I.A.A.; de Vries, A.J.; Goldbohm, R.A.; Tijburg, L.B.M.; Kardinaal, A.F.M.; van Poppel, G. Macular pigment density in

relation to serum and adipose tissue concentrations of lutein and serum concentrations of zeaxanthin. *Am. J. Clin. Nutr.* **2002**, *76*, 595–603.

66. Renzi, L.M.; Hammond, B.R., Jr.; Dengler, M.; Roberts, R. The relation between serum lipids and lutein and zeaxanthin in the serum and retina: Results from cross-sectional, case control and case study designs. *Lipids Health Dis.* **2012**, *11*, 33.
67. Conner, W.E.; Duell, P.B.; Kean, R.; Wang, Y. The prime role of HDL to transport lutein into the retina: Evidence from HDL-defiocient WHAM chickens having a mutant ABCA1 transporter. *Invest. Ophthalmol. Vis. Sci.* **2007**, *48*, 4226–4231.
68. Goodrow, E.F.; Wilson, T.A.; Houde, S.C.; Vishwanathan, R.; Scollin, P.A.; Handelman, G.; Nicholsi, R.J. Consumption of one egg per day increases serum lutein and lipoprotein concentrations in older adults without altering serum lipid and lipoprotein cholesterol concentrations. *J. Nutr.* **2006**, *136*, 2519–2524.
69. Blesso, C.N.; Andersen, C.J.; Bolling, B.W.; Fernandez, M.L. Egg intake improves carotenoid status by increasing plasma HDL, cholesterol in adults with metabolic syndrome. *Food Funct.* **2013**, *4*, 213–221.
70. Wang, Y.; Illingworth, D.R.; Conner, S.L.; Duell, P.B.; Conner, W.E. Competitive inhibition of carotenoids transport and tissue concentrations by high supplements of lutein, zeaxanthin and beta-carotene. *Eur. J. Nutr.* **2010**, *49*, 327–336.
71. Connolly, E.E.; Beatty, S.; Thurnham, D.I.; Loughman, J.; Howard, A.N.; Stack, J.; Nolan, M. Augmentation of macula pigment following supplementation with all three macular carotenoids: An exploratory study. *Curr. Eye Res.* **2010**, *35*, 335–351.
72. Wald, G.; Nathauson, N.; Jencks, W.P.; Tarr, E. Crustacyanin, the blue carotenoid protein of the lobster shell. *Biol. Bull.* **1948**, *95*, 249–250.
73. Bhosale, P.; Larson, A.J.; Frederick, J.M.; Southwick, K.; Thulin, C.D.; Bernstein, P.S. Identification and characterization of a Pi isoform of glutathione S-transferase (GST1) as a zeaxanthin-binding protein in the macula of the human eye. *J. Biol. Chem.* **2004**, *279*, 49447–49454.
74. Bhosale, P.; Li, B.; Sharifzadeh, M.; Gellermann, W.; Frederick, J.M.; Tscuchida, K.; Bernstein, P.S. Purification and partial characterization of a lutein-binding protein from human retina. *Biochemistry* **2009**, *48*, 4798–4807.
75. Li, B.; Vachali, P.; Frederick, J.M.; Bersntein, P.S. Identification of StARD3 as the lutein-binding protein in the macular of primate retina. *Biochemistry* **2011**, *50*, 2541–2549.
76. During, A.; Doraiswamy, S.; Harrison, E.H. Xanthophylls are preferentially taken up compared with β-carotene by retinal cells via a SRBI-dependent mechanism. *J. Lipid Res.* **2008**, *49*, 1715–1724.
77. Beatty, S.; Koh, H.; Phil, M.; Henson, D.D.; Boulton, M. The role of oxidative stress in the pathogenesis of age-related macular degeneration. *Surv. Ophthalmol.* **2000**, *45*, 115–134.
78. Chatterjee, A.; Milton, R.C.; Thyle, S. Prevalence and etiology of cataracts in Punjab. *Br. J. Ophthalmol.* **1982**, *66*, 35–42.
79. Das, B.N.; Thompson, J.R.; Patel, R.; Rosenthal, A.R. The prevalence of age-related cataracts in the Asian community of Leicester: A community based study. *Eye* **1990**, *4*, 723–726.

80. Wolf-Schnurrbusch, U.E.K.; Roosli, N.; Weyermann, E.; Heldner, M.R. Ethnic differences in macular pigment density and distribution. *Invest. Ophthalmol.* **2007**, *48*, 3783–3788.
81. Sommer, A.; Tielsch, J.M.; Katz, J.; Quigly, H.A.; Gottsch, J.D.; Javitt, J.C.; Martone, J.F.; Royall, R.M.; Witt, K.A.; Ezrine, S. Racial differences in the cause-specific prevalence of blindess in East Baltimore. *N. Engl. J. Med.* **1991**, *325*, 1412–1417.
82. Dherani, M.; Murthy, G.V.; Gupta, S.K.; Young, I.S.; Maraini, G.; Camparini, M.; Priuce, G.M.; John, N.; Chakravarthy, U.; Fletcher, A.E. Blood levels of vitamin C, carotenoids and retinol are inversely associated with cataract in a North Indian population. *Invest. Ophthalmol. Vis. Sci.* **2008**, *49*, 3328–3335.
83. Moeller, S.M.; Voland, R.; Tinker, L.; Blodi, B.A.; Klein, M.L.; Gehrs, M.; Johnson, E.J.; Snodderly, M.; Wallace, R.B.; Chappell, R.J.; *et al.* Associations between age-related nuclear cataract and lutein and zeaxanthin in the diet and serum in the carotenoids in the Age-Related Eye Disease Study, an ancillary study of the women's Health Institute Initiative. *Arch. Ophthalmol.* **2008**, *126*, 354–364.
84. Vu, H.T.; Robman, L.; Hodge, A.; McCarty, C.A.; Taylor, H.R. Lutein and zeaxanthin and the risk of cataract: The Melbourne visual impairment project. *Invest. Ophthalmol. Vis. Sci.* **2006**, *47*, 3783–3786.
85. Laitinen, A.; Laatikainen, L.; Harkanen, T.; Seppo, K.; Reunanen, A.; Aromaa, A. Prevalence of major eye diseases and causes of visual impairement in the adult Finnish population, a nationwide population-based survey. *Acta Ophtahlmol.* **2010**, *88*, 463–471.
86. Karppi, J.; Laukkanen, J.A.; Kurl, S. Plasma lutein and zeaxanthin and the risk of age-related nuclear cataract among the elderly Finnish population. *Br. J. Nutr.* **2012**, *108*, 148–154.
87. Augood, C.A.; Vingerling, J.R.; de Jong, P.T.; Chakravarthy, U.; Seland, J.; Soubrane, G.; Tomazzolis, L.; Topouzis, F.; Bentham, G.; Rahu, M.; *et al.* Prevalence of age-related maculopathy in older Europeans: The European Eye Study (EUREYE). *Arch. Ophthalmol.* **2006**, *124*, 529–535.
88. Li, Y.; Xu, L.; Jonas, J.B.; Yang, H.; Ma, Y.; Li, J. Prevalence of age-related maculopathy in the adult population in China: The Beijing Eye Study. *Am. J. Ophthalmol.* **2006**, *142*, 788–793.
89. Gupta, S.K.; Murthy, G.V.; Morrison, N.; Price, G.M.; Dherani, M.; John, N.; Fletcher, A.E.; Chakravarthy, U. Prevalence of early and late age-related macular degeneration in a rural population in north India: The INDEYE feasibility study. *Invest. Ophthalmol. Vis. Sci.* **2007**, *48*, 1007–1011.
90. Moon, B.G.; Joe, S.G.; Hwang, J.-U.; Kim, H.K.; Choe, J.; Yoon, Y.H. Prevalence and risk factors of early-stage, age-related macular degeneration in patients examined at a health promotion centre in Korea. *J. Korean Med. Sci.* **2012**, *27*, 537–541.
91. Mares-Perlman, J.A.; Klein, R. Diet and Age-related Macular Degeneration. In *Nutritional and Environmental Influences on the Eye*; Taylor, A., Ed.; Fla CRC Press: Boca Raton, FL, USA, 1999; pp. 181–214.
92. Moeller, S.M.; Jacques, P.F.; Blumberg, J.B. The potential role of dietary xanthophylls in cataract and age-related macular degeneration. *J. Am. Coll. Nutr.* **2000**, *19*, 522S–527S.
93. Carpentier, S.; Knaus, M.; Suh, M. Associations between lutein, zeaxanthin, and age-related macular degeneration. *Crit. Rev. Food Sci. Nutr.* **2009**, *49*, 313–326.

94. Frégeau-Reid, J.; Abdel-Aal, E.-S.M. Einkorn: A Potential Functional Wheat and Genetic Resource. In *Specialty Grains for Food and Feed*; Abdel-Aal, E.-S.M., Wood, P.J., Eds.; American Association of Cereal Chemists Inc.: St. Paul, MN, USA, 2005; pp. 37–61.
95. Abdel-Aal, E.-S.M.; Akhtar, M.H. Recent advances in the analyses of carotenoids and their role in human health. *Curr. Pharmaceut. Anal.* **2006**, *2*, 195–204.
96. Kean, E.G.; Hamaker, B.R.; Ferruzzi, M.G. Carotenoids bioaccessibility from whole grain and degermed maize meal products. *J. Agric. Food Chem.* **2008**, *56*, 9918–9926.
97. Abdel-Aal, E.-S.M.; Rabalski, I. Effect of baking on free and bound phenolic acids in wholegrain bakery products. *J. Ceral Sci*. 2013, in press.
98. Abdel-Aal, E.-S.M.; Rabalski, I. Antioxidant Properties of high-lutein grain-based functional foods in comparison with ferulic acid and lutein. *Am. J. Biomed. Sci.* 2013, in press.
99. De Oliveira, G.P.R.; Rodriguez-Amaya, D.B. Processed and prepared corn products as sources of lutein and zeaxanthin: Compositional variation in the food chain. *J. Food Sci.* **2007**, *72*, S79–S85.

4

Observation of Human Retinal Remodeling in Octogenarians with a Resveratrol Based Nutritional Supplement

Stuart Richer *, William Stiles, Lawrence Ulanski, Donn Carroll and Carla Podella

Eye Clinic 112e, Captain James Lovell Federal Health Care Center, 3001 Green Bay Rd, North Chicago, IL 60064, USA; E-Mails: ilovemabel@aol.com (W.S.); larry.ulanski@gmail.com (L.U.); donn.carroll@gmail.com (D.C.); cjpstella63@gmail.com (C.P.)

* Author to whom correspondence should be addressed; E-Mail: stuart.richer1@VA.Gov;

Abstract: *Purpose*: Rare spontaneous remissions from age-related macular degeneration (AMD) suggest the human retina has large regenerative capacity, even in advanced age. We present examples of robust improvement of retinal structure and function using an OTC oral resveratrol (RV) based nutritional supplement called Longevinex® or L/RV (*circa* 2004, Resveratrol Partners, LLC, Las Vegas, NV, USA). RV, a polyphenolic phytoalexin caloric-restriction mimic, induces hormesis at low doses with widespread beneficial effects on systemic health. RV alone inhibits neovascularization in the murine retina. Thus far, published evidence includes L/RV mitigation of experimentally induced murine cardiovascular reperfusion injury, amelioration of human atherosclerosis serum biomarkers in a human Japanese randomized placebo controlled trial, modulation of micro RNA 20b and 539 that control hypoxia-inducing-factor (HIF-1) and vascular endothelial growth factor (VEGF) genes in the murine heart (RV inhibited micro RNA20b 189-fold, L/RV 1366-fold). Little is known about the effects of L/RV on human ocular pathology. *Methods*: Absent FDA IRB approval, but with permission from our Chief of Staff and medical center IRB, L/RV is reserved for AMD patients, on a case-by-case compassionate care basis. Patients include those who progress on AREDS II type supplements, refuse intra-vitreal anti-VEGF injections or fail to respond to Lucentis®, Avastin® or Eylea®. Patients are clinically followed traditionally as well as with multi-spectral retinal imaging, visual acuity, contrast sensitivity, cone glare recovery and macular visual fields. Three cases are presented. *Results*: Observed dramatic short-term anti-VEGF type effect including anatomic restoration of retinal structure with a suggestion of improvement in choroidal blood flow by near IR multispectral imaging. The visual function improvement mirrors the effect seen anatomically. The effect is bilateral with the added benefit of better RPE function. Effects have lasted for one year or longer when taken daily, at which point one patient required initiation of anti-VEGF agents. Unanticipated systemic benefits were observed. *Conclusions*: Preliminary observations support previous publications in animals and humans. Restoration of structure and visual function in octogenarians with daily oral consumption of L/RV is documented. Applications include failure on AREDS II supplements, refusing or failing conventional anti-VEGF therapy, adjunct therapy to improve RPE function, and compassionate use in medically underserved or economically depressed third-world countries.

Keywords: macular degeneration; gene expression; epigenetics; RPE (retinal pigment epithelium) function; VEGF; pharmacogenomics

---

1. Introduction

These notable cases support our original publication as well as work presented in India and subsequently published [1,2]. Resveratrol (RV) was discovered in the US in the 1940s, and later found to be an anti-hyperlipidemic medicinal component of grapes and red wine, also extracted from dried roots of the common weed *Polygonum cuspidatum.* In the modern era, RV has been characterized as a promiscuous, gene regulating, small molecular weight, polyphenol phytoalexin demonstrating broad-spectrum cell receptor and microRNA activity. It protects cells against mitochondrial DNA mutations, has "anti-aging" SIRTUIN activation /deactivation properties, modulates inflammation and most recently mitigated the earliest atherosclerotic marker (loss of flow-mediated dilatation) in a Japanese human clinical trial [3]. The second international conference on the biology of RV [4] and two major literature reviews have broad medical interest [5,6]. There are nearly 3500 papers in PubMed concerning some aspect of RV's ability to inhibit carcinogenesis at all three stages of initiation, promotion, and progression.

The cardio-protective potential of RV, a major factor underlying the so called "*Red Wine French Paradox*" is equally impressive, in that RV itself can directly protect isolated hearts from ischemia reperfusion injury [7]. In fact, RV protects most vital organs including the kidney, heart, and brain from ischemic reperfusion injury. Broad based cardiac protection is conferred by RVs' diverse roles as intracellular antioxidant, anti-inflammatory modulator (decreasing COX-2, C-reactive protein and TNF), anti-hypertensive, anti-cholesterol, anti-platelet, nitric oxide synthase expression inductor as well as its ability to regulate angiogenesis in the heart and inhibit neovascularization in the rat retina [5–7]. A substantial body of evidence strongly supports the notion that RV mediated cardio-protection is achieved by a unique and often overlooked mechanism called preconditioning. This means the heart is protected prior to a myocardial infarction or chronic ischemia, largely via release of nitric oxide, but also heme oxygenase and adenosine.

RVs' vascular attributes have special clinical significance and promise for age-related macular degeneration (AMD), due to the debilitating eye diseases' association with cardiovascular disease risk factors and aging. The emerging importance of sub-retinal choroidal blood flow is now thought to play a pivotal role in AMD. By providing vascular enhancement, small molecular weight cytoprotective nutritionals provide additional vascular enhancement beyond other nutritional factors, *i.e.*, multivitamins, the carotenoids lutein and zeaxanthin. The latter have been studied by the US National Eye Institute, Age Related Eye Disease Study (AREDS) and within our clinic via three placebo controlled, double masked randomized controlled clinical studies involving multivitamins, lutein and most recently zeaxanthin, published during the last two decades [2,8,9].

2. Method

Selecting an oral OTC-RV AMD supplement: Given there are 432 brands of RV supplements listed at the *Natural Medicines Comprehensive Database*, careful selection of a non-prescription "*over the counter*" RV supplement was limited to brands that have undergone dosage or toxicity testing [10].

Likewise, there is concern over bioavailability and stability of RV as it can be photo-isomerized from *trans* to *cis* RV by exposure to ultraviolet radiation. Selection criteria included evaluating efforts taken to preserve and optimize the biological action of RV to come as close as possible to research-grade RV (frozen, sealed vial) or an alcohol extract of grapes (unfiltered red wine) sealed in a dark bottle. It has been experimentally determined in animals that RV based products provided with additional small natural molecules work synergistically rather than additively and therefore stand the best chance of working in severe and progressive chronic disease. Molecular synergism is believed to be the reason why red wine exerts such a profound biological effect at a relatively low dose of polyphenols—three to five glasses of red wine providing only 180–300 mg of total polyphenols.

A product called Longevinex® (Resveratrol Partners, LLC, Las Vegas, NV, USA)-hereafter L/RV, was selected that provides 100 mg micronized/microencapsulated *trans*-RV. Micronization dramatically increases the blood concentration of RV. Enfolded in plant starches and dextrins, microencapsulated supplements uniquely protect their components from light, heat and oxygen. The L/RV formulation includes a proprietary blend of other red wine polyphenols, namely quercetin and ferulic acid along with 1200 mg vitamin D3, and a copper/iron/calcium binding molecule called IP6 (inositol hexaphosphate). L/RV has demonstrated synergism at two academic centers and the National Institute of Health [11,12]. Studies show quercetin enhances the immediate bioavailability of RV. Vitamin D3 is important for its ability to exert control over a broad number of genes including those involved in innate immunity, inflammation and vascular calcification. RV increases sensitivity of the vitamin D receptor. Serum 25(OH)D3 liver reserve status is inversely associated with early AMD in the Third National Health and Nutrition Examination Survey, though doubts over that association have recently been expressed.

In animal models, L/RV demonstrated broad superior cardiovascular disease advantage by greater reduction of cardiac fibrosis (scar area), better coronary artery blood flow, far better aortic blood flow and left-ventricular pumping power (left ventricular pressure) compared to RV (or aspirin). In fact, L/RV exceeds the effect of RV in 15 of the 25 top microRNA's implicated in an excised rodent heart model of heart attack and largely restored the pre-event microRNA pattern [11]. MicroRNAs are short non-coding RNAs that mesh with messenger RNA to silence certain genes and are now considered the epigenetic "*guiding hand of the human genome*" [13]. With respect to the retina, L/RV was shown under microRNA analysis (rodent heart tissue) to exhibit many-fold greater down-regulation of microRNA that control HIF-1 hypoxia inducing factor and VEGF-vascular endothelial growth factor genes involved in choroidal neovascularization (angiogenesis), compared to RV alone [12]. These are the critical genes involved in exudative AMD.

In the first human RCT, L/RV produced favorable results (improvement of reduced flow-mediated dilatation, the first sign of atherosclerosis, while decreasing serum insulin, insulin resistance and C-reactive protein) without side effects [3].

Clinical Safety Considerations: In the event of inadvertent overdose there is concern that RV may turn from antioxidant to a pro-oxidant. RV characteristically exhibits a U or J shaped risk curve, being cardio-protective between 175 and 350 mg human equivalent dose (HED) in rodents, and cytotoxic (cell killing) at 10-times higher dose (between 1750 mg and 3500 mg HED)—3500 mg being universally lethal to rat hearts. Significantly, L/RV (Longevinex®) has been shown to exhibit an unparalleled margin of safety at high doses, exhibiting an L-shaped toxicity curve up to 2800 mg HED whereas 1750 mg becomes a potential pro-oxidant and increases scarring in an induced model of rodent heart attack. This is a margin of safety superior to RV alone.

As RV and L/RV bind to copper and iron, these supplements are contraindicated in growing children, pre-menopausal females and patients with anemia. After ruling out anemia, our octogenarian patients were prescribed one capsule daily L/RV and followed clinically. L/RV was compassionately provided when no other options were available beyond the Vision Impairment Service Team (low vision and blind-rehabilitation services).

Consent/IRB and Safety: The use of a marketed product as part of medical practice for an individual patient does not require the submission of an IND (Investigational New Drug). However, oversight was requested and approved by the Chief of Staff and IRB (Hines DVA, Chicago, IL, USA). The "medication" used has exhibited good safety and freedom from side effect at the recommended dosage (one capsule per day) among non-anemic subjects over eight years [14]. FDA animal and human toxicity data, unusual for a dietary supplement, has recently been completed (pending publication). Notations were made in the chart regarding the patients' willingness to take a nutriceutical pill every day and the fact they were out of options according to retinal specialist consultation. Patients secured L/RV on their own, except in the case of inpatients (*i.e.*, Case 2) who secured the product under the auspices of our Chief of Pharmacy.

Retinal Structure: *Retinal Spectral Separation Image* were obtained with an ARIS® automated retinal imaging system 110 (Visual Pathways, Inc., Prescott, AZ, USA) camera. Compared with traditional fundus photographs, we use spectral (visible/IR) separation images for AMD patients, because of their greater sensitivity in identifying intra-retinal pathology (*i.e.*, retinal drusen that increase in size and volume in AMD), the critical underlying blood supply underneath the retina (*i.e.*, the choroidal network that becomes less dense in AMD) and the macular pigment optical density distribution typically diminished in AMD patients.

Traditional colored fundus photographs were also derived through simple wavelength recombination. *Retinal Pigment Epithelium (RPE) auto fluorescent images* were obtained with the Canon CX1® clinical fundus camera (Canon Medical, Canon USA, Inc., Melville, NY, USA) employing 555 ± 25 nm excitation/640 nm barrier filters. Excessive accumulation of lipofuscin granules in the lysosomal compartment of RPE cells represents a common downstream pathogenetic pathway in various hereditary and complex retinal diseases including AMD [13]. Compared with fluorescein angiography, *in vivo Retinal Spectral Domain Optical Coherence Tomographic (SD OCT) images* were obtained with the RTVue® instrument (OptoVue, Freemont, CA, USA). OCT provides precisely aligned high-resolution *in vivo* histologic sagittal retinal section and thickness images. The OCT highlights retinal alterations in morphology, structure and reflectivity, facilitating baseline and serial clinical evaluation of the retinal layers.

Visual Function well known to be impaired in AMD, was measured with several clinical instruments. *Clinical best-refracted Snellen acuity* was taken in a semi-darkened room using a digital projection system (M & S Technologies, Skokie, IL, USA). The *contrast sensitivity function (CSF)*, a measure of how an eye sees large objects (low spatial frequencies at 1.5 and 3 cycles/degree) and small objects such as Snellen letters (higher spatial frequencies, *i.e.*, 18 cycles/degree)—*x* axis, at differing contrasts—*y* axis. The area under the curve of the resulting CSF at five spatial frequencies was measured with The Functional Vision Analyzer® (Stereo Optical, Chicago, IL, USA) with best refraction. *Photo-stress cone glare recovery in seconds* to a bright flash, a measure AMD induced retinal-RPE dysfunction, was measured with a clinical Macular Disease Detection MDD-2® device. (Health Research Science, LLC, Lighthouse Pt, FL, USA).

3. Results

Figures 1–3 present octogenarian L/RV AMD patients for whom all other therapeutic measures had been exhausted (ARED and AREDS II supplements, anti-VEGF treatments *etc.*), or the patient either refused intra-vitreal injections or were classified as non-candidates by conventional retinal ophthalmologic evaluation. Subjects (two males and one female) were either US WW II veterans or veterans of the Korean Conflict (Case 2) and Vietnam Era (Case 3) receiving eye care at the James A Lovell Federal Health Care Facility, North Chicago, IL, USA.

Figure 1. *Case 1.* An 86 y/o morbidly obese male with multiple co morbidities and advanced AMD who is able to read again by three weeks, and whose Snellen visual acuity improves by seven lines at the six weeks visit. Interestingly, in addition to better IR choroidal circulatory images, his bilateral topographic corneal distortions and hearing exam both improve during the same time period.

(A)

Baseline | 6 weeks | 12 weeks

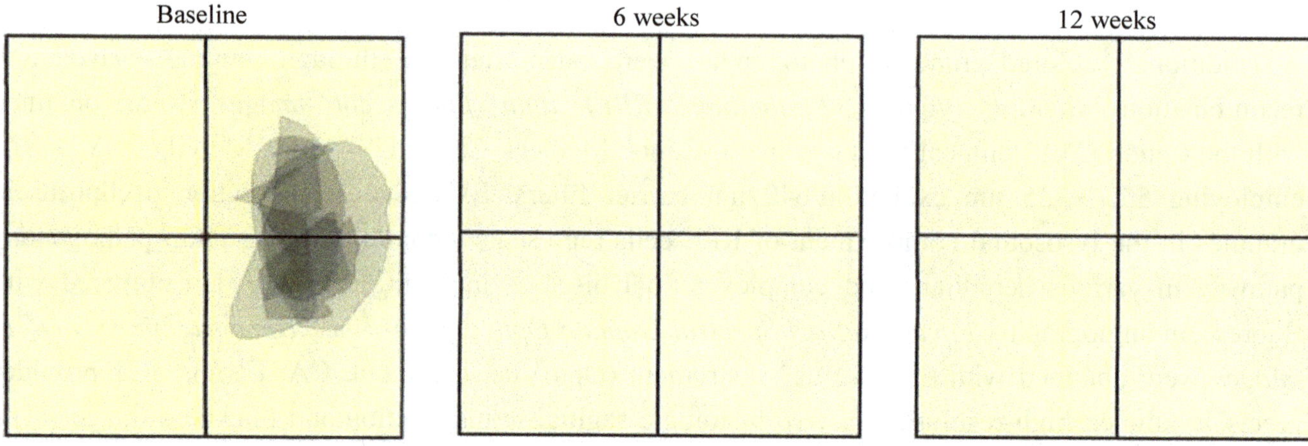

Resolved central scotomas.

(B)

Baseline | 6 weeks | 12 weeks

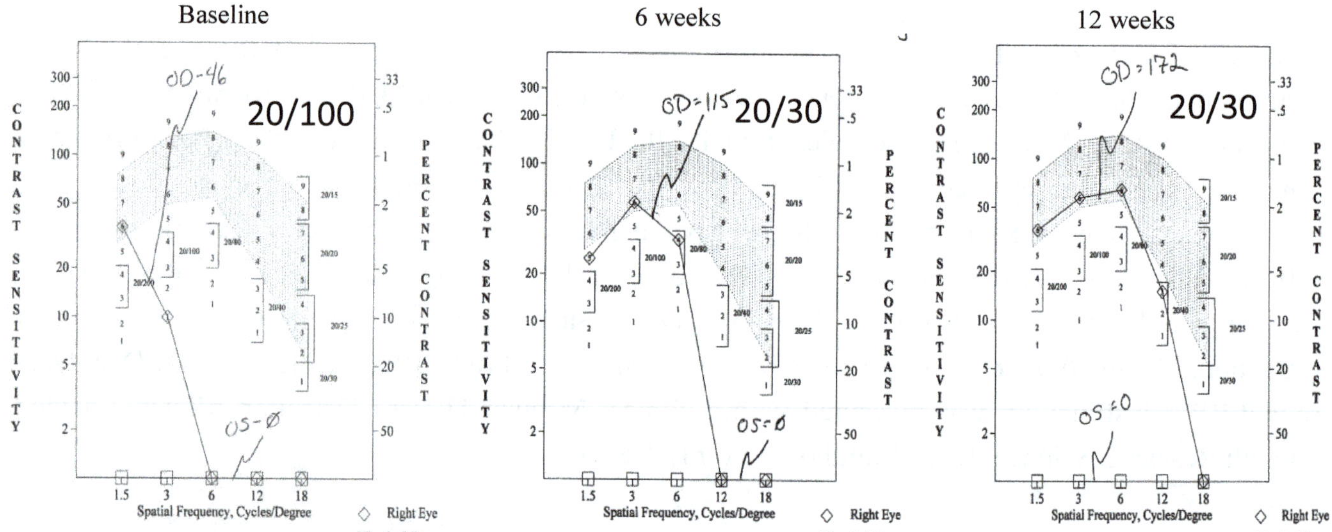

Glare recovery: MDD2-Red

Baseline

Right eye: 35 s

Left eye: not possible

Better contrast sensitivity and cone glare recovery.

Glare recovery: KOWA

6 weeks

Right eye: 18 s

Left eye: not possible

Glare recovery: KOWA

12 weeks

Right eye: 18 s

Left eye: not possible

Figure 1. *Cont.*

(C)

Baseline | 6 weeks | 12 weeks

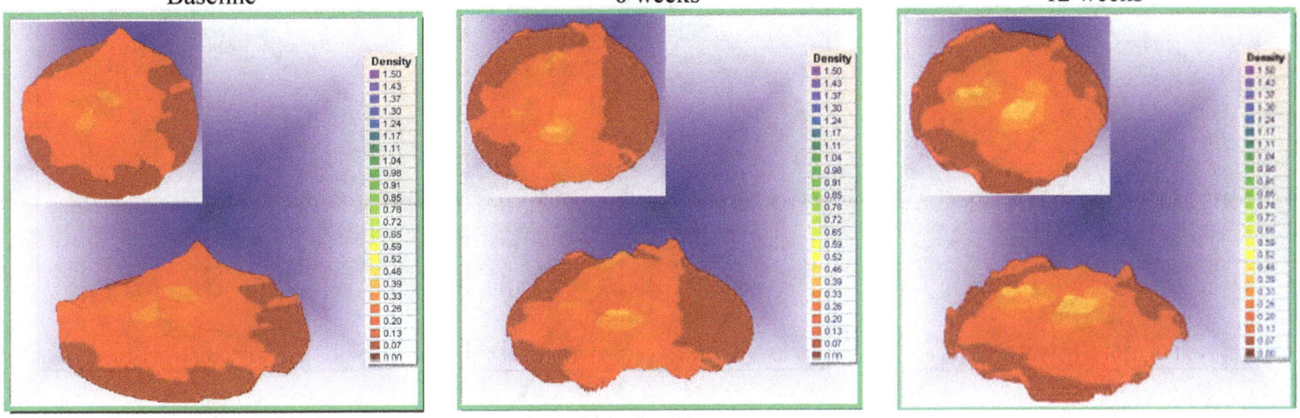

Measures:	Measures:	Measures:
Peak = 0.33 du	Peak = 0.35 du	Peak = 0.41 du
Volume = 1813	Volume = 1712	Volume = 2272
2 DEG Mean MP = 0.22	2 DEG Mean MP = 0.18	2 DEG Mean MP = 0.26
Right eye only.	*Right eye only.*	*Right eye only.*

(D)

Baseline | 6 weeks | 12 weeks

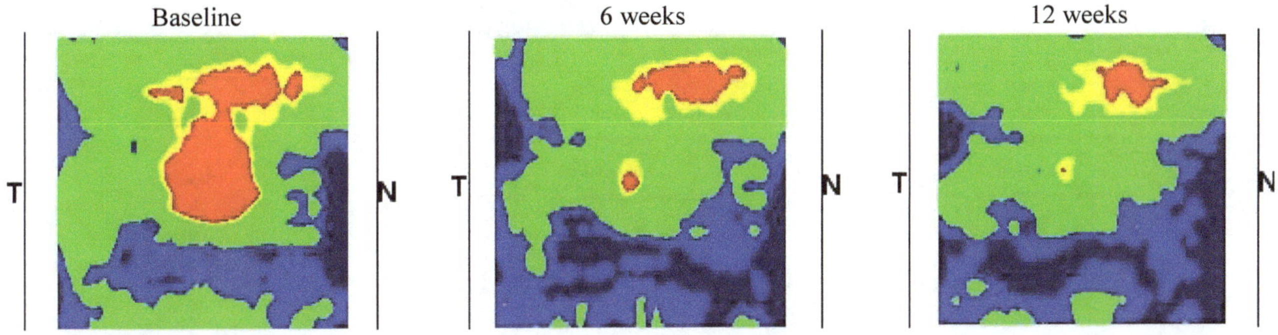

Red = elevation; Blue = depression.

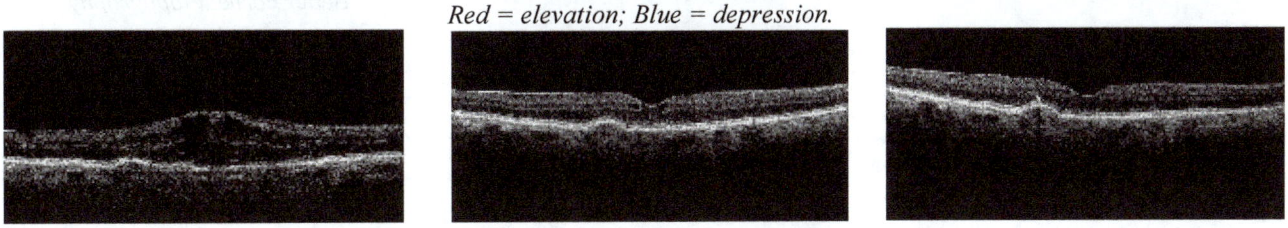

Similar macula pigment but resolved anterior and posterior retinal edema.

Figure 1. *Cont.*

(E)

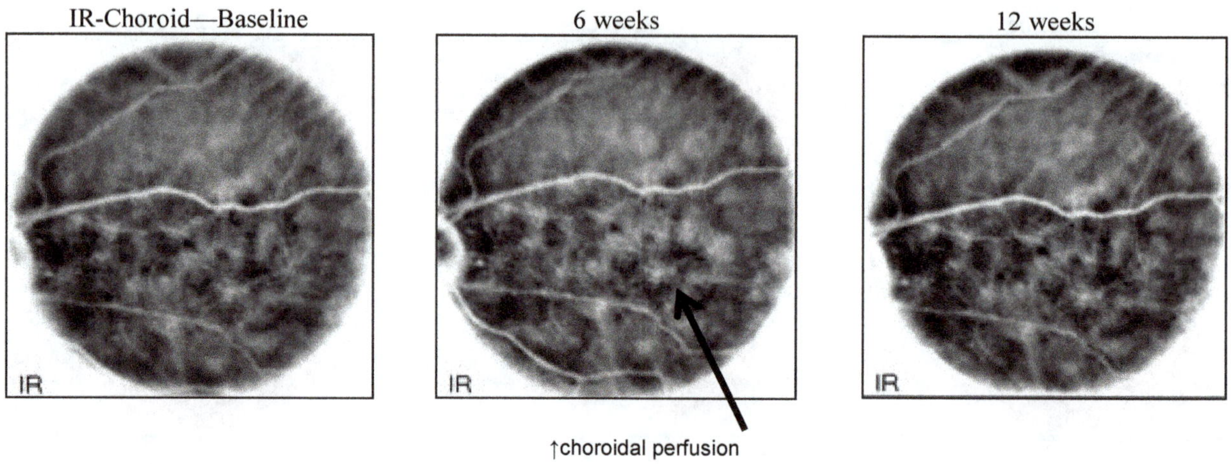

(F)

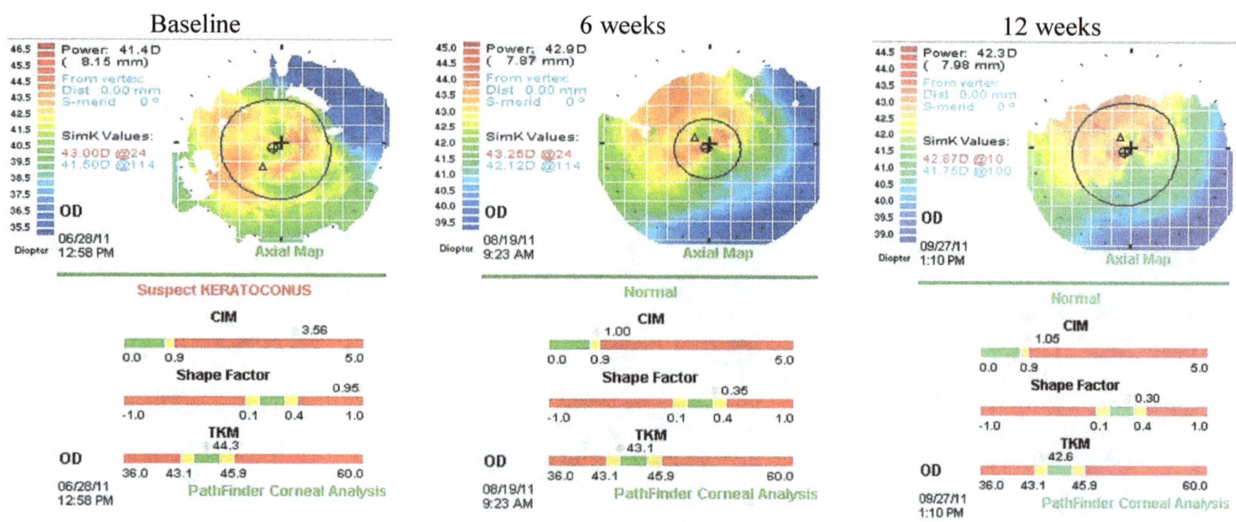

Better corneal topography

(G)

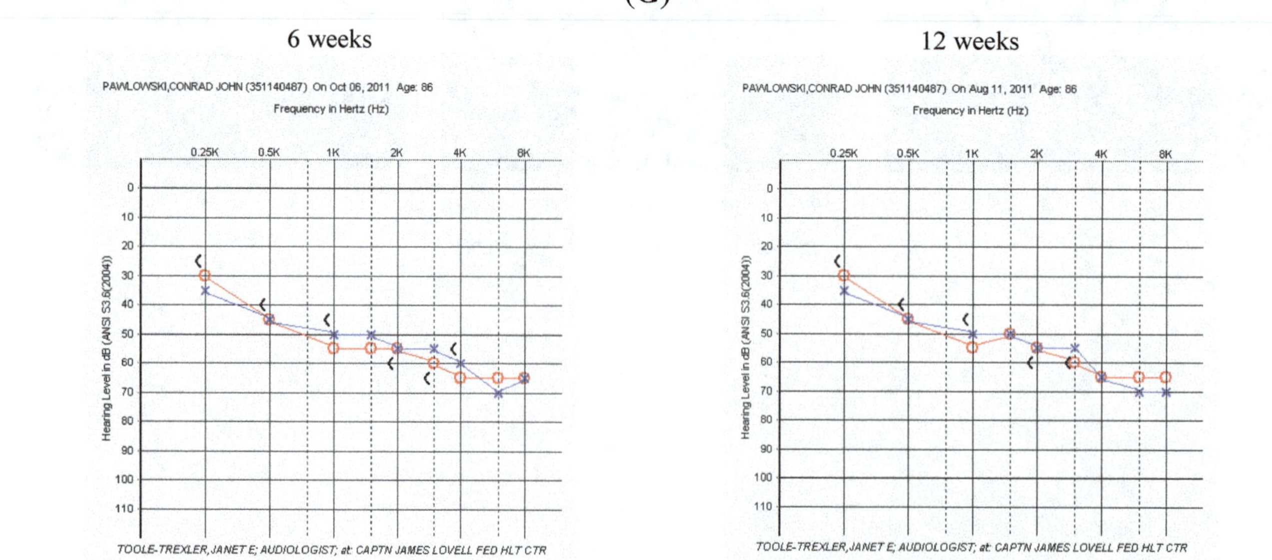

Better hearing on audiogram

Figure 2. *Case 2.* An 88 y/o female with bilateral wet AMD, who cannot read or identify faces. She adamantly refused intravitreal anti-VEGF treatments, after appeals by two ophthalmologists. Four days after beginning RV/L, she reports a hole opening up in the vision in her better eye, allowing her to see faces. Subsequent measurement at two weeks shows bilateral improvement in visual function and near resolution of retinal fluid. Interestingly, her unremitting hypotension and syncope have not been symptomatic, nor has she experienced chronic migraines since she started L/RV some five months ago.

(A)

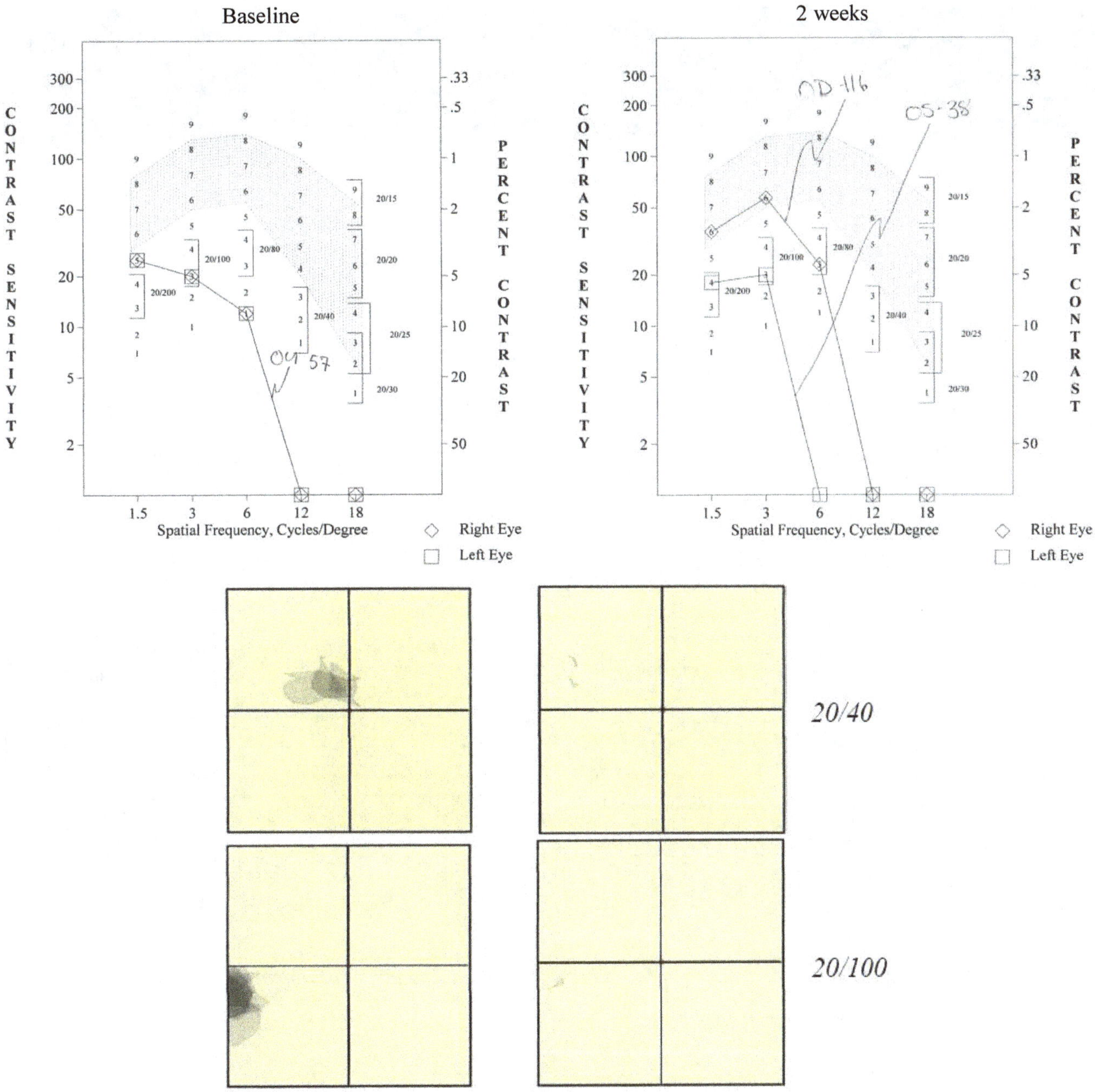

Bilateral improvement in contrast sensitivity and bilateral resolution of visual scotomas.

Figure 2. *Cont.*

(B)

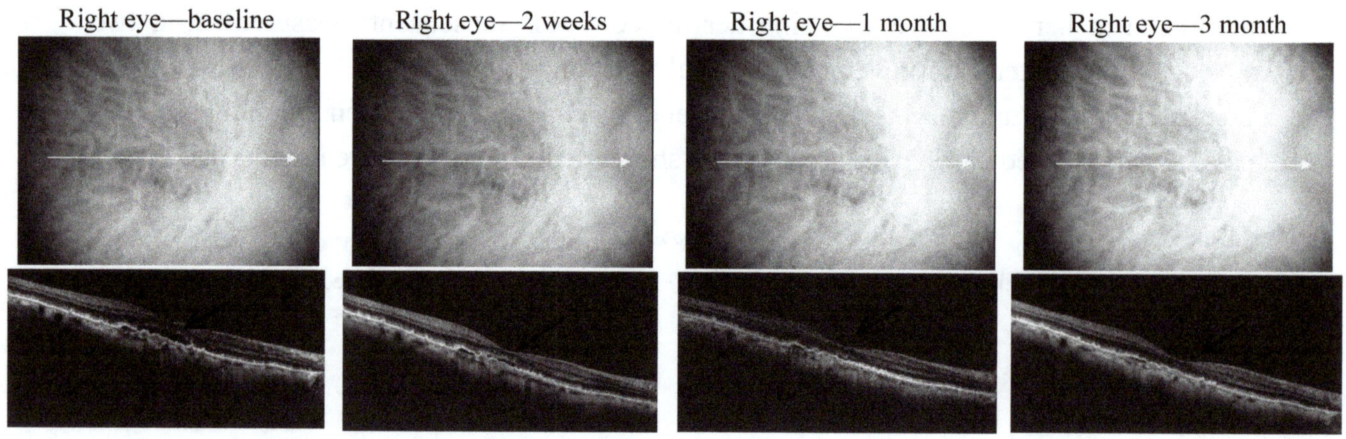

Resolved sub-retinal edema

(C)

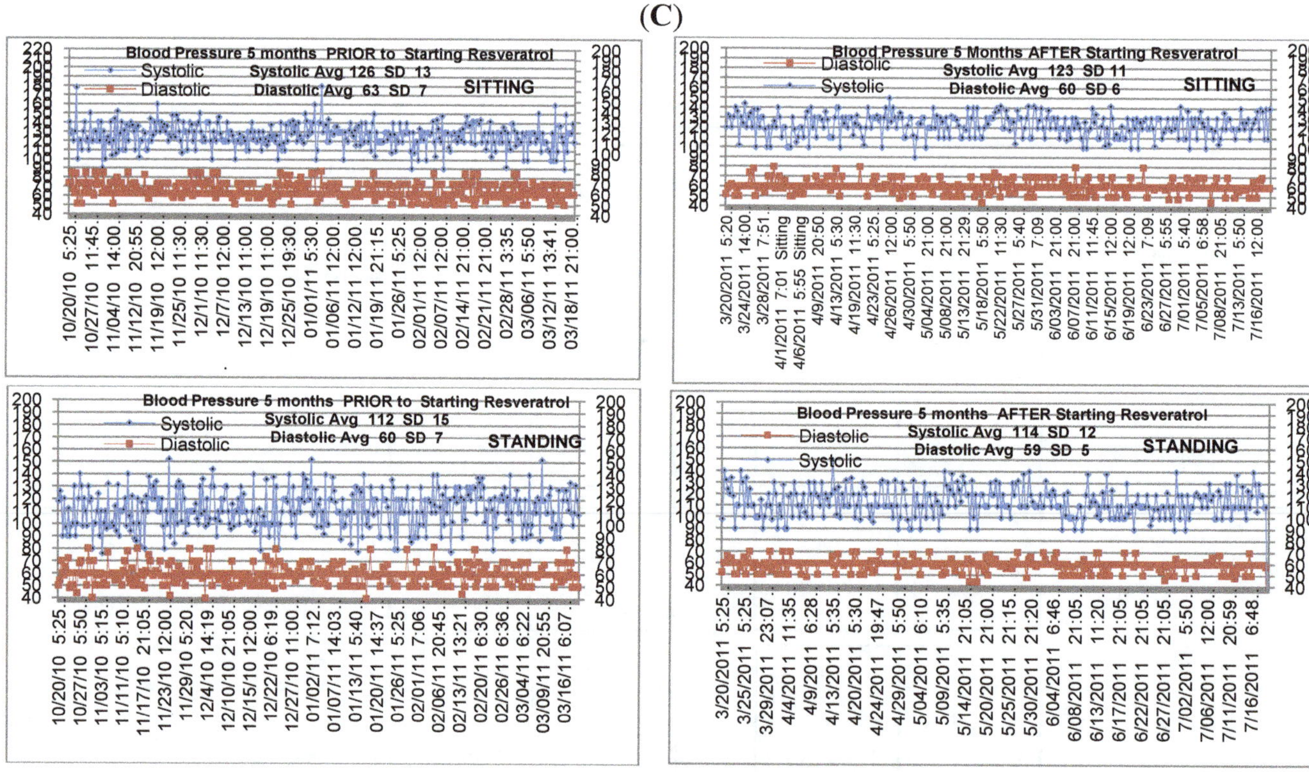

Serial sitting and standing blood pressure. Note improved blood pressure in standing position as evidenced by tighter systolic / diastolic ranges, and improved standard deviations.

Figure 3. *Case 3*. A younger 75 y/o Vietnam Veteran w prolonged post-traumatic stress disorder, diabetes and dry AMD × 10 years who developed wet AMD in his left eye six months ago but adamantly refused repeated requests to do invasive diagnostic (fluorescein angiography) and intravitreal Lucentis® injections or any other type of injection(s). He started L/RV and reported better vision in five days and passed his driver's license after seven capsules. At his two week clinical appointment, we see objective retinal and visual restoration, similar to anti-VEGF therapy.

(A)

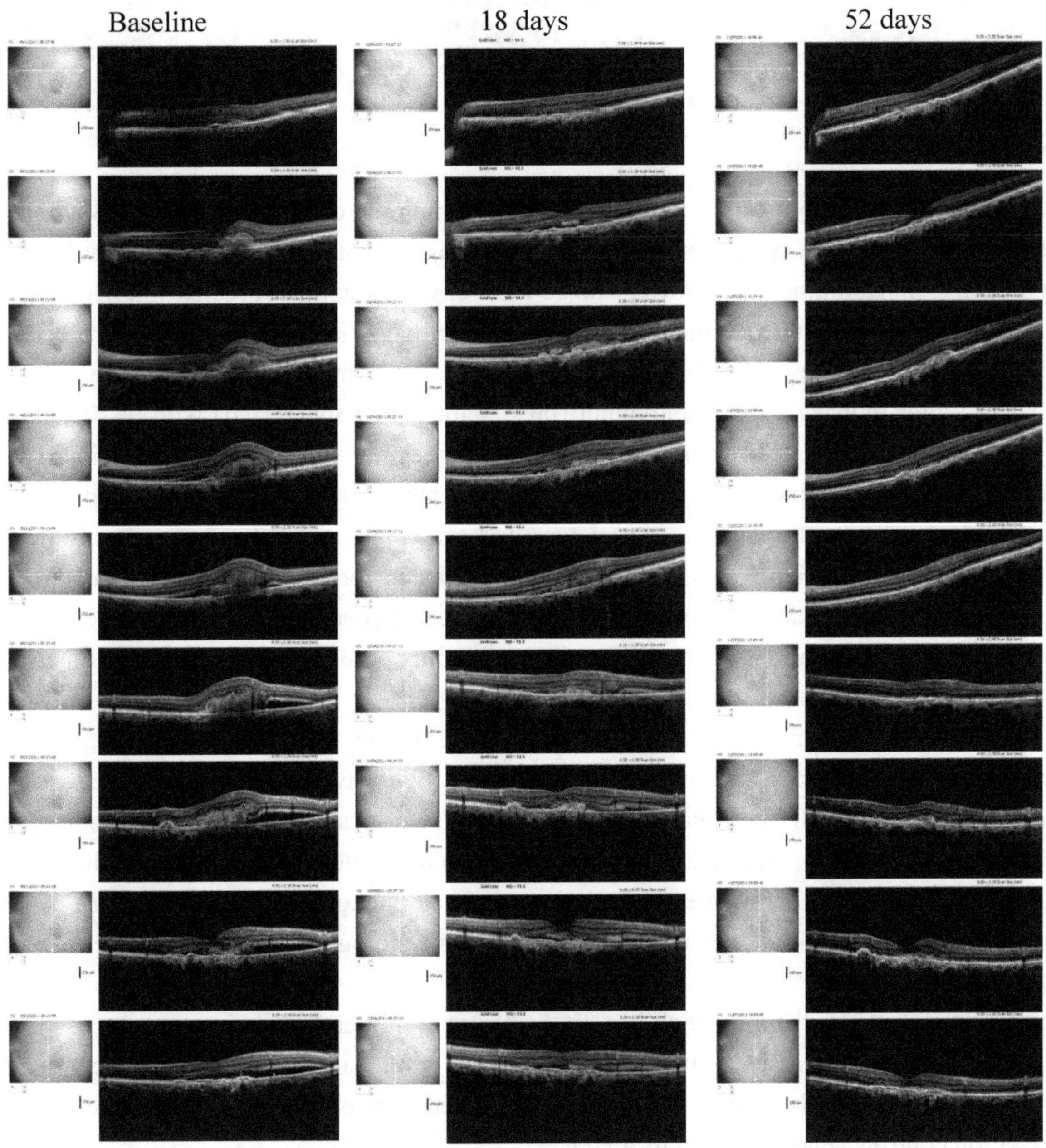

Serial SDOCT scans of left retina, documenting restoration of retinal architecture on all 10 scans (5 horizontal and 5 vertical scans) centered on the fovea, with registration verification to the left of each image.

Figure 3. *Cont.*

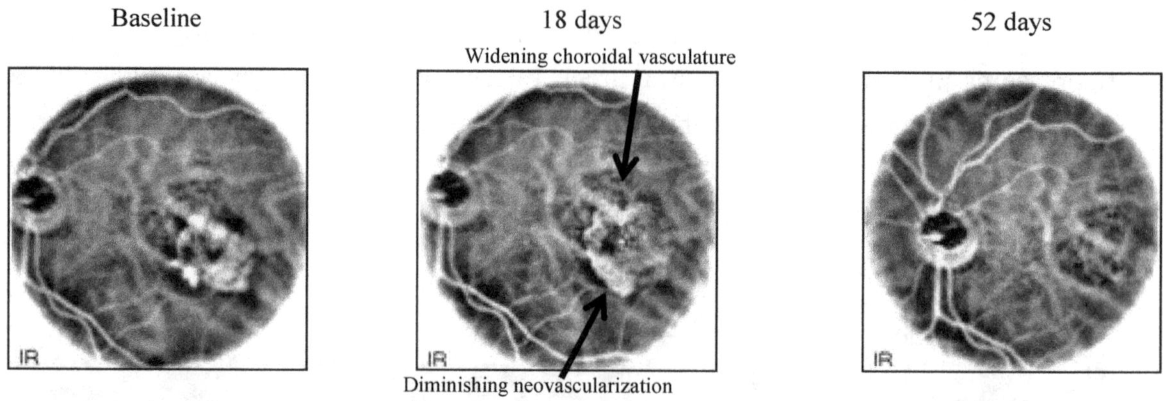

4. Discussion

L/RV, a nutritional supplement, demonstrated wide-ranging ocular, visual and systemic health benefit(s) in octogenarian AMD patients with no medical options other than "*wait and see*", low-vision care and blind rehabilitation. In AMD, objective retinal imaging revealed higher intra-retinal reflectivity denoting distinct differentiation of individual retinal striatum and retinal microstructure [2]. Specifically, we have observed a brighter IS/OS junction (perhaps mitochondrial renewal) and a brighter and flatter retinal pigment epithelium (presumably more melanized) with less shadowing of underlying structures as visualized by OCT imaging, suggesting both improved anterior retinal and posterior retinal photoreceptor/RPE health. There were rapid Avastin®, Lucentis® and EyLea®-like anti-VEGF effects. This improvement in structure was accompanied in all cases not only by broadly superior conventional Snellen Visual Acuity, but also greater comprehensive visual function: better contrast sensitivity, scotoma resolution/improvement and quickened photo-stress glare recovery. In all cases, bilateral improvements were observed - albeit with only modest improvements in function in the more severely diseased eye.

Octogenarians report an improvement in physical stamina shortly after starting L/RV with Medical-center documented co-morbidity improvements. We have observed improved audiograms (patient 1, another unpublished). Patient 1 also demonstrated an unanticipated smoother corneal epithelial topographic scan. Patient 2 improved her systemic hypotension and syncope the very reason she has been hospitalized for two years. Collectively, these phenomena suggest a return of structure and function in the "*oldest-old*" toward a more youthful physiological state and support our previous two publications [1,2].

These cases illustrate the potential benefit of using a mineral-chelating matrix to thwart the accumulation of redox-reactive divalent copper and iron, since age-related accumulation of these minerals parallels the onset of age-related retinal disease. Significantly, age-related over mineralization controls genes involved in AMD.

Hypoxia/ischemia/angiogenesis-related damage, seen in aged and diseased retinal tissues, are controlled by "*master ischemic*" micro RNAs. In this context, RV and more so L/RV in murine heart tissue, were found to exert a profound effect over micro RNAs, restoring expression to pre-event profiles largely via control of the hypoxia-inducing-factor gene (HIF-1: micro RNA-20b) and the vascular endothelial growth factor gene (VEGF: micro RNA-539), though L/RVs epigenetic effects were not limited to these genes. L/RV exhibits a 1.82 times greater differentiation over micro RNA-539 (up +314.6 compared to plain RV, up +172.4) and a 7.22 times greater down-regulation over micro RNA-20b (down −1366.0 compared to plain RV, down −189.0) [11]. Therefore, plain RV may not produce results equivalent to those demonstrated in these subjects, and higher doses are not recommended as this theoretically induces a pro-oxidant effect.

The metabolically active retina is uniquely characterized by daily disc shedding, renewal of photoreceptors, high oxygen/blood perfusion levels and exposure to radiation. This suggests a regenerative capacity likely hindered by local inflammation and oxidation. In some cases we see serous elevation of the retina with altered photoreceptor outer segments and highly reflective outer-plexiform degenerative bodies, thought to represent cone distress and rod engorgement. We have observed these phenomena to often disappear after starting L/RV. Despite the capacity for repair and regeneration, once photoreceptors or inner retinal neurons have degenerated severely, they are not spontaneously replaced in mammals, as seen in the worse functioning eyes in this case series. However, we unexpectedly observed diminished RPE auto fluorescence in several patients taking L/RV, as reported by others, with RV, *in vitro* suggesting innate regenerative capacity. We have had AF images independently verified.

Is it possible that we are seeing hormesis sustained nascent stem cell regeneration? The retina retains a regenerative/repair capacity for replacement of lost neurons via differentiation of Müller glia cells to a progenitor (stem-cell like) state. Non-telomeric double-strand DNA breaks may exhaust the stem cell pool, impairing cellular repair. Small nutriceutical molecules are essential for double-strand DNA-break repair. Furthermore, RV may exert a surprising ability to facilitate stem cell survival and thus tissue renewal. Stem cells are normally generated at sites of tissue damage. Recent studies suggest certain small antioxidant molecules like RV, via their ability to quell free radicals, enable endogenously produced or injected stem cells to survive rather than die. Obvious restoration of retinal layers as visualized on digital SD-OCT images suggest the observed retinal cell repopulation and tissue regeneration in these octogenarian patients were likely facilitated by stem cell survival.

In the heart, RV remarkably normalizes vascularization and promotes capillary budding in damaged cardiomyocytes that have a slow-cell turnover rate [12]. In the retina, RV inhibits new blood vessel outcropping in retinal tissues that have a fast cell turnover rate. RV alone and we believe more so RV combined with other potentiating small molecules, activates autophagy, a catabolic renewal process which involves degradation of a cell's own debris through lysosomal enzymes, facilitating a coordinated genomic response and eventual greater differentiation (gene expression or silencing) of several longevity proteins. The previously demonstrated beneficial low-dose epigenetic effects of RV and the L/RV nutriceutical multi-molecule mix is believed to mimic that observed with studies involving modest-dose red wine that prompts activation of adenosine receptors. Adenosine, a cell-protective/vaso-dilative nucleoside, is known to prevent damage in tissues deprived of oxygen (hypoxia, ischemia), as typically occurs in AMD.

Treatment-resistant AMD patients, even the oldest-old, may not be "beyond hope". Only treatment of a larger number of cases, within a research protocol, will reveal with what reliability. However, there is reason to believe that the clinical phenomena we observe are curative and not due to placebo effects. We have observed recurrence of visual decline and altered retinal morphology with temporary cessation of L/RV, suggesting cause and effect relationship. Of course, unknown mechanisms and explanations for these phenomena might be at play. Retinal drusen can spontaneously resolve in 15% of AMD patients. However, one of us (DC) has observed diminution of drusen volume in as little as one week after starting L/RV, albeit in younger patients. He also has documented regeneration of glial tissue and improvement in visual function in a case of familial vitelliform (hereditary) retinal dystrophy. Diseased retinas typically worsen. See Appendix Figure A1.

While this report herald hopes for patients with otherwise intractable cases of neovascular or geographic AMD, much needs to be learned. These three cases represent the most demonstrable visual and structural improvement we have seen, all of whom were non-candidates for anti-VEGF therapy. The oldest patient treated is age 92. L/RV appears to stabilize AMD disease progression and has produced modest improvements in multiple clinical aspects of vision (acuity, contrast, fields, glare recovery). There are no reported side effects.

It is our hope that a nutritional supplement modulating inflammation, inducing micro RNA 20b and 539, mitochondrial renewal and redox reactive mineral sequestration be added to the ophthalmologist's toolbox. It appears some of the enigmatic biological mechanisms responsible for cases of spontaneous remission of retinal disease are of environment—gene interactive epigenetic origin. Compassionate use, pilot studies and fast track FDA Phase 2 randomized clinical trial of L/RV, all appear warranted.

Anti-VEGF therapy is the prevailing treatment for the fast-progressive "*wet*" form of AMD. Elevated vascular endothelial growth factor (VEGF) appears to be a local problem in the retina rather than a systemic issue. While injected monoclonal antibodies narrowly block VEGF, molecular medicine exerts broader epigenetic control over neovascularization, inflammation, RPE health, blood-flow and possibly tissue regeneration. Because of the broad genomic action of RV and more so L/RV, the health benefits of these small molecules cannot be confined to any particular retinal layer. In these cases notable improvement in vision, but curiously also hearing, blood pressure and vigor were observed among octogenarians. While broad biological action by RV has been exhibited in the animal lab, this may be the first documented presentation of positive tissue-wide and system-wide biological effects in humans.

We have observed speedy anatomic and bilateral visual benefit with ingestion of a red wine extract combined with vitamin D and a redox-active divalent metal sequestering agent. In AMD, we conjecture that L/RV may reduce the number of required injections, benefit some patients that fail anti-VEGF therapy, as well be useful to patients who are averse to needle infusion or cannot afford standard therapy. Side effects were not reported.

5. Conclusions

In our ongoing clinical experience, treatment-resistant macular degeneration patients are not beyond hope, unless scarring or absolute wide spread retinal/choroidal histopathologic tissue destruction has occurred. Furthermore, there is reason to believe the beneficial nutrient—induced retinal structural and functional visual effects in these case presentations, are not due to a placebo effect. Nonetheless, randomized placebo controlled molecular medicine clinical studies, to confirm the proposed beneficial effects of low dose epigenetic nutriceutical intervention beyond AREDS 2 supplementation, are warranted.

Declaration

Presented at the Association for Research in Vision and Ophthalmology Meeting (ARVO), Fort Lauderdale, FL, USA, poster #286, 6 May 2012.

Acknowledgements

These medical case reports are based on original clinical work supported by the Optometry/Ophthalmology sections of Captain James Lovell Federal Health Care Facility, DVA-Naval Medical Center, North Chicago, IL, USA. Further peer-reviewed scientific studies are available at [14].

References

1. Richer, S.; Stiles, W. Molecular medicine in ophthalmic care. *Optometry* **2009**, *80*, 695–671.
2. Harris, G.; Pratt, S.; Richer, S. Section I. Conditions of the Ears, Eyes, Nose, and Throat. Chapter 1: Age-Related Macular Degeneration. In *Food and Nutrients in Disease Management*, 2nd ed.; Kohlstadt, I., Ed.; CRC Press: New York, NY, USA, 2012.
3. Fujitaka, K.; Otani, H.; Jo, F.; Jo, H.; Nomura, E.; Iwasaki, M.; Nishikawa, M.; Iwasaka, T.; Das, D.K. Modified resveratrol Longevinex improves endothelial function in adults with metabolic syndrome receiving standard treatment. *Nutr. Res.* **2011**, *31*, 842–847.
4. The 2nd International Scientific Conference on Resveratrol and Health. Available online: http://www.resveratrol2012.eu/index.php/Resveratrol-2012/2/0/ (accessed on 15 May 2013).
5. Vang, O.; Ahmad, N.; Baile, CA.; Baur, J.A.; Brown, K.; Csiszar, A.; Das, D.K.; Delmas, D.; Gottfried, C.; Lin, H.-Y.; *et al.* What is new for an old molecule? Systematic review and recommendations on the use of resveratrol. *PLoS One* **2011**, *6*, e19881.
6. Pezzuto, J.M. The phenomenon of resveratrol: Redefining the virtues of promiscuity. *Ann. N. Y. Acad. Sci.* **2011**, *1215*, 123–130.
7. Juhasz, B.; Mukherjee, S.; Das, D.K. Hormetic response of resveratrol against cardioprotection. *Exp. Clin. Cardiol.* **2010**, *15*, e134–e138.
8. Richer, S.; Stiles, W.; Graham-Hoffman, K.; Levin, M.; Ruskin, D.; Wrobel, J.; Park, D.W.; Thomas, C. Randomized, double-blind, placebo-controlled study of zeaxanthin and visual function in patients with atrophic age-related macular degeneration: The Zeaxanthin and Visual Function Study (ZVF) FDA IND #78, 973. *Optometry* **2011**, *82*, 687–680.
9. Age-Related Eye Disease Study 2 (AREDS 2). Available online: http://www.nei.nih.gov/areds2/ (accessed on 5 May 2013).
10. Search Natural Medicines Comprehensive Database. Available online: http://naturaldatabase.therapeuticresearch.com/home.aspx?cs=&s=ND&AspxAutoDetectCookieSupport=1 (accessed on 5 May 2013).
11. Barger, J.L.; Kayo, T.; Pugh, T.D.; Prolla, T.A.; Weindruch, R. Short-term consumption of

a resveratrol-containing nutriceutical mixture mimics gene expression of long-term caloric restriction in mouse heart. *Exp. Gerontol.* **2008**, *43*, 859–866.

12. Mukhopadhyay, P.; Mukherjee, S.; Ahsan, K.; Baqchi, A.; Pacher, P.; Das, D.K. Restoration of altered microRNA expression in the ischemic heart with resveratrol. *PLoS One* **2010**, *5*, e15705.
13. Brunk, U.T.; Terman, A. Lipofuscin: Mechanisms of age-related accumulation and influence on cell function. *Free Radic. Biol. Med.* **2002**, *33*, 611–619.
14. Home Page of Longevinex®. Available online: http://www.longevinex.com/ (accessed on 5 May 2013).

Appendix

Figure A1. (**A**) SD OCT horizontal left macula retinal scan of a 60 y/o male with Stage 2 Adult Foveo-Macular Dystrophy, a variant of Vitelliform Macular Dystrophy. The L retina is more effected with 20/70 VA and central 4 degree foveal Amsler grid distortion. (The R eye is 20/20 with form fruste findings—not shown). Diagnosis made in 2007 by William KM Shields, Retina & Macula Specialists, Olympia, WA, USA. A sister and both parents similarly affected. (**B**) After 5 days on Longevinex®, patient reports darkening and less distortion of the central Amsler grid with 1 line VA improvement to 20/60 with the same eyeglasses. (**C**) At 6 weeks, the Amsler grid shows continual darkening and the patient reports that the central distorted area has moved to the right side of the grid. Vision is now 20/50, 2 lines better than baseline. The SDOCT images show increasing tissue mass and reformation of the fovea, denoting possible *in vivo* stem cell activity. Note images are registered, within the fovea, according to the 840 nm IR ETDRS grid (left) simultaneously imaged on the retina. (Images courtesy of Donn Carroll, Private Practice, WA Medical Vision Center, Morton, WA, USA).

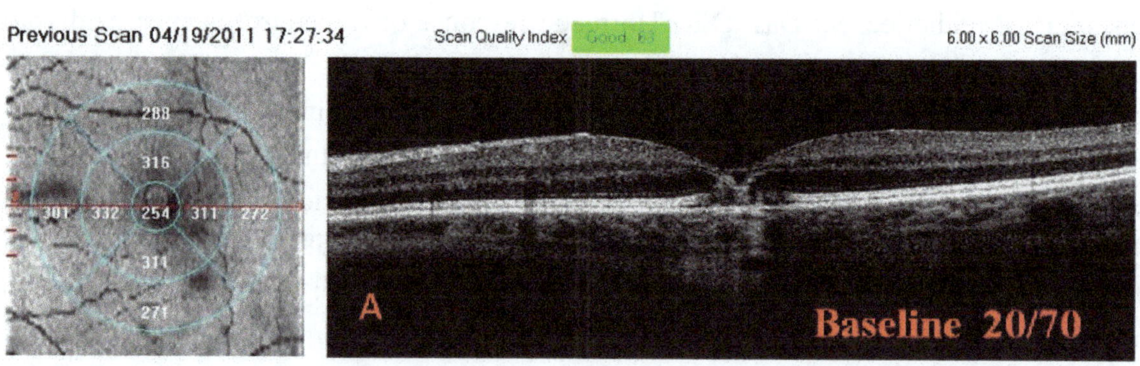

Figure A1. *Cont.*

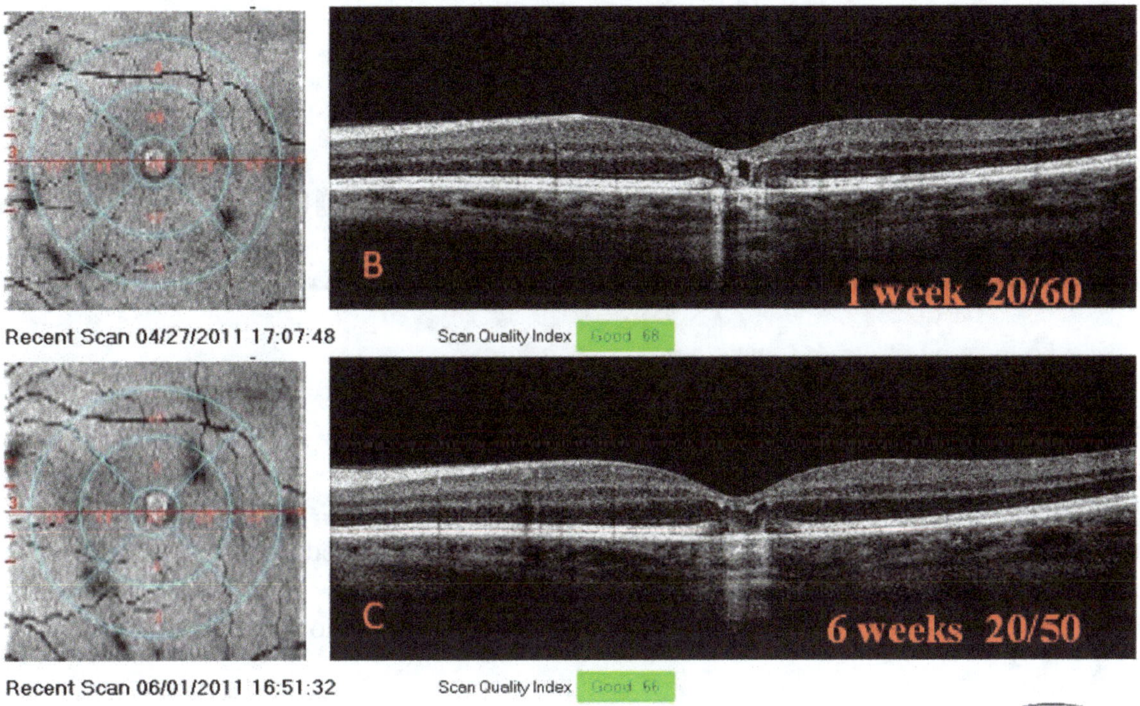

5

Vitamin A Derivatives as Treatment Options for Retinal Degenerative Diseases

Lindsay Perusek and Tadao Maeda *

Department of Ophthalmology & Visual Sciences, School of Medicine, Case Western Reserve University, Cleveland, OH 44106-4965, USA; E-Mail: lxp106@case.edu

* Author to whom correspondence should be addressed; E-Mail: tadao.maeda@case.edu;

Abstract: The visual cycle is a sequential enzymatic reaction for vitamin A, all-*trans*-retinol, occurring in the outer layer of the human retina and is essential for the maintenance of vision. The central source of retinol is derived from dietary intake of both retinol and pro-vitamin A carotenoids. A series of enzymatic reactions, located in both the photoreceptor outer segment and the retinal pigment epithelium, transform retinol into the visual chromophore 11-*cis*-retinal, regenerating visual pigments. Retina specific proteins carry out the majority of the visual cycle, and any significant interruption in this sequence of reactions is capable of causing varying degrees of blindness. Among these important proteins are Lecithin:retinol acyltransferase (LRAT) and retinal pigment epithelium-specific 65-kDa protein (RPE65) known to be responsible for esterification of retinol to all-*trans*-retinyl esters and isomerization of these esters to 11-*cis*-retinal, respectively. Deleterious mutations in these genes are identified in human retinal diseases that cause blindness, such as Leber congenital amaurosis (LCA) and retinitis pigmentosa (RP). Herein, we discuss the pathology of 11-*cis*-retinal deficiency caused by these mutations in both animal disease models and human patients. We also review novel therapeutic strategies employing artificial visual chromophore 9-*cis*-retinoids which have been employed in clinical trials involving LCA patients.

Keywords: vitamin A; all-*trans*-retinol; 11-*cis*-retinal; retina; visual cycle; carotenoids; 9-*cis*-retinyl acetate; retinal pigmented epithelium; photoreceptor; Leber congenital amaurosis

---

1. Introduction

Vitamin A is an essential vitamin for vertebrates and therefore must be obtained from dietary sources. Intake of adequate vitamin A is required in adults to maintain immune system integrity, vision, and the regulation of gene transcription, while in embryo development it is required for organogenesis, tissue differentiation and hematopoiesis [1–3]. Total vitamin A intake consists of many dietary forms including retinyl esters, β-carotene and free retinol. The various ingested forms of vitamin A are then processed, stored in the liver and can be released into the systemic circulation upon demand.

The various functions of vitamin A are carried out by several metabolically active derivatives including 11-*cis*-retinal and all-*trans*-retinoic acid, which are required for vision and transcriptional gene regulation respectively [4,5]. Enzymatic activity and gene regulation within many tissues is dependent upon a consistent supply of vitamin A, therefore tissues such as the eye, possess cyclic series of reactions to regenerate biologically active vitamin A such as a visual chromophore 11-*cis*-retinal. The efficient renewal of vitamin A is termed the visual cycle, and is indispensable for normal vision in humans. Genetic mutations which result in faulty enzymes required for the eye specific processing of vitamin A may cause early onset retinal degeneration due to the lack of 11-*cis*-retinal chromophore and ultimately can lead to complete loss of vision. Retinoid therapies utilize specific isomers of vitamin A and have proven to be effective at alleviating progressive tissue damage in animal models of retinal degeneration. Retinoid treatment maintains functional responses as well as tissue integrity both of which are observed to decline significantly with age in animal models of retinal diseases. Similar phenotypic pathology and age related degeneration trends are seen in human patients suffering from blinding diseases such as Leber congenital amaurosis (LCA) and retinitis pigmentosa (RP). Retinoid therapies therefore have the potential to improve the quality of life in patients suffering from genetic retinal diseases by delaying progressive vision loss.

2. Absorption and Distribution of Dietary Vitamin A as Retinyl Esters and Provitamin A Carotenoids

De novo synthesis of vitamin A is limited to plants and some microorganisms, therefore all vertebrates, including humans, must obtain vitamin A from dietary sources either as preformed vitamin A or provitamin A carotenoids [6]. The majority of vitamin A in the mammalian diet is not present in the free retinol form, but instead as both retinyl esters in animal tissues, and carotenoids contained in plant material. Preformed vitamin A, in the form of retinol or retinyl esters, is found almost exclusively in animal goods such as dairy products and organ meats such as liver [7,8]. Conversely provitamin A carotenoids, such as β-carotene, can be found in green leafy vegetables, such as spinach, as well as a variety of fruits such as apricots and papaya [9]. The intestinal mucosa is the active site for the uptake of free retinol, cleavage of carotenoids, and the hydrolysis of retinyl esters in vertebrates [10].

2.1. Intestinal Uptake and Metabolism of Pro-Vitamin A Carotenoids

Carotenoids are naturally occurring isoprenoid compounds (C40) produced by plants and some microorganisms. Carotenoids contain conjugated double bonds in the form of a polyene hydrocarbon chain, which is responsible for a variety of red and orange pigments that absorb light in the range of

300–600 nm [11]. Carotenoids in nature commonly contain a terminal benzene ring, which is either oxygenated or unoxygenated to yield molecules termed xanthophylls and carotenes respectively. Carotenoids serve many functions in mammalian biology including inherent antioxidant capabilities, incorporation into the macular region of the central human retina, and conversion into retinoid signaling molecules involved in development and gene regulation [12–14].

When ingested by mammalians carotenes are considered pro-vitamin A compounds since vertebrates have the ability to enzymatically transform various dietary carotenes into vitamin A. The first step in vitamin A metabolism begins with the symmetric cleavage of a carotene, such as β-carotene, by an enzyme at the intestinal brush boarder termed β,β-carotene 15,15′-monooxygenase (BCMO1) (Figure 1). BCMO1 cleaves carotenes at C15′/C15′ of the carbon backbone yielding two retinaldhyde molecules. BCMO1 converts a limited number of carotenoids to retinoid products *in vivo*, while a related protein BCDO2 (β,β-carotene 9,10-dioxygenase) cleaves carotenoids asymmetrically at the C9′/C10′ bond, and displays a broader substrate specificity [15]. Studies in BCMO1 knockout mice demonstrate that BCDO2 cannot compensate for the loss in carotene cleavage and vitamin A production, demonstrating the non-overlapping role of the two oxygenases [16].

Cell culture studies have suggested that the uptake of β-carotene, a common carotenoid in the human diet, is a saturable and regulated process controlled by the intestine-specific homeobox transcription factor (ISX) [17,18]. In a previous study, large doses of β-carotene were administered to healthy volunteers and less than half of the provitamin was reported to be converted to retinol, suggesting that the enzymatic cleavage of β-carotene to retinol is regulated in a dose dependent manner [19].

2.2. Intestinal Uptake of Retinyl Esters and Reesterification of Retinol by LRAT

Dietary retinoids are efficiently absorbed in the small intestine, but must be converted to the alcohol form of vitamin A before cellular transport. Dietary retinyl esters are hydrolyzed to retinol in the intestinal lumen or at the brush broader of enterocytes by pancreatic lipase or phospholipase B respectively [15,20]. Enterocyte specific uptake of free retinol or recently hydrolyzed retinyl ester is facilitated by cellular retinol binding protein II (CRBP-II) which binds the hydrophobic molecule with high affinity and transports it within the cytosol [21]. Three distinct retinol binding proteins exist in mammalians, CRBP-I is expressed ubiquitously in tissues while CRBP-II is both primarily and highly expressed in the jejuna mucosa suggesting its unique role in retinol absorption in the intestine, while CRBP-III primarily is found in heart, muscle, adipose and mammary tissue [22–24].

Following enterocyte uptake, free retinol is reesterified with long chain fatty acids, such as palmitate, and is secreted into the lymphatic system in the form of chylomicrons (Figure 1). Reesterification is accomplished by an acyltransferase enzyme, lecithin: retinol acyltransferase (LRAT), before incorporation into nascent chylomicrons [25]. Nascent chylomicrons include newly formed retinyl esters as well as other dietary lipids such as cholesterol, and enter the general circulation through the thoracic duct where they are further metabolized into smaller particles termed chylomicron remnants and distributed to the liver and other tissues [26]. The majority of absorbed free retinyl esters are also packaged into chylomicrons and secreted in the lymphatic system [27]. The remaining unabsorbed retinyl esters are systemically circulated and taken up by target tissues such as adipose, heart, muscle and lung tissue [28].

Figure 1. The metabolism of carotenoids and retinoids begin in the intestinal lumen, where provitamin A and retinoid molecules are absorbed. Retinyl esters are transported to the liver via the lymphatic system, while retinol is transported through the bloodstream before delivery to target tissues, such as the retina.

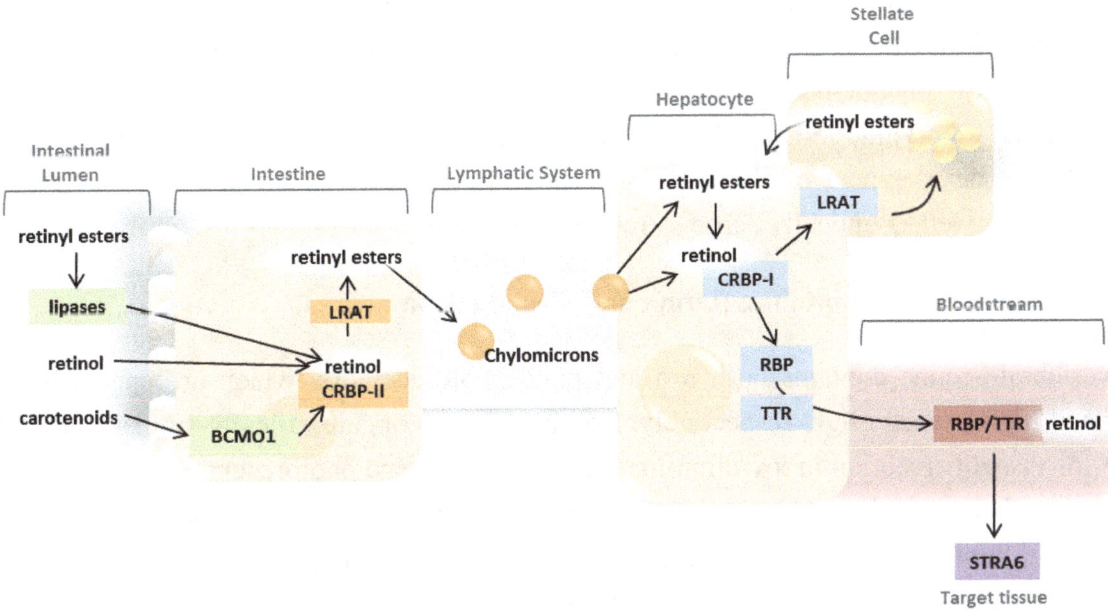

2.3. Systemic Circulation and Cellular Uptake by STRA6

Following hepatic uptake of retinyl esters hydrolysis of the ester linkage forms a retinol molecule, which binds immediately to the intercellular retinol-binding protein CRBP-I. A portion of retinol remains bound to intracellular CRBP-I, but the majority quickly becomes reesterified by LRAT, and stored within liver stellate cells [29]. Retinol stored as retinyl esters accumulate in the highest amounts in the liver but are also stored in tissues such as adipose, lung, and retinal pigment epithelium [30–33]. Secretion of retinol from these organs, with the exception of the RPE, into the systemic blood stream maintains normal blood retinol levels, even under times of diet insufficiency. Circulating plasma retinol is transported via a retinol-binding protein (RBP) and transthyretin (TTR) complex, and is required for transport since the retinol molecule alone is highly lipophilic (Figure 1). Genetic knockouts of *Rbp* in mice show that without the RBP transport protein these animals are exceedingly sensitive to vitamin A deficiency because of the inability to mobilize hepatic stores, and continue to have low serum retinol concentrations even after supplementing the diet [34]. In humans a deficiency of RBP results in a progressive atrophy of the retinal pigment epithelium and difficulty in dark adaptation, but patients are otherwise unaffected in other organs, perhaps due to the delivery of retinyl esters to tissues by chylomicron remnants [35]. TTR on the other hand may play a minor role in the transport of retinol since studies with TTR deficient mice show that mutants are healthy and fertile, despite extremely low retinol and circulating RBP levels [36]. However, the binding of TTR is believed to reduce the glomeruli filtration rate of RBP by increasing the molecular weight of the complex and therefore decreasing vitamin A urinary excretion [37].

Binding of the RBP-TTR-retinol complex to the plasma membrane receptor stimulated by retinoic acid gene 6 (STRA6) of a target cell releases the vitamin from its carrier and facilitates cellular uptake

(Figure 1). STRA6 is highly expressed in cells or tissues, which depend on vitamin A for proper function. In the eye, retinal pigment epithelium cells highly express STRA6 near the basolateral membrane, allowing for efficient transport of vitamin A from the choroidal blood circulation, therefore allowing retinol to enter the visual cycle. Suppressing STRA6 expression in RPE cells has been observed to cause a decrease in the uptake of vitamin A in the eye, whereas up regulation of STRA6 by retinoic acid stimulation enhances vitamin A uptake [38]. Clinically, mutations in STRA6 cause various pathological phenotypes in humans including anophthalmia, mental retardation, congenital heart defects and embryonic lethality [39,40]. In the mouse retina specifically mutations in the *Stra6* gene lead to the development of short rod and cone photoreceptors, reduced scotopic and photopic ERG responses as well as optically dense vitreous humor [41].

3. Incorporation of Retinol into the Retina and Visual Cycle

The vertebrate retina contains both rod and cone photoreceptors, which are specialized for low intensity and high intensity light respectively. Rod photoreceptors are efficient single-photon detectors allowing for visual perception in low illumination. However, cone photoreceptors are far less sensitive but because of the varying sensitivities of opsin molecules these cells can distinguish various wavelengths of light allowing for the perception of color (reviewed in [42]).

Visual perception relies on the cyclic processing of 11-*cis*-retinal and its binding to a special class of light sensing GPCRs within photoreceptors cells, termed opsins to form visual pigments as rhodopsin or cone opsins. The light sensitive component of the human retina is comprised mainly of rod and cone photoreceptors cells, both, which utilize the 11-*cis*-retinal chromophore for visual transduction. The steady supply of 11-*cis*-retinal is maintained by cooperative enzymatic processing occurring between outer segments of both types of photoreceptor cells and the RPE layer, or between cone outer segments and Müller cells. Collectively these processes are referred to as the visual cycle. In many human retinal diseases these cyclic processes are disturbed resulting in an inability to either produce an adequate supply of 11-*cis*-retinal or a failure to remove the build-up of various retinoid products.

3.1. RPE and the Photoreceptor Visual Cycle

The RPE contains a cascade of proteins required for the enzymatic isomerization of all-*trans*-retinol into the light sensitive chromophore 11-*cis*-retinal (Figure 2). All-*trans*-retinol is transported to RPE through the choridal blood circulation or photoreceptor outer segments. All-*trans*-retinol is subsequently absorbed on the basolateral side of the cell by the receptor STRA6 from the choridal blood circulation, which is facilitated by membrane bound LRAT. All-*trans*-retinol is transported though the interface of photoreceptor outer segments and microvilli of RPE via interphotoreceptor matrix and interphotoreceptor retinoid-binding protein (IRBP) (Figures 1 and 2). In both transport pathways, LRAT is necessary for the efficient uptake and usage of retinol in the RPE since it supplies esterified retinoid substrates for the formation of 11-*cis*-retinol via retinal pigment epithelium-specific 65 kDa protein (RPE65). In addition, retinyl esters not catalyzed by RPE65 accumulate to form retinyl esters used for retinoid storage in RPE specific organelles termed retinosomes [31,38,43,44]. Genetic knockout of the *Lrat* gene in mice has been observed to hinder vitamin A uptake in the gut, abolish the production of retinyl esters in most tissues (excluding adipose tissue which utilizes a different pathway for retinyl ester formation), and severely impair visual function [45,46]. In the retina a complete lack of retinyl ester formation results in the absence of 11-*cis*-retinal and therefore impairs the regeneration of rhodopsin, consequently this deficiency leads to progressive retinal degeneration manifested by the shortening of rod outer segments.

Figure 2. Visual cycle. Absorption of light by visual pigments (rhodopsin or cone opsin) causes isomerization of 11-*cis*-retinal to all-*trans*-retinal, resulting in phototransduction. Decay of activated rhodopsin yields opsin and all-*trans*-retinal, which is released and pumped out into the cytosol by a photoreceptor specific ATP-binding transporter (ABCA4) and reduced to all-*trans*-retinol by all-*trans*-retinal dehydrogenases (RDH8 and RDH12). All-*trans*-retinol diffuses into the RPE where it is esterified by lecithin:retinol acyltransferase (LRAT) to all-*trans*-retinyl esters, which are stored in retinosomes. All-*trans*-retinyl esters are isomerized to 11-*cis*-retinol in a reaction involving a 65 kDa RPE-specific protein (RPE65). To complete the visual cycle, 11-*cis*-retinol is then oxidized by 11-*cis*–retinal specific RDH (RDH5) to 11-*cis*-retinal, which then diffuses back into the photoreceptor where it combines with opsin to regenerate visual pigments. IRBP, interphotoreceptor retinoid-binding protein; Stra6, stimulated by retinoic acid gene 6.

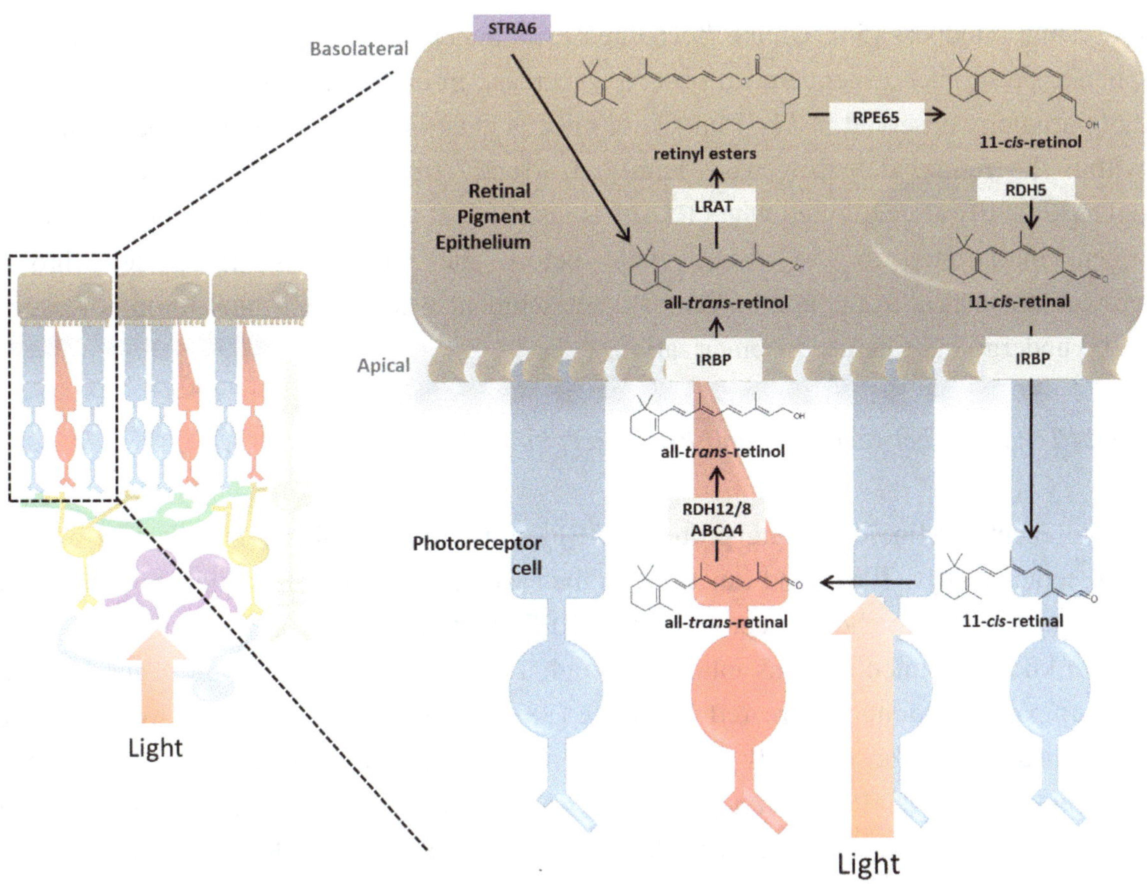

3.2. *Müller Cells and the Cone Visual Cycle*

Cone photoreceptor cells utilize a second pathway to regenerate chromophore independent of the RPE. The existence of this second cycle allows for rapid cone pigment regeneration under constant and bright illumination where pigment is rapidly bleached [47]. Unlike rod cells which solely rely on the RPE to convert all-*trans*-retinol to 11-*cis*-retinol, evidence from various species have suggested that Müller cells in the neural retina have the ability to perform this isomerization step autonomously from the RPE [48,49]. In addition, recent biochemical evidence has suggested that cones cells oxidize 11-*cis*-retinol to 11-*cis*-retinal thus allowing for faster chromophore recycling than seen in rod photoreceptors [42,50]. The cone specific visual cycle is evolutionarily conserved in numerous rod dominated and cone dominated species signifying the importance of this cycle despite the photoreceptor ratio variation seen between species [50].

3.3. Enzymatic Processing of Retinol in the RPE

The next step in the visual cycle after retinol esterification is the combined isomerization and hydrolysis of retinyl esters by the isomerohydrolase protein RPE65 [46,51,52]. This reaction yields 11-*cis*-retinol which further becomes oxidized by 11-*cis*-retinol dehydrogenase (RDH5) to 11-*cis*-retinal, additional dehydrogenases are also known to be involved in this oxidation including RDH11 and RDH10 (reviewed in [53]). Analogous to the *Lrat* deletion, genetic deletion or mutation of the *Rpe65* gene produces an intrinsic 11-*cis*-retinoid deficiency leading to the rapid onset of retinal degeneration and blindness [54]. Unlike *Rpe65* and *Lrat*, genetic knockout of *Rdh5* does not produce a drastic phenotype in mice except for an observed increase in *cis*-retinols and retinyl esters [43]. The absence of pathology observed in *Rhd5* knockout mice is most likely explained by the redundancy that exists within the retinol dehydrogenase family. Currently the view is that other proteins in the dehydrogenase family are exploited when RDH5 is insufficient [55]. The formation of 11-*cis*-retinal is the last enzymatic step in the visual cycle before the retinoid is transported through the interphotoreceptor matrix to the photoreceptor outer segment where it will bind to one of many opsin proteins and undergo light induced isomerization.

3.4. Retinoid Transport between RPE and Photoreceptor Cells

Interphotoreceptor retinoid-binding protein (IRBP) is the major soluble protein that exists in the interphotoreceptor matrix (IPM), and functions as the two-way carrier of retinoids, both from the RPE to photoreceptors and from photoreceptors back to RPE [56,57] (Figure 2). Surprisingly the rod visual cycle in *Irbp* knockout mice remains intact, although 11-*cis*-retinal regeneration occurs at a reduced rate when compared to identically reared WT mice [58]. Recently IRBP has been found to be crucial for the cone visual cycle most notably for proper cone function, maintenance of cone outer segments and eye development [58–60]. In *Xenopus* IRBP was found to bind specifically to the pericellular matrix of cone outer segments and Müller cell microvilli, suggesting that IRBP plays a significant role in the transport of retinoids to these cell types [61]. It is unknown whether other proteins are involved in this transport, and some potential candidates have been investigated, though the data are not conclusive [62]. Efficient transport is certainly necessary for the proper recycling of retinoids during the visual cycle because of their hydrophobicity, thus undiscovered secondary and compensatory transport mechanisms existing in the interphotoreceptor matrix may still remain to be uncovered.

3.5. Photoreceptor Cells and Visual Transduction

Once inside the photoreceptor cell the newly formed 11-*cis*-retinal forms a covalent schiff base bond with an opsin molecule contained within an outer segment disc membrane [63,64]. Incoming photons must pass through all layers of the retina before reaching photoreceptor outer segments and initiating phototransduction (Figure 2). Photon absorption by 11-*cis*-retinal changes the bound retinoid configuration from *cis* to *trans*, and allows the opsin molecule to activate the regulatory protein transducin through its own conformation change to MetaII. Transducin activation is accomplished by the catalytic exchange of GDP for GTP facilitated by photoactivated opsin. This exchange leads to a decrease of cytoplasmic cGMP concentrations, and eventually a nerve response is propagated to the brain and perceived as vision (phototransduction and visual processing reviewed in [65–67]). Rod and cones cells bind distinct transducin proteins, however by employing comparable genomics it was found that all forms of vertebrate opsin contain the same functional domains for binding transducin, confirming the importance of this signaling pathway in vision [68].

During transducin activation the schiff base bond between the opsin molecule and the newly isomerized all-*trans*-retinal is hydrolyzed. This hydrolysis forms free all-*trans*-retinal which subsequently becomes reduced to all-*trans*-retinol and binds to the cytosolic protein cellular retinol-binding protein type-1 (CRBP1) where it is transported out of the photoreceptor cell and back to the RPE for regeneration [69]. Excessive exposure to light, or a genetic mutation in one of the many essential visual cycle proteins can cause the accumulation of all-*trans*-retinal leading to the formation of condensation products, such as A2E, and cell toxicity [70–72].

4. Deficiencies in 11-*cis*-Retinal and Associated Retinal Degenerative Diseases

Mouse models of 11-*cis*-retinal deficiency have provided invaluable data regarding the importance of sustained retinoid cycling between the RPE and photoreceptor cells in vision; in addition, these models have provided biologically similar models of human retinal degeneration diseases for study. Both *Lrat* and *Rpe65* knockout mouse models have been employed in this field of research because of their inability to produce the essential chromophore 11-*cis*-retinal, and thus these animals develop retinal pathology similarly to what is observed in certain human retinal dystrophies.

*4.1. Pathophysiology of 11-*cis*-Deficient Retinal Diseases in Mouse Models of Retinal Degeneration*

The progressive loss of rod photoreceptors and shortening of rod outer segments with age has been reported in mice lacking functional *Lrat* or *Rpe65* [45,52]. Additionally both mouse models show rapid degeneration of cone photoreceptors, with complete degeneration of M/L and S opsin occurring at P28 and P42 respectively [73,74]. Both knockout mice display mislocalization of cone opsin at P28 and upon repeated administration of 11-*cis*-retinal opsin trafficking can be partially corrected in young *Lrat*$^{-/-}$ and *Rpe65*$^{-/-}$ mice, emphasizing the importance of 11-*cis*-retinal for proper cone opsin conformation and trafficking [54,74,75]. Recently, mounting evidence supports the hypothesis that mislocalization of cone opsin results in increased endoplasmic reticulum stress and induces the early cone cell death seen in LCA mouse models. Pharmacological studies in *Lrat*$^{-/-}$ and *Rpe65*$^{-/-}$ mice have demonstrated that cone cell death can be ameliorated by both the ER chemical chaperone tauroursodeoxycholic acid, and proteasome inhibitor MG-132 respectively, suggesting a central role for ER in opsin protein degradation [76,77].

Rod opsin on the other hand is observed to traffic normally in the absence of 11-*cis*-retinal, both in *Lrat* and *Rpe65* knockout mice, suggesting that rod pigment does not necessarily need its chromophore for proper photoreceptor localization [74], whereas 11-*cis*-retinal deficiency can induce abnormality of length and morphological structures of rod outer segments in LCA mouse models [74,78]. Experiments in P23H mutant mice have shown that the 11-*cis*-retinal or 9-*cis*-retinal chromophore is important for increasing protein stability and intracellular transportation of mutant rod opsin, providing evidence that specific protein sequences may also be important for proper functioning and transport of rod opsin [79–81].

The cyclic processing of chromophore can be blocked by removal or mutation in any one of the enzymes required for regeneration. Furthermore cycle interruption may result not only in cessation of 11-*cis*-retinal chromophore production but also in the accumulation of products from the previous steps, leading to cell disruption and death. Mutations in *Lrat* and *Rpe65* disrupt the visual cycle at distinct steps in regeneration and therefore knockout animals present differences in retinoid composition in the eye. The loss of functional RPE65 prevents the conversion of stored retinyl esters to 11-*cis*-retinal and causes the unrestrained accumulation of retinyl esters in the RPE, leading to a nonfunctioning visual cycle [52]. Excessive ester accumulation, appearing as retinosomes, can be clearly seen in young *Rpe65*$^{-/-}$ mice, while such structures are rare in either *Lrat*$^{-/-}$ or wild-type mice (Figure 3). In addition noninvasive two-photon imaging techniques have revealed analogous fluorescent structures in RPE of 3 months old *Rpe65*$^{-/-}$ mice, while these structures were completely absent from *Lrat*$^{-/-}$, and minimal in wild-type mice [44].

Figure 3. (**A**) Horizontal EM images of RPE in 3 month old *Rpe65*$^{-/-}$, *Lrat*$^{-/-}$ and wild-type mice. Of particular interest are the large retinosomes present around the perimeter of RPE cells in *Rpe65*$^{-/-}$ mice (black arrows), these formations are indicative of excessive ester accumulation in the retina. (**B**) Two photon imaging of the RPE in 3 month old *Rpe65*$^{-/-}$, *Lrat*$^{-/-}$ and wild-type mice. Large autofluorescent spots are observed in the RPE of *Rpe65*$^{-/-}$ mice (white arrows), while such spots are absent in *Lrat*$^{-/-}$ mice, and are minimally observed in wild type mice. Scale bar 5.0 μm.

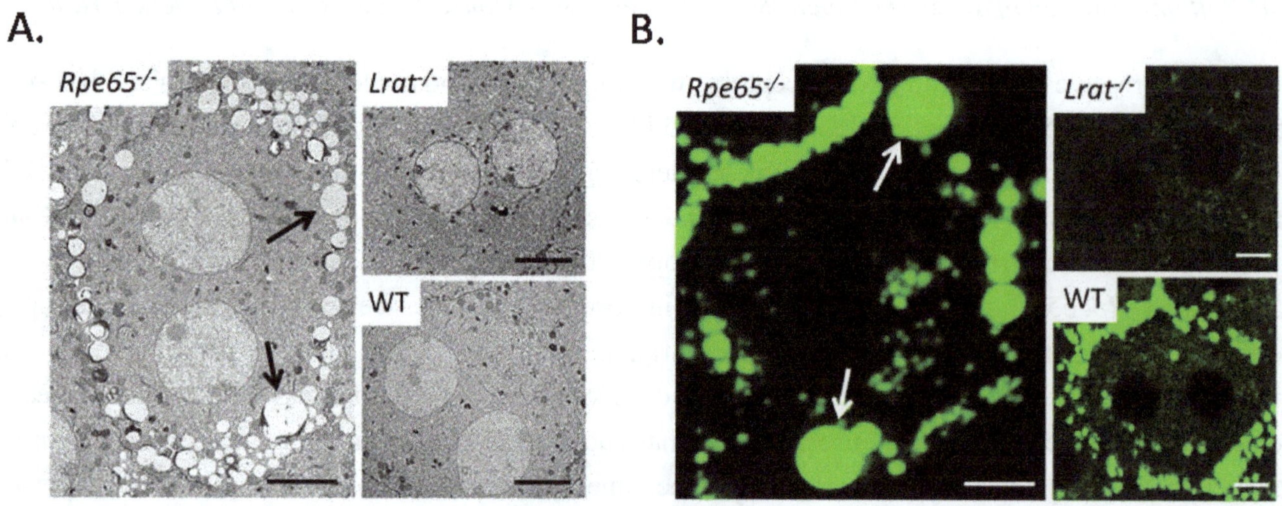

Whereas *Rpe65*$^{-/-}$ mice exhibit extremely high concentrations of retinyl ester, mice lacking the enzyme LRAT possess only trace amounts of retinyl esters in the RPE, but likewise have a no detectable 11-*cis*-retinal in the retina, indicating that LRAT is essential for the esterification step of the visual cycle [74]. Furthermore, LRAT activity is required for storage of retinyl esters in other tissues, such as the liver and lungs, thus in addition to the retinal degenerative phenotype *Lrat*$^{-/-}$ mice are highly susceptible to vitamin A deficiency [30,82]. In conclusion, because of the pathological similarities shared between select human retinal degenerative diseases and both *Rpe65*$^{-/-}$ and *Lrat*$^{-/-}$ mice these models provide practical avenues for comprehensively studying aspects of human disease progression and potential treatments.

*4.2. 11-*cis*-Retinal Deficiency and Leber Congenital Amaurosis*

Defects in 11-*cis*-retinal regeneration are seen in a number of human inherited degenerative retinopathies including early childhood onset Leber congenital amaurosis (LCA). Diagnosis of LCA is usually confirmed early in life by irregular electroretinographic and papillary responses, and vision commonly declines with age until complete blindness is observed by the third or fourth decade of life [83,84]. Numerous gene mutations have been reported to cause LCA in humans including RPE65, LRAT, CRX (Homeodomain transcription factor), CRB1 (Crumbs like protein 1), TULP1 (Tubby-like protein), AIPL1 (aryl hydrocarbon interacting protein), and various other genes [84]. LCA typically is an autosomal recessive inherited disease, though autosomal dominant patterns have been reported [85]. The early-onset rod-cone dystrophy phenotype is observed in human patients diagnosed with LCA, but also in *Rpe65*$^{-/-}$ and *Lrat*$^{-/-}$ mice, as discussed above [45,52,86]. Early in life patients with LCA exhibit visual impairment with attenuated rod and cone function, macular atrophy, severely delayed or minimal ERG responses, nystagmus, and retinal cell degeneration [83,84,87,88]. LCA is currently considered an incurable disease but several promising therapies are presently being investigated, including gene therapy and chromophore replacement therapy [89–91].

5. Artificial Visual Chromophore Therapeutics and Further Applications

Pharmacological replacement of 11-*cis*-retinal has been shown to be highly effective at reconstituting functional visual pigment, increasing ERG responses and reducing the rate of retinal degeneration in animals with *Rpe65* or *Lrat* mutations [89,91]. 9-*cis* isomers have proven to be the most successful isomer in replacing the native 11-*cis* chromophore *in vivo*. Moreover 9-*cis*-retinal is preferred over 11-*cis*-retinal for chromophore replacement therapy because of its increased stability, ease of synthesis and ability to form light sensitive isorhodopsin *in vivo* [91]. Once incorporated into the rod outer segment 9-*cis*-retinal forms a schiff base with residue K296 of opsin producing a chromophore molecule analogous to 11-*cis*-retinal bound chromophore, and reducing the amount of endogenous opsin apoprotein [92] (Figure 4).

Figure 4. Isomers of the opsin chromophore. Both 11-*cis*-retinal and 9-*cis*-retinal form a Schiff base with residue K296 of the opsin molecule forming the light sensitive chromophore used in vision.

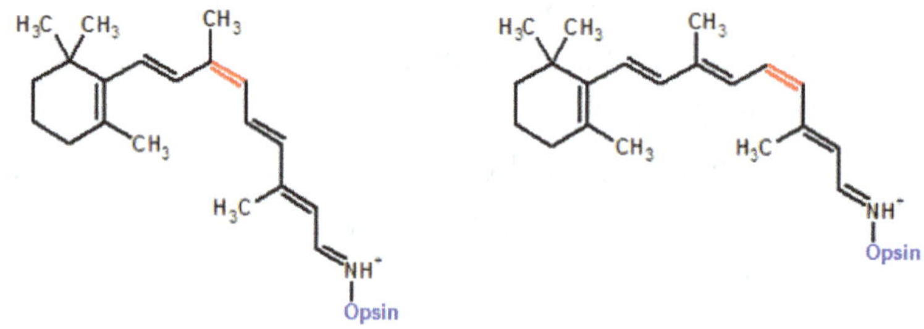

Opsin bound 9-*cis*-retinal Chromophore

Opsin bound 11-*cis*-retinal Chromophore

9-*cis*-retinoids taken orally, are converted to pro-drug forms *in vivo*, stored in the liver, transported in the blood, and eventually taken up into retinal tissue similar to dietary vitamin A. The capability to store 9-*cis* retinoids in tissues that naturally sequester vitamin A is especially important in producing a continuous therapeutic effect with retinoid drug administration. To avoid potential negative effects of administering large doses of retinoids future development of targeted delivery systems may lead to lower toxicity and improved effectiveness [93,94].

*5.1. Prevention of the LCA Phenotype with Administration of 9-*cis*-Retinoids in Animal Models*

The *Lrat*$^{-/-}$ and *Rpe65*$^{-/-}$ mouse provide useful disease models for studying the efficacy and toxicity of chromophore replacement therapy, since these mice lack visual chromophore and develop retinopathy that closely resembles LCA in humans. In *Rpe65*$^{-/-}$ mice oral gavage of 9-*cis*-retinal, the biologically active form, which binds with opsin, has been shown to produce functional isorhodopsin, restore rod function, increase light sensitivity, and reduce RPE ester concentration *in vivo* [89,91]. Likewise, intravitreal injections of 9-*cis*-retinal increased ERG responses and improved obstacle avoidance in a RPE65 deficient canine model of LCA [95]. 9-*cis*-retinal treatment in both *Lrat*$^{-/-}$ and *Rpe65*$^{-/-}$ mice demonstrate the ability of this retinal isomer to bypass essential steps in retinoid regeneration, fully integrate into photoreceptor outer segments and form isorhodopsin capable of sensing light (Figure 5).

Various analogs of 9-*cis*-retinal have been investigated that theoretically provide better stability in gastric acidity when ingested and are further metabolized in the liver to produce storage forms of 9-*cis*-retinyl esters, such as 9-*cis*-retinyl palmitate [93,96]. Prolonged improvements in ERG responses in 9-*cis* retinyl acetate treated *Rpe65*$^{-/-}$ mice implies that 9-*cis*-retinoids are stored in the liver, mobilized, taken up by RPE cells through the circulation as 9-*cis*-retinol and incorporated into the visual cycle similar to the all-*trans* isomer [97]. Uptake of retinol from the circulation into the RPE of *Rpe65*$^{-/-}$ mice remains functional despite the presence of an abnormally large quantity of retinyl esters, implying that circulating 9-*cis*-retinoids can be absorbed by the RPE even though a functional visual cycle does not exist [98]. Prodrugs, which can be stored by the body, provide a practical approach to 9-*cis*-retinal delivery in humans by increasing drug bioavailability and decreasing the need for frequent dosing.

Figure 5. Normal phase HPLC analysis of retinoids in dark adapted mouse models of retinal degeneration. Concentrations of *cis*-retinoids and retinyl esters in the retina differ before and after 9-*cis*-retinoid treatment. Control *Rpe65* knockout mice exhibit significantly increased concentrations of retinyl esters and are devoid of 11-*cis*-retinal. *Rpe65*$^{-/-}$ mice treated with 9-*cis*-retinoids show increase 9-*cis*-retinal bound to rhodopsin. Likewise, untreated *Lrat* knockout mice lack both 11-*cis*-retinal and retinyl esters, while treated *Lrat* knockout mice show an increase 9-*cis*-retinal bound to rhodopsin. WT mice show normal concentrations of 11-*cis*-retinal, as well as small amounts of retinyl esters.

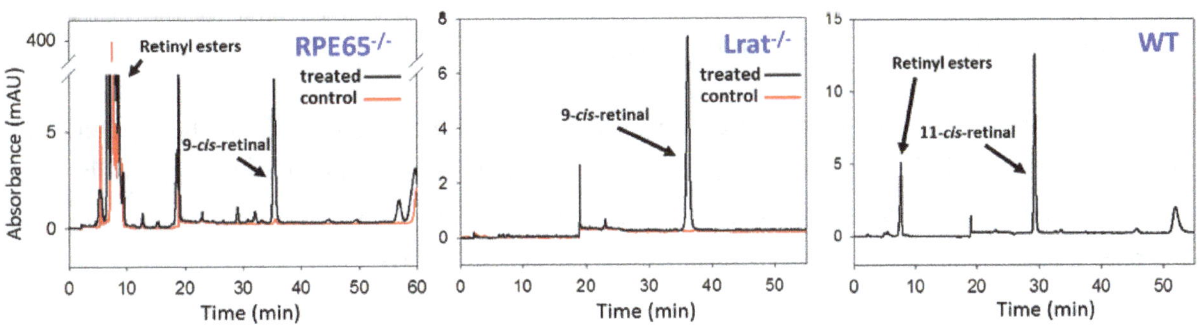

9-*cis*-retinyl acetate is one such prodrug, since it must be metabolized to the active 9-*cis*-retinal by the liver and then delivered to the eye via the bloodstream. Analogous to 9-*cis*-retinal therapy 9-*cis*-retinyl acetate treatment in *Lrat*$^{-/-}$ and *Rpe65*$^{-/-}$ mice generates functional isorhodopsin, maintains retinal thickness, and attenuates the decrease in ERG scotopic and photopic responses consistently seen with increasing age [71,99]. Similar to rod photoreceptors, the rate of age related cone photoreceptor cell death was slowed in 9-*cis*-retinyl acetate treated *Rpe65*$^{-/-}$ and *Lrat*$^{-/-}$ mice compared to untreated counterparts [100,101]. Furthermore significantly improved pure cone cell ERG responses were recorded in 9-*cis*-retinyl acetate treated *Rpe65*$^{-/-}$ and *Lrat*$^{-/-}$ mice lacking the functional transducin protein required for continued phototransduction in only rod cells. These data suggest that chromophore replacement therapy may be beneficial for also rescuing cone photoreceptor cells in LCA patients, which tend to be lost earlier in disease progression than rod photoreceptor cells [100]. Pharmacokinetic and systemic retinal toxicity studies demonstrated that WT, *Rpe65*$^{-/-}$, and *Lrat*$^{-/-}$ mice administered various dosing regimens of 9-*cis*-retinyl acetate displayed no toxicity at therapeutic dosing [97,99]. A recent study demonstrated that retinas of *Rpe65*$^{-/-}$ and *Lrat*$^{-/-}$ mice were well tolerated to continuous exposure of high levels of QLT091001, a 9-*cis*-retinyl acetate drug, without the accumulation of toxic retinoid byproducts, such as A2E, and obvious pathological changes in neural retina and RPE [99]. Importantly QLT091001, developed by QLT, Inc., has been tested in preliminary human clinical trials (ClinicalTrials.gov number, NCT01014052).

More recently, subcutaneous implantations of microparticle-hydrogels loaded with 9-*cis*-retinyl acetate have improved ERG responses and maintained retinal morphology in *Lrat*$^{-/-}$ mice, suggesting that the use of such implants can reduce the frequency of dosing and therefore decrease the risk of hypervitaminosis A in patients [94,102–107]. The side effects observed from extreme over supplementation of vitamin A derivatives have prompted extensive research and development of chemically modified retinoids, as well as novel delivery systems that decrease toxicity and increase drug effectiveness. Excess natural or synthetic retinoids pose serious teratogenic risks and can possibly lead to craniofacial, cardiac, thymic, and central nervous system malformations in infants [106–108]. In adults chronic hypervitaminosis A, caused by long-term retinoid administration, can result in fibrosis and cirrhosis of the liver, hypercalcemia and bone loss [102–104]. The severe side effects observed from over supplementing vitamin A derivatives have recently prompted extensive research and development of chemically modified retinoids, as well as novel delivery systems that decrease toxicity and increase drug effectiveness. Advancements in slow release therapies may in the future reduce the necessity for frequent dosing allowing patients to visit clinicians less frequently, while providing a consistent dosing of the drug.

*5.2. Therapeutics of 9-*cis*-Carotenoids in the Treatment of LCA*

Proretinoid compounds, such as carotenoids, have also been investigated for their potential use in treating chromophore deficiency in retinal diseases. Of particular interest is the naturally occurring carotenoid isomer 9-*cis*-β-carotene, because if metabolized and cleaved symmetrically by BCMO1, this carotene isomer has the potential to produce 9-*cis*-retinal *in vivo*. In addition substituting carotenes in place of retinoid supplements is particularly appealing since it eliminates the risk of developing hypervitaminosis A, given that β-carotene uptake and catabolic cleavage is negatively regulated by dietary vitamin A intake [17,109].

Recently a clinical study in patients with fundus albipunctatus, a congenital form of night blindness resulting from a genetic mutation in gene RDH5 required for the oxidation of 11-*cis*-retinol to 11-*cis*-retinal, demonstrated that administration of 9-*cis*-carotene rich supplements improved ERG responses and enhanced patients mean visual field score [110,111]. Conversely, a similar experiment was performed in both the *Lrat*$^{-/-}$ and *Rpe65*$^{-/-}$ mouse and demonstrated extremely limited delivery of 9-*cis*-retinal to the eye when these animals were administrated 9-*cis*-β-carotene isolated from *D. barawil* extracts [112]. Furthermore it was demonstrated *in vitro* that a second carotenoid cleavage enzyme, β-carotene dioxygenase 2 (BCDO2), exists in the intestine and favorably cleaves 9-*cis*-β-carotene asymmetrically, producing products which are further metabolized into all-*trans*-retinal by BCMO1 [112]. The results from the latter study provide evidence that *cis*-carotenoids are far less effective than 9-*cis*-retinoids for delivery of 9-*cis*-retinal to the eye because of the different catabolic pathways used to produce active retinoid compounds from proretinoids. The above mentioned clinical study included a small sample size of seven patients, and did not contain a control or placebo group; therefore the results observed in this study could be attributed to the increase in the overall intake of dietary vitamin A and not the specific action of the 9-*cis* isomer of β-carotene.

6. Conclusions

To sustain vision vertebrates require the continued cyclic regeneration of the vitamin A derivative 11-*cis*-retinal. Prolonged insufficient dietary supply of vitamin A, select genetic defects in genes required for the production of 11-*cis*-retinal chromophore or discontinuous retinoid cycling may have devastating effects on the overall health of the retina and the quality of vision. Particular human diseases, such as LCA, lack the functional enzymatic reactions to regenerate 11-*cis*-retinal, and therefore patients with these defects exhibit decreased visual responses at an early age, which additionally decline steadily throughout life.

Supplementation with preformed *cis*-retinoid derivatives has been show to bypass defective steps in the visual cycle, and regenerate pigments necessary for vision in animal models of retinal degenerative diseases. The main caveats to retinoid treatment are the myriad of toxic effects seen with administration of pharmacological doses of vitamin A derivatives for prolonged lengths of time. Therefore novel methods for reducing the risk of vitamin A toxicity, improving drug effectiveness, and reducing the frequency of dosing are absolutely necessary for designing a safe retinoid derived drug for treatment of retinal degenerative diseases associated with chromophore deficiency.

Acknowledgments

The authors would like to kindly thank H. Fujioka and M. Hitomi for electron microscopy images. Additionally the authors would like to thank A. Maeda, K. Palczewski, S. Howell and D. Peck for critically reviewing the manuscript. This work was supported in part by funding from the National Institutes of Health (K08EY019880, P30 EY11373); the Research to Prevent Blindness Foundation; Foundation Fighting Blindness; Midwest Eye Bank and the Ohio Lions Eye Research Foundation.

References

1. Sommer, A.; Vyas, K.S. A global clinical view on vitamin A and carotenoids. *Am. J. Clin. Nutr.* **2012**, *96*, 1204S–1206S.
2. Duester, G. Retinoic acid synthesis and signaling during early organogenesis. *Cell* **2008**, *134*, 921–931.
3. Oren, T.; Sher, J.A.; Evans, T. Hematopoiesis and retinoids: Development and disease. *Leuk. Lymphoma* **2003**, *44*, 1881–1891.
4. Wald, G. Molecular basis of visual excitation. *Science* **1968**, *162*, 230–239.
5. Rhinn, M.; Dolle, P. Retinoic acid signalling during development. *Development* **2012**, *139*, 843–858.
6. Plack, P.A. Occurrence, absorption and distribution of vitamin A. *Proc. Nutr. Soc.* **1965**, *24*, 146–153.
7. Gaucheron, F. Milk and dairy products: A unique micronutrient combination. *J. Am. Coll. Nutr.* **2011**, *30*, 400S–409S.
8. Thurnham, D.I.; Northrop-Clewes, C.A. Optimal nutrition: Vitamin A and the carotenoids. *Proc. Nutr. Soc.* **1999**, *58*, 449–457.
9. Allen, L.H. To what extent can food-based approaches improve micronutrient status? *Asia Pac. J. Clin. Nutr.* **2008**, *17*, 103–105.
10. Dew, S.E.; Ong, D.E. Specificity of the retinol transporter of the rat small intestine brush border. *Biochemistry* **1994**, *33*, 12340–12345.

11. Vachali, P.; Bhosale, P.; Bernstein, P.S. Microbial carotenoids. *Methods Mol. Biol.* **2012**, *898*, 41–59.
12. Bernstein, P.S.; Yoshida, M.D.; Katz, N.B.; McClane, R.W.; Gellermann, W. Raman detection of macular carotenoid pigments in intact human retina. *Investig. Ophthalmol. Vis. Sci.* **1998**, *39*, 2003–2011.
13. Moore, T. Vitamin A and carotene: The absence of the liver oil vitamin A from carotene. VI. The conversion of carotene to vitamin A *in vivo*. *Biochem. J.* **1930**, *24*, 692–702.
14. Amengual, J.; Lobo, G.P.; Golczak, M.; Li, H.N.; Klimova, T.; Hoppel, C.L.; Wyss, A.; Palczewski, K.; von Lintig, J. A mitochondrial enzyme degrades carotenoids and protects against oxidative stress. *FASEB J.* **2011**, *25*, 948–959.
15. Hu, K.Q.; Liu, C.; Ernst, H.; Krinsky, N.I.; Russell, R.M.; Wang, X.D. The biochemical characterization of ferret carotene-9′,10′-monooxygenase catalyzing cleavage of carotenoids *in vitro* and *in vivo*. *J. Biol. Chem.* **2006**, *281*, 19327–19338.
16. Lietz, G.; Oxley, A.; Boesch-Saadatmandi, C.; Kobayashi, D. Importance of beta,beta-carotene 15,15′-monooxygenase 1 (BCMO1) and beta,beta-carotene 9′,10′-dioxygenase 2 (BCDO2) in nutrition and health. *Mol. Nutr. Food Res.* **2012**, *56*, 241–250.
17. Lobo, G.P.; Hessel, S.; Eichinger, A.; Noy, N.; Moise, A.R.; Wyss, A.; Palczewski, K.; von Lintig, J. ISX is a retinoic acid-sensitive gatekeeper that controls intestinal β,β-carotene absorption and vitamin A production. *FASEB J.* **2010**, *24*, 1656–1666.
18. Seino, Y.; Miki, T.; Kiyonari, H.; Abe, T.; Fujimoto, W.; Kimura, K.; Takeuchi, A.; Takahashi, Y.; Oiso, Y.; Iwanaga, T.; *et al.* Isx participates in the maintenance of vitamin A metabolism by regulation of beta-carotene 15,15′-monooxygenase (Bcmo1) expression. *J. Biol. Chem.* **2008**, *283*, 4905–4911.
19. O'Neill, M.E.; Thurnham, D.I. Intestinal absorption of beta-carotene, lycopene and lutein in men and women following a standard meal: Response curves in the triacylglycerol-rich lipoprotein fraction. *Br. J. Nutr.* **1998**, *79*, 149–159.
20. Rigtrup, K.M.; Kakkad, B.; Ong, D.E. Purification and partial characterization of a retinyl ester hydrolase from the brush border of rat small intestine mucosa: Probable identity with brush border phospholipase B. *Biochemistry* **1994**, *33*, 2661–2666.
21. Ong, D.E. Cellular transport and metabolism of vitamin A: Roles of the cellular retinoid-binding proteins. *Nutr. Rev.* **1994**, *52*, S24–S31.
22. Li, E.; Norris, A.W. Structure/function of cytoplasmic vitamin A-binding proteins. *Annu. Rev. Nutr.* **1996**, *16*, 205–234.
23. Newcomer, M.E.; Jamison, R.S.; Ong, D.E. Structure and function of retinoid-binding proteins. *Subcell. Biochem.***1998**, *30*, 53–80.
24. Piantedosi, R.; Ghyselinck, N.; Blaner, W.S.; Vogel, S. Cellular retinol-binding protein type III is needed for retinoid incorporation into milk. *J. Biol. Chem.* **2005**, *280*, 24286–24292.
25. Blomhoff, R.; Green, M.H.; Berg, T.; Norum, K.R. Transport and storage of vitamin A. *Science* **1990**, *250*, 399–404.
26. Redgrave, T.G. Chylomicron metabolism. *Biochem. Soc. Trans.* **2004**, *32*, 79–82.
27. Goodman, D.W.; Huang, H.S.; Shiratori, T. Tissue distribution and metabolism of newly absorbed vitamin A in the rat. *J. Lipid Res.* **1965**, *6*, 390–396.

28. Van Bennekum, A.M.; Kako, Y.; Weinstock, P.H.; Harrison, E.H.; Deckelbaum, R.J.; Goldberg, I.J.; Blaner, W.S. Lipoprotein lipase expression level influences tissue clearance of chylomicron retinyl ester. *J. Lipid Res.* **1999**, *40*, 565–574.
29. MacDonald, P.N.; Ong, D.E. Evidence for a lecithin-retinol acyltransferase activity in the rat small intestine. *J. Biol. Chem.* **1988**, *263*, 12478–12482.
30. O'Byrne, S.M.; Wongsiriroj, N.; Libien, J.; Vogel, S.; Goldberg, I.J.; Baehr, W.; Palczewski, K.; Blaner, W.S. Retinoid absorption and storage is impaired in mice lacking lecithin: Retinol acyltransferase (LRAT). *J. Biol. Chem.* **2005**, *280*, 35647–35657.
31. Orban, T.; Palczewska, G.; Palczewski, K. Retinyl ester storage particles (Retinosomes) from the retinal pigmented epithelium resemble lipid droplets in other tissues. *J. Biol. Chem.* **2011**, *286*, 17248–17258.
32. Frey, S.K.; Vogel, S. Vitamin A metabolism and adipose tissue biology. *Nutrients* **2011**, *3*, 27–39.
33. Chytil, F. The lungs and vitamin A. *Am. J. Physiol.* **1992**, *262*, L517–L527.
34. Quadro, L.; Blaner, W.S.; Salchow, D.J.; Vogel, S.; Piantedosi, R.; Gouras, P.; Freeman, S.; Cosma, M.P.; Colantuoni, V.; Gottesman, M.E. Impaired retinal function and vitamin A availability in mice lacking retinol-binding protein. *EMBO J.* **1999**, *18*, 4633–4644.
35. Seeliger, M.W.; Biesalski, H.K.; Wissinger, B.; Gollnick, H.; Gielen, S.; Frank, J.; Beck, S.; Zrenner, E. Phenotype in retinol deficiency due to a hereditary defect in retinol binding protein synthesis. *Investig. Ophthalmol. Vis. Sci.* **1999**, *40*, 3–11.
36. Wolf, G. Retinol transport and metabolism in transthyretin-"knockout" mice. *Nutr. Rev.* **1995**, *53*, 98–99.
37. Zanotti, G.; Berni, R. Plasma retinol-binding protein: Structure and interactions with retinol, retinoids, and transthyretin. *Vitam. Horm.* **2004**, *69*, 271–295.
38. Kawaguchi, R.; Yu, J.; Honda, J.; Hu, J.; Whitelegge, J.; Ping, P.; Wiita, P.; Bok, D.; Sun, H. A membrane receptor for retinol binding protein mediates cellular uptake of vitamin A. *Science* **2007**, *315*, 820–825.
39. Pasutto, F.; Sticht, H.; Hammersen, G.; Gillessen-Kaesbach, G.; Fitzpatrick, D.R.; Nürnberg, G.; Brasch, F.; Schirmer-Zimmermann, H.; Tolmie, J.L.; Chitayat, D.; *et al.* Mutations in STRA6 cause a broad spectrum of malformations including anophthalmia, congenital heart defects, diaphragmatic hernia, alveolar capillary dysplasia, lung hypoplasia, and mental retardation. *Am. J. Hum. Genet.* **2007**, *80*, 550–560.
40. White, T.; Lu, T.Y.; Metlapally, R.; Katowitz, J.; Kherani, F.; Wang, T.Y.; Tran-Viet, K.N.; Young, T.L. Identification of STRA6 and SKI sequence variants in patients with anophthalmia/microphthalmia. *Mol. Vis.* **2008**, *14*, 2458–2465.
41. Ruiz, A.; Mark, M.; Jacobs, H.; Klopfenstein, M.; Hu, J.; Lloyd, M.; Habib, S.; Tosha, C.; Radu, R.A.; Ghyselinck, N.B.; *et al.* Retinoid content, visual responses, and ocular morphology are compromised in the retinas of mice lacking the retinol-binding protein receptor, STRA6. *Investig. Ophthalmol. Vis. Sci.* **2012**, *53*, 3027–3039.
42. Saari, J.C. Vitamin A metabolism in rod and cone visual cycles. *Annu. Rev. Nutr.* **2012**, *32*, 125–145.
43. Maeda, A.; Maeda, T.; Imanishi, Y.; Golczak, M.; Moise, A.R.; Palczewski, K. Aberrant metabolites in mouse models of congenital blinding diseases, formation and storage of retinyl esters. *Biochemistry* **2006**, *45*, 4210–4219.

44. Imanishi, Y.; Batten, M.L.; Piston, D.W.; Baehr, W.; Palczewski, K. Noninvasive two-photon imaging reveals retinyl ester storage structures in the eye. *J. Cell Biol.* **2004**, *164*, 373–383.
45. Batten, M.L.; Imanishi, Y.; Maeda, T.; Tu, D.C.; Moise, A.R.; Bronson, D.; Possin, D.; van Gelder, R.N.; Baehr, W.; Palczewski, K. Lecithin-retinol acyltransferase is essential for accumulation of all-*trans*-retinyl esters in the eye and in the liver. *J. Biol.Chem.* **2004**, *279*, 10422–10432.
46. Gollapalli, D.R.; Rando, R.R. All-*trans*-retinyl esters are the substrates for isomerization in the vertebrate visual cycle. *Biochemistry* **2003**, *42*, 5809–5818.
47. Wang, J.S.; Estevez, M.E.; Cornwall, M.C.; Kefalov, V.J. Intra-retinal visual cycle required for rapid and complete cone dark adaptation. *Nat. Neurosci.* **2009**, *12*, 295–302.
48. Jones, G.J.; Crouch, R.K.; Wiggert, B.; Cornwall, M.C.; Chader, G.J. Retinoid requirements for recovery of sensitivity after visual-pigment bleaching in isolated photoreceptors. *Proc. Natl. Acad. Sci. USA* **1989**, *86*, 9606–9610.
49. Kefalov, V.J. Rod and cone visual pigments and phototransduction through pharmacological, genetic, and physiological approaches. *J. Biol. Chem.* **2012**, *287*, 1635–1641.
50. Wang, J.S.; Kefalov, V.J. The cone-specific visual cycle. *Prog. Retin. Eye Res.* **2011**, *30*, 115–128.
51. Trehan, A.; Canada, F.J.; Rando, R.R. Inhibitors of retinyl ester formation also prevent the biosynthesis of 11-*cis*-retinol. *Biochemistry* **1990**, *29*, 309–312.
52. Redmond, T.M.; Yu, S.; Lee, E.; Bok, D.; Hamasaki, D.; Chen, N.; Goletz, P.; Ma, J.X.; Crouch, R.K.; Pfeifer, K. Rpe65 is necessary for production of 11-*cis*-vitamin A in the retinal visual cycle. *Nat. Genet.* **1998**, *20*, 344–351.
53. Parker, R.O.; Crouch, R.K. Retinol dehydrogenases (RDHs) in the visual cycle. *Exp. Eye Res.* **2010**, *91*, 788–792.
54. Rohrer, B.; Lohr, H.R.; Humphries, P.; Redmond, T.M.; Seeliger, M.W.; Crouch, R.K. Cone opsin mislocalization in Rpe65(−/−) mice: A defect that can be corrected by 11-*cis* retinal. *Investig. Ophthalmol. Vis. Sci.* **2005**, *46*, 3876–3882.
55. Driessen, C.A.; Winkens, H.J.; Hoffmann, K.; Kuhlmann, L.D.; Janssen, B.P.; van Vugt, A.H.; van Hooser, J.P.; Wieringa, B.E.; Deutman, A.F.; Palczewski, K.; *et al.* Disruption of the 11-*cis*-retinol dehydrogenase gene leads to accumulation of *cis*-retinols and *cis*-retinyl esters. *Mol. Cell. Biol.* **2000**, *20*, 4275–4287.
56. Gonzalez-Fernandez, F. Interphotoreceptor retinoid-binding protein—An old gene for new eyes. *Vis. Res.* **2003**, *43*, 3021–3036.
57. Wu, Q.; Blakeley, L.R.; Cornwall, M.C.; Crouch, R.K.; Wiggert, B.N.; Koutalos, Y. Interphotoreceptor retinoid-binding protein is the physiologically relevant carrier that removes retinol from rod photoreceptor outer segments. *Biochemistry* **2007**, *46*, 8669–8679.
58. Jin, M.; Li, S.; Nusinowitz, S.; Lloyd, M.; Hu, J.; Radu, R.A.; Bok, D.; Travis, G.H. The role of interphotoreceptor retinoid-binding protein on the translocation of visual retinoids and function of cone photoreceptors. *J. Neurosci.* **2009**, *29*,1486–1495.
59. Parker, R.O.; Fan, J.; Nickerson, J.M.; Liou, G.I.; Crouch, R.K. Normal cone function requires the interphotoreceptor retinoid binding protein. *J. Neurosci.* **2009**, *29*, 4616–4621.

60. Wisard, J.; Faulkner, A.; Chrenek, M.A.; Waxweiler, T.; Waxweiler, W.; Donmoyer, C.; Liou, G.I.; Craft, C.M.; Schmid, G.F.; Boatright, J.H.; *et al.* Exaggerated eye growth in IRBP-deficient mice in early development. *Investig. Ophthalmol. Vis. Sci.* **2011**, *52*, 5804–5811.
61. Garlipp, M.A.; Gonzalez-Fernandez, F. Cone outer segment and Muller microvilli pericellular matrices provide binding domains for interphotoreceptor retinoid-binding protein (IRBP). *Exp. Eye Res.* **2013**, doi:10.1016/j.exer.2013.02.003.
62. Gonzalez-Fernandez, F. Evolution of the visual cycle: The role of retinoid-binding proteins. *J. Endocrinol.* **2002**, *175*, 75–88.
63. Matsumoto, H.; Yoshizawa, T. Existence of a beta-ionone ring-binding site in the rhodopsin molecule. *Nature* **1975**, *258*, 523–526.
64. Bownds, D. Site of attachment of retinal in rhodopsin. *Nature* **1967**, *216*, 1178–1181.
65. Jastrzebska, B.; Debinski, A.; Filipek, S.; Palczewski, K. Role of membrane integrity on G protein-coupled receptors: Rhodopsin stability and function. *Prog. Lipid Res.* **2011**, *50*, 267–277.
66. Masland, R.H. The neuronal organization of the retina. *Neuron* **2012**, *76*, 266–280.
67. Wassle, H. Parallel processing in the mammalian retina. *Nat. Rev. Neurosci.* **2004**, *5*, 747–757.
68. Carleton, K.L.; Spady, T.C.; Cote, R.H. Rod and cone opsin families differ in spectral tuning domains but not signal transducing domains as judged by saturated evolutionary trace analysis. *J. Mol. Evol.* **2005**, *61*, 75–89.
69. Saari, J.C.; Nawrot, M.; Garwin, G.G.; Kennedy, M.J.; Hurley, J.B.; Ghyselinck, N.B.; Chambon, P. Analysis of the visual cycle in cellular retinol-binding protein type I (CRBPI) knockout mice. *Investig. Ophthalmol. Vis. Sci.* **2002**, *43*, 1730–1735.
70. Rozanowska, M.; Handzel, K.; Boulton, M.E.; Różanowski, B. Cytotoxicity of all-*trans*-retinal increases upon photodegradation. *Photochem. Photobiol.* **2012**, *88*, 1362–1372.
71. Maeda, A.; Maeda, T.; Golczak, M.; Chou, S.; Desai, A.; Hoppel, C.L.; Matsuyama, S.; Palczewski, K. Involvement of all-*trans*-retinal in acute light-induced retinopathy of mice. *J. Biol. Chem.* **2009**, *284*, 15173–15183.
72. Sparrow, J.R.; Boulton, M. RPE lipofuscin and its role in retinal-pathobiology. *Exp. Eye Res.* **2005**, *80*, 595–606.
73. Znoiko, S.L.; Rohrer, B.; Lu, K.; Lohr, H.R.; Crouch, R.K.; Ma, J.X. Downregulation of cone-specific gene expression and degeneration of cone Photoreceptors in the Rpe65(−/−) mouse at early ages. *Investig. Ophthalmol. Vis. Sci.* **2005**, *46*, 1473–1479.
74. Fan, J.; Rohrer, B.; Frederick, J.M.; Baehr, W.; Crouch, R.K. Rpe65(−/−) and Lrat(−/−) mice: Comparable models of Leber congenital amaurosis. *Investig. Ophthalmol. Vis. Sci.* **2008**, *49*, 2384–2389.
75. Zhang, H.; Fan, J.; Li, S.; Karan, S.; Rohrer, B.; Palczewski, K.; Frederick, J.M.; Crouch, R.K.; Baehr, W. Trafficking of membrane-associated proteins to cone photoreceptor outer segments requires the chromophore 11-*cis*-retinal. *J. Neurosci.* **2008**, *28*, 4008–4014.
76. Zhang, T.; Baehr, W.; Fu, Y. Chemical chaperone TUDCA preserves cone photoreceptors in a mouse model of Leber congenital amaurosis. *Investig. Ophthalmol. Vis. Sci.* **2012**, *53*, 3349–3356.
77. Sato, K.; Ozaki, T.; Ishiguro, S.; Nakazawa, M. M-opsin protein degradation is inhibited by MG-132 in Rpe65(−/−) retinal explant culture. *Mol. Vis.* **2012**, *18*, 1516–1525.

78. Batten, M.L.; Imanishi, Y.; Yu, D.C.; Doan, T.; Zhu, L.; Pang, J.J.; Glushakova, L.; Moise, A.R.; Baehr, W.; van Gelder, R.N.; *et al.* Pharmacological and rAAV gene therapy rescue of visual functions in a blind mouse model of Leber congenital amaurosis. *PLoS Med.* **2005**, *2*, e333.

79. Deretic, D. A role for rhodopsin in a signal transduction cascade that regulates membrane trafficking and photoreceptor polarity. *Vis. Res.* **2006**, *46*, 4427–4433.

80. Noorwez, S.M.; Malhotra, R.; McDowell, J.H.; Smith, K.A.; Krebs, M.P.; Kaushal, S. Retinoids assist the cellular folding of the autosomal dominant retinitis pigmentosa opsin mutant P23H. *J. Biol. Chem.* **2004**, *279*, 16278–16284.

81. Sakami, S.; Maeda, T.; Bereta, G.; Okano, K.; Golczak, M.; Sumaroka, A.; Roman, A.J.; Cideciyan, A.V.; Jacobson, S.G.; Palczewski, K. Probing mechanisms of photoreceptor degeneration in a new mouse model of the common form of autosomal dominant retinitis pigmentosa due to P23H opsin mutations. *J. Biol. Chem.* **2011**, *286*, 10551–10567.

82. Liu, L.; Gudas, L.J. Disruption of the lecithin:retinol acyltransferase gene makes mice more susceptible to vitamin A deficiency. *J. Biol. Chem.* **2005**, *280*, 40226–40234.

83. Perrault, I.; Rozet, J.R.; Gerber, S.; Ghazi, I.; Leowski, C.; Ducroq, D.; Souied, E.; Dufier, J.L.; Munnich, A.; Kaplan, J. Leber congenital amaurosis. *Mol. Genet. Metab.* **1999**, *68*, 200–208.

84. Hufnagel, R.B.; Ahmed, Z.M.; Corrêa, Z.M.; Sisk, R.A. Gene therapy for Leber congenital amaurosis: Advances and future directions. *Graefes Arch. Clin. Exp. Ophthalmol.* **2012**, *250*, 1117–1128.

85. Perrault, I.; Hanein, S.; Gerber, S.; Barbet, F.; Dufier, J.L.; Munnich, A.; Rozet, J.M.; Kaplan, J. Evidence of autosomal dominant Leber congenital amaurosis (LCA) underlain by a CRX heterozygous null allele. *J. Med. Genet.* **2003**, *40*, e90.

86. Den Hollander, A.I.; Roepman, R.; Koenekoop, R.K.; Cremers, F.P. Leber congenital amaurosis: Genes, proteins and disease mechanisms. *Prog. Retin. Eye Res.* **2008**, *27*, 391–419.

87. Aleman, T.S.; Jacobson, S.G.; Chico, J.D.; Scott, M.L.; Cheung, A.Y.; Windsor, E.A.; Furushima, M.; Redmond, T.M.; Bennett, J.; Palczewski, K; *et al.* Impairment of the transient pupillary light reflex in Rpe65(−/−) mice and humans with leber congenital amaurosis. *Investig. Ophthalmol. Vis. Sci.* **2004**, *45*, 1259–1271.

88. Lorenz, B.; Gyürüs, P.; Preising, M.; Bremser, D.; Gu, S.; Andrassi, M.; Gerth, C.; Gal, A. Early-onset severe rod-cone dystrophy in young children with RPE65 mutations. *Investig. Ophthalmol .Vis. Sci.* **2000**, *41*, 2735–2742.

89. Van Hooser, J.P.; Aleman, T.S.; He, Y.G.; Cideciyan, A.V.; Kuksa, V.; Pittler, S.J.; Stone, E.M.; Jacobson, S.G.; Palczewski, K. Rapid restoration of visual pigment and function with oral retinoid in a mouse model of childhood blindness. *Proc. Natl. Acad. Sci. USA* **2000**, *97*, 8623–8628.

90. Bainbridge, J.W.; Smith, A.J.; Barker, S.S.; Robbie, S.; Henderson, R.; Balaggan, K.; Viswanathan, A.; Holder, G.E.; Stockman, A.; Tyler, N.; *et al.* Effect of gene therapy on visual function in Leber's congenital amaurosis. *N. Engl. J. Med.* **2008**, *358*, 2231–2239.

91. Van Hooser, J.P.; Liang, Y.; Maeda, T.; Kuksa, V.; Jang, G.F.; He, Y.G.; Rieke, F.; Fong, H.K.; Detwiler, P.B.; Palczewski, K. Recovery of visual functions in a mouse model of Leber congenital amaurosis. *J. Biol. Chem.* **2002**, 277, 19173–19182.

92. Palczewski, K.; Kumasaka, T.; Hori, T.; Behnke, C.A.; Motoshima, H.; Fox, B.A.; Le, T.I.; Teller, D.C.; Okada, T.; Stenkamp, R.E; *et al.* Crystal structure of rhodopsin: A G protein-coupled receptor. *Science* **2000**, *289*, 739–745.
93. Palczewski, K. Retinoids for treatment of retinal diseases. *Trends Pharmacol. Sci.* **2010**, *31*, 284–295.
94. Gao, S.Q.; Maeda, T.; Okano, K.; Palczewski, K. A microparticle/hydrogel combination drug-delivery system for sustained release of retinoids. *Investig. Ophthalmol. Vis. Sci.* **2012**, *53*, 6314–6323.
95. Gearhart, P.M.; Gearhart, C.; Thompson, D.A.; Petersen-Jones, S.M. Improvement of visual performance with intravitreal administration of 9-*cis*-retinal in Rpe65-mutant dogs. *Arch. Ophthalmol.* **2010**, *128*, 1442–1448.
96. Collins, M.D.; Tzimas, G.; Hummler, H.; Bürgin, H.; Nau, H. Comparative teratology and transplacental pharmacokinetics of all-*trans*-retinoic acid, 13-*cis*-retinoic acid, and retinyl palmitate following daily administrations in rats. *Toxicol. Appl. Pharmacol.* **1994**, *127*, 132–144.
97. Maeda, T.; Maeda, A.; Casadesus, G.; Palczewski, K.; Margaron, P. Evaluation of 9-*cis*-retinyl acetate therapy in Rpe65−/− mice. *Investig. Ophthalmol .Vis. Sci.* **2009**, *50*, 4368–4378.
98. Qtaishat, N.M.; Redmond, T.M.; Pepperberg, D.R. Acute radiolabeling of retinoids in eye tissues of normal and rpe65-deficient mice. *Investig. Ophthalmol. Vis. Sci.* **2003**, *44*, 1435–1446.
99. Maeda, T.; Dong, Z.; Jin, H.; Sawada, O.; Gao, S.; Utkhede, D.; Monk, W.; Palczewska, G.; Palczewski, K. QLT091001, a 9-*cis*-retinal analog, is well-tolerated by retinas of mice with impaired visual cycles. *Investig. Ophthalmol. Vis. Sci.* **2013**, *54*, 455–466.
100. Maeda, T.; Cideciyan, A.V.; Maeda, A.; Golczak, M.; Aleman, T.S.; Jacobson, S.G.; Palczewski, K. Loss of cone photoreceptors caused by chromophore depletion is partially prevented by the artificial chromophore pro-drug, 9-*cis*-retinyl acetate. *Hum. Mol. Genet.* **2009**, *18*, 2277–2287.
101. Hamann, S.; Schorderet, D.F.; Cottet, S. Bax-induced apoptosis in leber's congenital amaurosis: A dual role in rod and cone degeneration. *PLoS One* **2009**, *4*, e6616.
102. Baxi, S.C.; Dailey, G.E. Hypervitaminosis A—A Cause of Hypercalcemia. *West. J. Med.* **1982**, *137*, 429–431.
103. Guarascio, P.; Portmann, B.; Visco, G.; Williams, R. Liver damage with reversible portal-hypertension from vitamin A intoxication: Demonstration of ito cells. *J. Clin. Pathol.* **1983**, *36*, 769–771.
104. Nollevaux, M.C.; Guiot, Y.; Horsmans, Y.; Leclercq, I.; Rahier, J.; Geubel, A.P.; Sempoux, C.; Hypervitaminosis A-induced liver fibrosis: Stellate cell activation and daily dose consumption. *Liver Int.* **2006**, *26*, 182–186.
105. Jirillo, E.; Jirillo, F.; Magrone, T. Healthy effects exerted by prebiotics, probiotics, and symbiotics with special reference to their impact on the immune system. *Int. J. Vitam. Nutr. Res.* **2012**, *82*, 200–208.
106. Soprano, D.R.; Soprano, K.J. Retinoids as teratogens. *Annu. Rev. Nutr.* **1995**, *15*, 111–132.
107. Collins, M.D.; Mao, G.E. Teratology of retinoids. *Annu. Rev. Pharmacol. Toxicol.* **1999**, *39*, 399–430.

108. Rothman, K.J.; Moore, L.L.; Singer, M.R.; Nguyen, U.D.T.; Mannino, S.; Milunsky, A. Teratogenicity of high vitamin A intake. *N. Engl. J. Med.* **1995**, *333*, 1369–1373.
109. Lobo, G.P.; Amengual, J.; Baus, D.; Shivdasani, R.A.; Taylor, D.; von Lintig, J. Genetics and diet regulate vitamin A production via the homeobox transcription factor ISX. *J. Biol. Chem.* **2013**, *288*, 9017–9027.
110. Rotenstreich, Y.; Harats, D.; Shaish, A.; Pras, E.; Belkin, M. Treatment of a retinal dystrophy, fundus albipunctatus, with oral 9-*cis*-β-carotene. *Br. J. Ophthalmol.* **2010**, *94*, 616–621.
111. Ajmal, M.; Khan, M.I.; Neveling, K.; Khan, Y.M.; Ali, S.H.; Ahmed, W.; Iqbal, M.S.; Azam, M.; den Hollander, A.I.; Collin, R.W.; *et al.* Novel mutations in RDH5 cause fundus albipunctatus in two consanguineous Pakistani families. *Mol. Vis.* **2012**, *18*, 1558–1571.
112. Maeda, T.; Perusek, L.; Amengual, J.; Babino, D.; Palczewski, K.; von Lintig, J. Dietary 9-*cis*-β,β-carotene fails to rescue vision in mouse models of leber congenital amaurosis. *Mol. Pharmacol.* **2011**, *80*, 943–952.

6

Diminishing Risk for Age-Related Macular Degeneration with Nutrition

Molly Schleicher [1], Karen Weikel [2], Caren Garber [1] and Allen Taylor [1,*]

[1] Laboratory for Nutrition and Vision Research, JM USDA Human Nutrition Research Center on Aging Tufts University, 711 Washington St, Boston, MA 02111, USA; E-Mails: molly.schleicher@tufts.edu (M.S.); caren.garber@tufts.edu (C.G.)

[2] Boston Medical Center, 650 Albany Street, Boston, MA 02118, USA; E-Mail: karen.weikel@bmc.org

* Author to whom correspondence should be addressed; E-Mail: allen.taylor@tufts.edu;

Abstract: Age-related macular degeneration (AMD) is the leading cause of blindness in the elderly. Clinical hallmarks of AMD are observed in one third of the elderly in industrialized countries. Preventative interventions through dietary modification are attractive strategies, because they are more affordable than clinical therapies, do not require specialists for administration and many studies suggest a benefit of micro- and macro-nutrients with respect to AMD with few, if any, adverse effects. The goal of this review is to provide information from recent literature on the value of various nutrients, particularly omega-3 fatty acids, lower glycemic index diets and, perhaps, some carotenoids, with regard to diminishing risk for onset or progression of AMD. Results from the upcoming Age-Related Eye Disease Study (AREDS) II intervention trial should be particularly informative.

Keywords: AMD; antioxidants; carotenoids; nutrition; glycemic index; aging

---

1. Introduction

Age-related macular degeneration (AMD) is the leading cause of blindness worldwide, affecting 30–50 million people. AMD affects over two million individuals of all ages and races in the United

States and 11% of those above the age of 80 [1]. Globally, costs associated with AMD are over $340 billion USD, and the majority of AMD patients are not eligible for clinical treatments [2–4]. Along with the burgeoning population of elderly, the prevalence of AMD is projected to grow over the next 20–30 years, with over five million individuals being affected by 2050 [5].

AMD is an eye disorder that gradually destroys the macula, the part of the retina with a high density of photoreceptors that is responsible for sharp, high-resolution vision. This part of the retina is able to receive light signals and quickly turn such signals into chemical and then electrical signals that are sent to the brain via the optic nerve. The brain then converts these electrical signals into the images we see. However, if the photoreceptors in the macula are damaged or prematurely shed, as in AMD, the central field of vision is distorted or lost [5].

Photoreceptors are exposed to extensive oxidative stress in the form of light and oxygen [6]. As a result, the outer 10% of photoreceptor segments are shed each night. These must be engulfed, degraded and the debris removed by the retinal pigment epithelium (RPE), which lies posterior to the photoreceptors [7]. Since one RPE cell services 30 photoreceptors, the RPE has among the highest degradative burdens in the body. In addition, the RPE is involved in maintaining the nutriture of the photoreceptors. Since photoreceptors do not have their own blood supply, it is crucial for nutrients from the choroidal blood supply to cross Bruch's membrane and enter the RPE and photoreceptors [6,8,9]. Adequate nutritional support to the RPE also facilitates efficient turnover of photoreceptors.

The combination of inadequate nutrition and the inability to properly degrade and dispose of cellular debris may contribute to the formation of deposits in the RPE-Bruch's membrane region. Basal laminar deposits accumulate between the RPE basement membrane and the RPE plasma membrane [10]. These are thought to precede the formation of drusen, which are established clinical indicators for early AMD [11–14]. Drusen are often found between the RPE and the choroid and contain a variety of lipids and proteins, including ubiquitin and advanced glycation end products, as well as inflammatory mediators [11].

There are two forms of AMD, commonly referred to as dry and wet. Approximately 90% of AMD patients in the US have dry AMD [5]. Dry AMD has three stages, early AMD, intermediate AMD and advanced AMD, which are characterized in part by the size and number of drusen [5]. Early AMD is indicated by small (<63 μm) and/or a few medium-sized (<125 μm) drusen. Intermediate AMD is indicated by many medium-sized or one or more large-sized drusen. Advanced dry AMD, also known as geographic atrophy, is diagnosed when there is focal, round depigmentation with sharp margins and, in some cases, visible choroidal vessels, as well [15]. In addition, there are often large and abundant drusen, as well as RPE and photoreceptor death in the macula. Consequently, patients with geographic atrophy experience significant vision loss.

Approximately 10% of AMD patients in the US have the more visually debilitating neovascular, or wet, form of AMD [5]. Neovascular AMD is manifested by formation of exudates and/or neovascularization of the retina. The latter is characterized by the development of aberrant blood vessels, originating from the choroid, that penetrate Bruch's membrane, causing damage to the RPE and overlying photoreceptors. These aberrant vessels are prone to leak, thus the designation "wet AMD". Such bleeding can cause the macula to swell and bulge, causing straight lines to appear curved [16].

Risk factors for AMD include age, gender, race, family history, genetics, weight and smoking. As individuals age, the risk for AMD increases [5]. Gender also appears to influence risk for AMD, with women having a slightly higher risk for AMD than men. Non-Hispanic blacks have less risk for non-exudative AMD at age 80 than Caucasians, and Asians have a higher rate of non-exudative AMD at age 60 than Caucasians [17]. Genetic analyses have shown that a primary relative who has AMD can increase one's own risk of the disease. Several single nucleotide polymorphisms have been associated with AMD risk in certain populations, with the most widely known polymorphism found on the Complement Factor H gene [18–22]. Obesity is another significant, yet modifiable risk factor, and it has been shown that a 3% reduction in the waist-to-hip ratio decreases risk for AMD by 20% [23]. The most consistently reported risk factor for AMD is smoking, as it increases the risk for AMD up to seven-fold [3].

Currently, there are no therapies to treat dry AMD [24]. There are available treatments for some neovascular AMD patients. However, they are used only after the patients have lost some vision. Clearly, there is a critical need for preventative measures against AMD.

2. Reader's Guide

There have been dozens of studies during the past 40 years. The following sections summarize data that relate relationships between particular nutrients and risk for AMD. Readers are referred to an exhaustive review by Weikel *et al.* [25] for a complete summary in text of the data collected up to 2011 regarding risk for onset or progress of AMD and intake, blood levels or supplement use of specific nutrients.

For clarity, this review will only use the term AMD, as AMD and age-related maculopathy (ARM) are used interchangeably. Furthermore, those studies that used the term "exudative AMD" will be described here as "neovascular", since both terms refer to the same condition. Those studies which used the term "severe AMD" will be described here as "late AMD", as per the majority of studies. Often, this refers to geographic atrophy or exudative, wet AMD.

Data in the figures is organized by type of exposure (intake, plasma level, *etc.*) and outcome measure (early AMD, late AMD, *etc.*). We further divide our discussion by study design, because there are different limitations inherent in each type of study. For each of the nutrients, the figures present risk for "any" type of AMD, early AMD indicators, early AMD, late AMD, followed by geographic atrophy and neovascular AMD, if these specific types of late AMD were analyzed. Data regarding "risk" are separated from data regarding "risk for progression". Information about the latter is crucial, because it addresses the opportunity to delay early AMD from progressing to vision-compromising disease. In order to present a comprehensive view, results of studies that found beneficial associations of a particular nutrient are reported in the figures with studies that found null associations and studies that found harmful associations of that same nutrient on the same outcome. Data from studies that do not indicate odds or hazard ratios are referenced in the text, but not indicated in the figures.

3. Dietary Carbohydrate

Most of the research investigating the role of carbohydrates in AMD risk relates to glycemic index. Glycemic index is the measure of the ability of 50 g of a certain food to raise blood glucose levels, relative to the ability of 50 g of a standard food (e.g., glucose) to raise blood glucose levels [26]. High glycemic foods result in higher levels of glucose in the blood within two hours of consumption. All epidemiologic data published to date indicates that consuming higher glycemic index foods is associated with a greater risk for AMD or AMD progression [27,28].

Cross-sectional analysis of baseline Age-Related Eye Disease Study (AREDS) data found that compared to those with dietary glycemic indexes in the first quintile, those with intakes in the fourth (OR (odds ratio) = 1.31; 95% CI (confidence interval): 1.02, 1.66) or fifth quintile (OR = 1.42; 95% CI: 1.09, 1.84) were at an increased risk for the appearance of large drusen [29] (Figure 1). There was also a trend for increasing glycemic index with increasing risk for large drusen (p = 0.001) [29]. Increasing dietary glycemic index increased risk for neovascular AMD (p = 0.005), and there was a statistically significant trend of increasing dietary glycemic index with advancement of AMD stage (p < 0.001) [29]. These observations corroborated findings from a cross-sectional analysis of the Nutrition and Vision Project (NVP), which found that after multivariate adjustment, those who had dietary glycemic indices in the highest tertile had an increased risk for AMD compared to the lowest tertile (OR = 2.71; 95% CI:1.24,5.93; p = 0.01, for trend) (Figure 1). Glycemic index did not affect risk for drusen in this population [30] (Figure 1).

Figure 1. Odds or risk ratio for early age-related macular degeneration (AMD) indicators (DRUSEN), late AMD indicators (LG DRUSEN) or AMD with intake of a high glycemic index diet: cross-sectional studies.

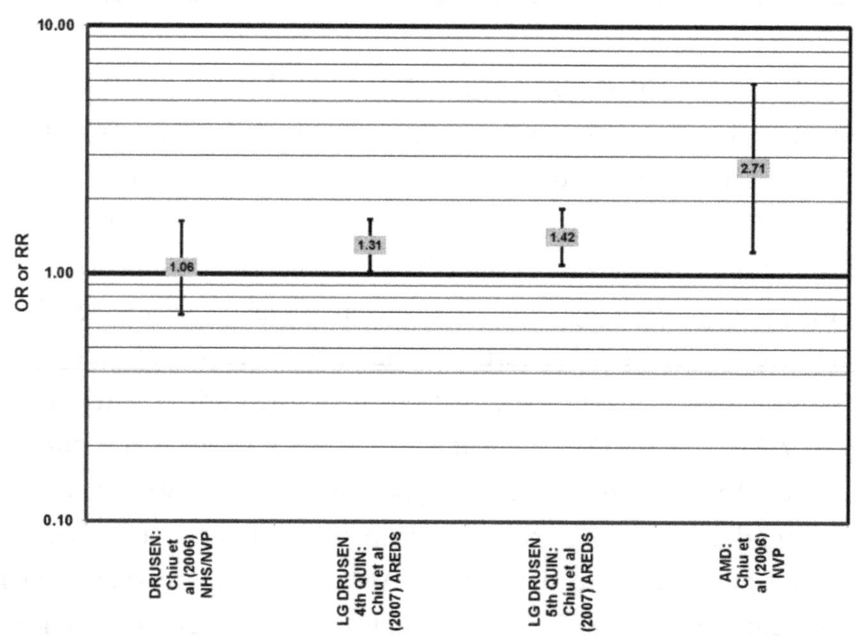

Prospective studies also indicate that higher glycemic index foods increase risk for AMD. In AREDS, risk of progression of AMD over an eight-year period was higher in those with a higher glycemic index diet (RR (relative risk)= 1.10; 95% CI: 1.00, 1.20; p = 0.047) [31] (Figure 2). Those at later stages of the disease had a greater risk of progression on the higher glycemic index diet (p < 0.001), and compared to those with the lowest quintile of dietary glycemic index, those in the highest quintile of dietary glycemic index had a 39% higher risk of progressing to advanced AMD (95% CI: 1.08, 1.79) [31] (Figure 2). The authors calculated that 20% of the prevalent AMD cases would have been eliminated if participants consumed a diet with a glycemic index below the median and predicted that by changing the dietary glycemic index only slightly, approximately 100,000 cases of AMD would be avoided in five years [29]. Additional analyses including data regarding intake of eicosapentaenoic acid (EPA) and docosahexaenoic acid (DHA) from 2924 AREDS participants revealed that consumption of high glycemic index diets increased the progression to advanced AMD by 32% (95% CI: 1.16, 1.52), and those who consumed a low glycemic index diet along with a high consumption of DHA were at even lower risk for progression to advanced AMD ($p < 0.001$) [32] (Figure 2).

Figure 2. Odds or risk ratio for early AMD indicators (PIG AB), late AMD indicators (SOFT DRUSEN), early AMD, or progression to late AMD, with intake of a high glycemic index diet: prospective studies.

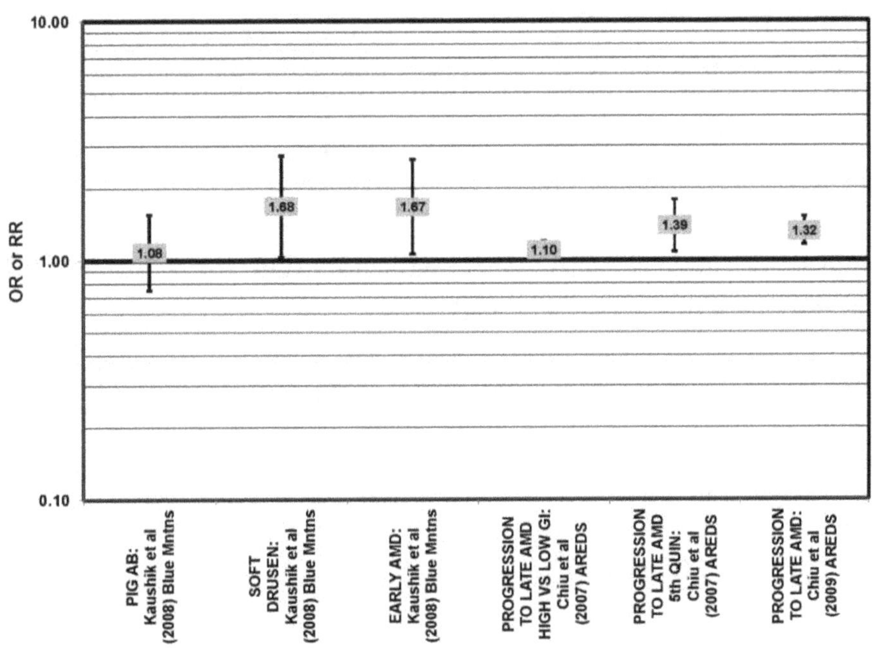

The Blue Mountains Eye Study corroborated the data from the Nurses' Health Study (NHS) and AREDS, showing that among 3654 participants 10 years after baseline, those with a dietary glycemic index in the highest quartile were at an increased risk for early AMD compared to those in the lowest quartile, after adjusting for age, sex, BMI (body mass index) smoking, blood pressure, history of cardiovascular disease and vegetable, fruit and fat intake (RR = 1.67; 95% CI: 1.06, 2.64; $p = 0.04$, for trend) (Figure 2). A significant trend of decreasing risk for early AMD with increased consumption of cereal fiber ($p = 0.05$) and breads and grains ($p = 0.03$) was found (Figure 3). Those consuming the highest amounts of cereal fiber, breads and grains had a reduced risk of soft drusen (RR = 0.61; 95% CI: 0.39, 0.96; $p = 0.01$, for trend) and pigment abnormalities (RR = 0.61; 95% CI: 0.43, 0.85; $p = 0.04$, for trend) (Figure 3). Comparison of the highest to lowest quartile of glycemic index also showed an increased risk for soft drusen over 10 years (RR = 1.68; 95% CI: 1.03, 2.74; $p = 0.04$, for trend) (Figure 2). In general, measures of the amount of carbohydrate were not associated with risk for early or late AMD [33] (Figure 4).

Figure 3. Odds ratio for early AMD indicators (PIG AB), late AMD indicators (SOFT DRUSEN), or early AMD; high *vs.* low intake of low glycemic index foods: prospective study.

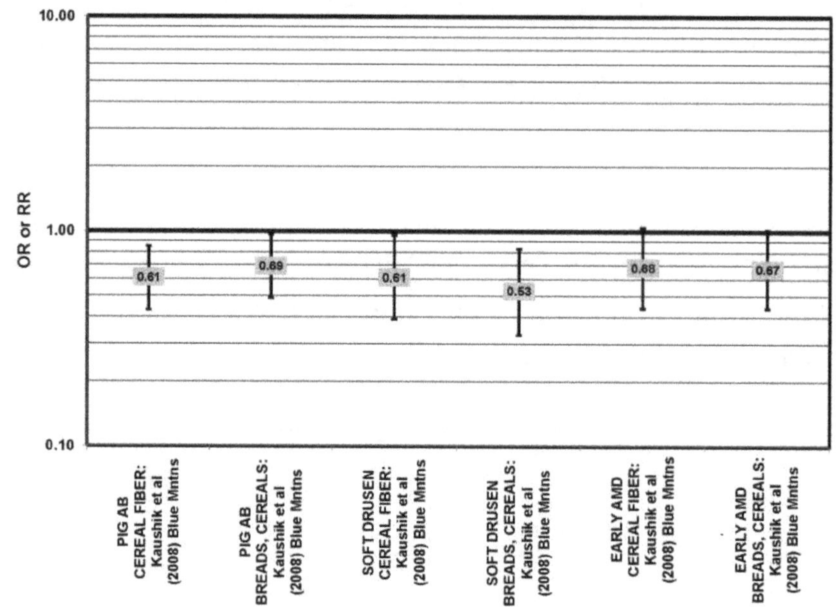

Figure 4. Odds or risk ratio for early AMD indicators (DRUSEN) or AMD; high *vs.* low intake of total carbohydrates: cross-sectional studies.

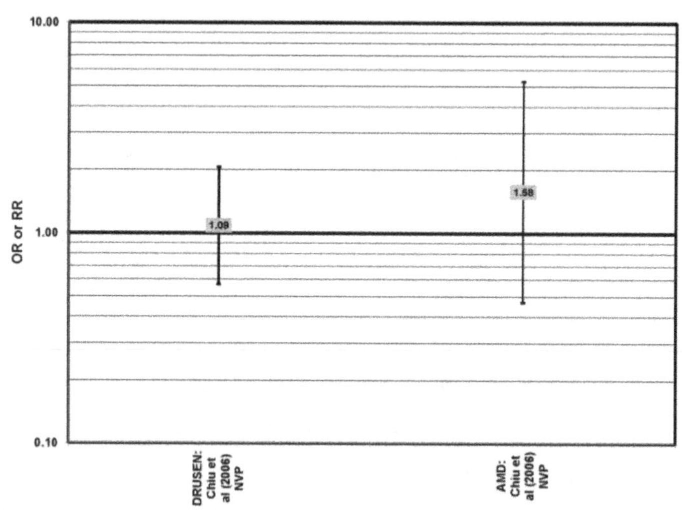

Three cohorts have examined the role of carbohydrates in AMD risk. Albeit a limited number of cohorts, they were large cohorts, and the evidence indicates that consumption of carbohydrates of a low glycemic index appears to lower risk for AMD and AMD progression. In comparison, total carbohydrate intake does not appear to be related to risk for or progression of AMD. Controlled laboratory studies have corroborated the data and propose the pathophysiologic mechanisms of the relationship between glycemic index and AMD [34,35]. These data indicate that glycoxidative stress results in accumulation of elevated levels of intracellular glycated proteins and compromised protein editing capacities. This leads to a viscous cycle of glycative damage, diminished proteolytic capacity, accumulation of glycated proteins, cytotoxicity and tissue dysfunction [25].

The above findings are consistent with data supporting consumption of lower glycemic index diets to decrease risk for obesity, a risk factor for AMD [36]. Several intervention studies have found that energy-restricted diets based on low glycemic index foods contribute to greater weight loss than calorically equivalent diets based on high glycemic index foods [37]. Taken together, these observational data encourage use of low glycemic index diets to lower the risk for AMD and AMD progression.

4. Dietary Fats and Fish

4.1. Omega-3 and Omega-6 Fatty Acids

Increased intake of omega-3 fatty acids, especially long-chain omega-3 fatty acids, such as DHA and EPA, found in fish, has been associated with amelioration of a number of chronic diseases, including AMD [38,39].

The Eye Disease Case Control Study (EDCC), which consisted of 349 cases and 504 controls, found that, in subjects with a low linoleic acid (omega-6 fatty acid) intake, there was a trend of retinal protection in those with higher intake of omega-3 fatty acids ($p = 0.05$). Without adjusting for omega-6 intake, this trend became non-significant ($p = 0.29$). This trend suggests that omega-6 and omega-3 fatty acids may be in a state of metabolic competition. However, while biochemical studies continue to suggest competition, further epidemiologic analysis did not support such competition. When comparing those with the highest and lowest EPA and DHA consumption, EPA and DHA did not confer significant protection from neovascular AMD before adjusting for linoleic acid intake (OR = 0.75; 95% CI: 0.44, 1.25) or in those with low (OR = 0.61; 95% CI: 0.26, 1.42) or high linoleic acid intake (OR = 0.78; 95% CI: 0.39, 1.56) [40] (Figure 5).

Figure 5. Neovascular AMD odds or risk ratio, high *vs.* low intake of omega-3 fatty acids: retrospective and cross-sectional studies.

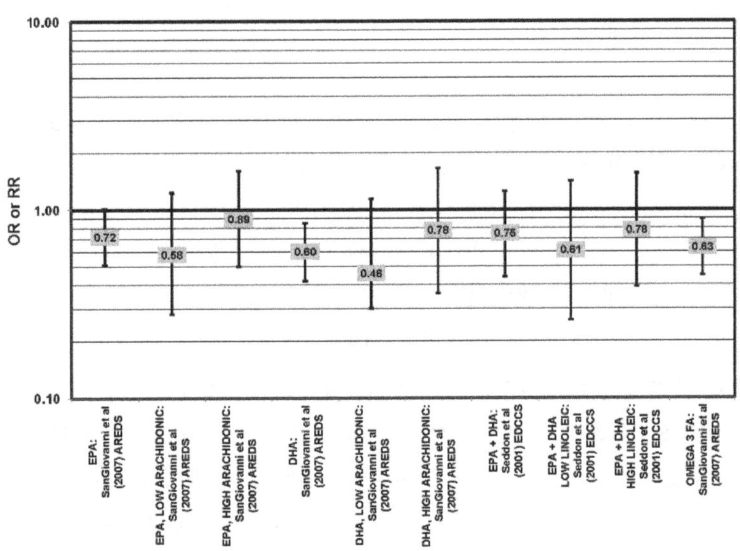

Strong evidence for a beneficial role of omega-3 fatty acids in eye health is found in two cross-sectional studies, the US Twin Study of Age-Related Macular Degeneration ("US Twin") and AREDS. The US Twin study found that compared to those consuming the least amount of omega-3

fatty acids, those consuming the highest amount had a reduced risk for any stage of AMD (OR = 0.55; 95% CI: 0.32, 0.95). This association was driven mostly by those with a low linoleic and omega-6 fatty acid intake ($p < 0.001$), as the association disappeared in those with an intake of linoleic acid above the median [41] (Figure 6). Analysis of the baseline data from 4519 participants in AREDS revealed that compared to those in the lowest quintile of intake, those in the highest quintile of intake for EPA (OR = 0.72; 95% CI: 0.51, 1.01; $p < 0.05$), DHA (OR = 0.60; 95% CI: 0.42, 0.85) and total long-chain omega-3 fatty acids (OR = 0.63; 95% CI: 0.45, 0.89) were at a reduced risk for neovascular AMD [42] (Figure 5). However, sub-group analysis of the population found that the reduction of risk associated with high consumption of EPA and DHA became non-significant when the cohort was separated by intake of arachidonic acid, another omega-6 fatty acid [42] (Figure 5).

Figure 6. Odds or risk ratio for early AMD indicators (DRUSEN), early AMD or LATE AMD and OR AMD; high *vs.* low intake of omega-3 fatty acids: retrospective and cross-sectional studies.

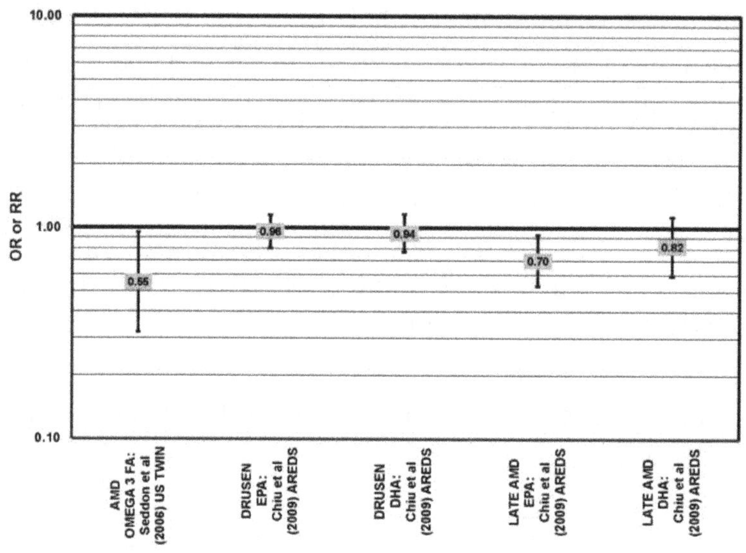

Data from prospective studies support a beneficial role of omega-3 fatty acids. Analysis of 1837 participants of AREDS found that increasing intake of DHA + EPA was associated with a decreased rate of progression to central geographic atrophy over 12 years ($p = 0.026$), and progression to central geographic atrophy was lowest in subjects with intakes in the highest quintiles of intake of DHA (OR = 0.68; 95% CI: 0.47, 0.99), EPA (OR = 0.70; 95% CI: 0.49, 1.00) and DHA + EPA (OR = 0.66; 95% CI: 0.46, 0.94) (Figure 7). Increasing intakes of DHA alone ($p = 0.001$) or DHA + EPA ($p = 0.032$) were also associated with a decrease in risk of progression to neovascular AMD ($p = 0.001$). Analysis of 2,924 AREDS participants revealed that those consuming more than 64 mg/day of DHA, compared to less than 26 mg/day, had a reduced risk for progression to advanced AMD (HR (hazard ratio) = 0.73; 95% CI: 0.57, 0.94) (Figure 7). Those consuming at least 42.3 mg EPA per day, compared to less than 12.7 mg/day, were at a reduced risk for progression to advanced AMD (HR = 0.74; 95% CI: 0.57, 0.94) (Figure 7). Participants who were healthy at baseline benefitted from a high DHA diet, as indicated by reduced progression of early AMD (HR = 0.58; 95% CI: 0.37, 0.92) [32] (Figure 8). Prospective analysis of 38,022 women from the Women's Health Study observed that women in the highest tertile of DHA intake, compared to those with the lowest DHA intake, had a 38% reduced risk for AMD (RR = 0.62, 95% CI: 0.45, 0.85) (p = 0.003 for trend). Similar relationships were found for higher intake of EPA (RR = 0.64, 95% CI: 0.46, 0.88) (p for trend = 0.004), and for DHA + EPA (RR, 0.62, 95% CI: 0.45–0.86) (p for trend = 0.03) [43]. A study of over 72,000 participants from the NHS and Health Professionals' Follow-Up Study (HPFUS) indicated that those with the highest intakes of DHA were at a reduced risk for AMD (RR = 0.70; 95% CI: 0.52, 0.93) [44] (Figure 9). Analysis of 6339 participants from the Melbourne Collaborative Cohort ("Melbourne") indicated that those consuming the highest amounts of omega-3 fatty acids were at a slightly reduced risk for early AMD (OR = 0.85; 95% CI: 0.71, 1.02; p = 0.03, for trend) (Figure 8), but there was no association between particular fatty acids, such as EPA, DHA and alpha-linolenic acid, and early or late AMD [45]. Benefits of omega-3 fatty acids in general were seen in 2454 participants of the Blue Mountains Eye Study. Compared to those with the lowest intakes of omega-3 fatty acids, those with the highest intakes were at reduced risk for incidence of early AMD (RR = 0.63; 95% CI: 0.42, 0.95) [46] (Figure 8) and such findings were corroborated in follow-up analysis (OR = 0.41; 95% CI: 0.22, 0.75) [47] (Figure 8). Finally, data from a European prospective cohort, EUREYE (The European Eye Study), indicated that among 2275 participants, those with consumption levels of DHA (OR = 0.32; 95% CI: 0.12, 0.87) and EPA (OR = 0.29, 95% CI: 0.11, 0.73) in the highest quartile had a reduced risk for neovascular AMD [48] (Figure 10).

Figure 7. Odds or risk ratio for progression to late AMD, geographic atrophy (GA) or neovascular AMD (NEO); high *vs.* low intake of omega-3 fatty acids: prospective studies.

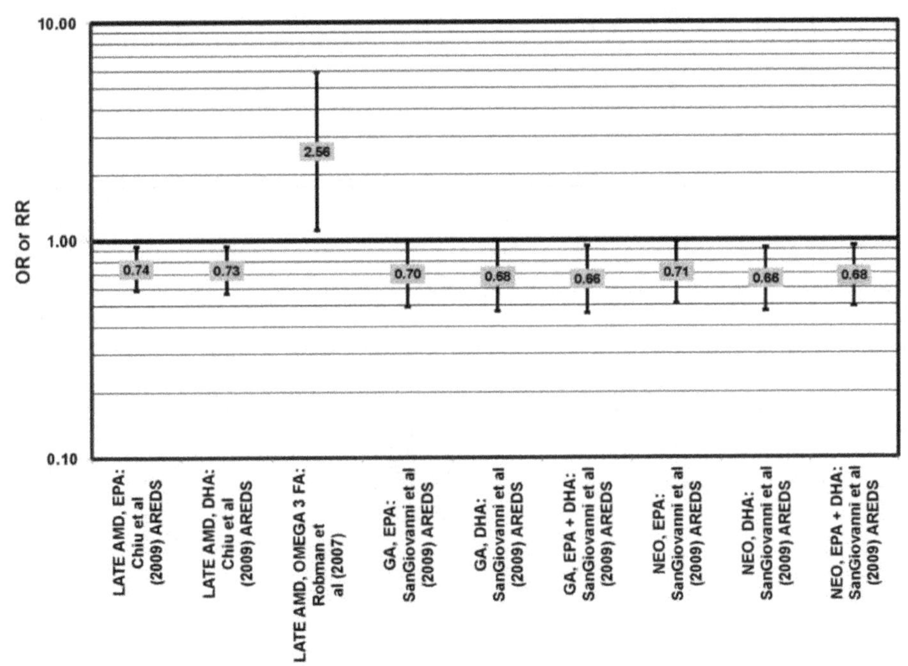

Figure 8. Odds or risk ratio for early AMD or progression to early AMD; high *vs.* low intake of omega-3 fatty acids: prospective studies.

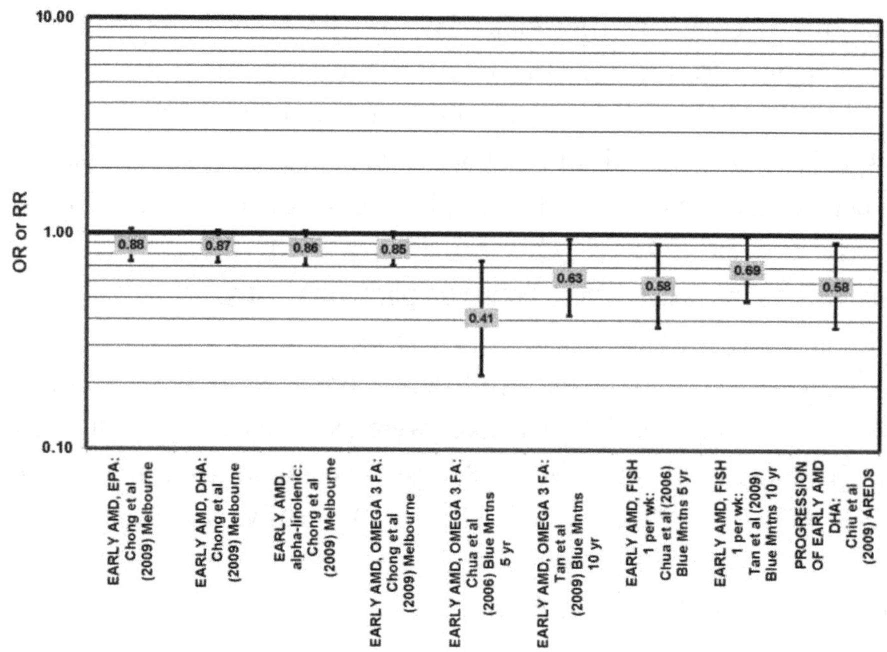

Figure 9. Odds or risk ratio for AMD or intermediate AMD; high *vs.* low intake of omega-3 fatty acids: prospective studies.

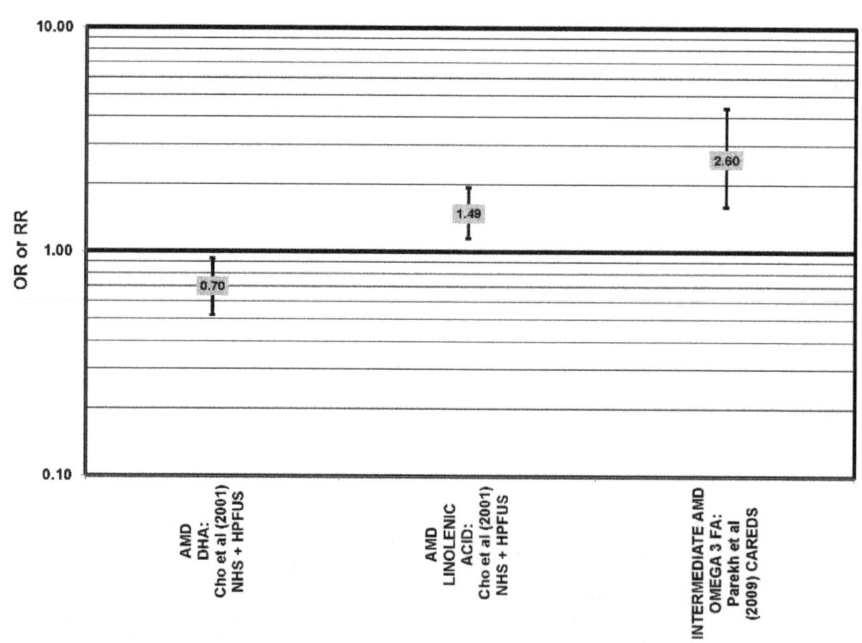

Figure 10. Odds or risk ratio for late, neo AMD; high *vs.* low intake of omega-3 fatty acids: prospective studies.

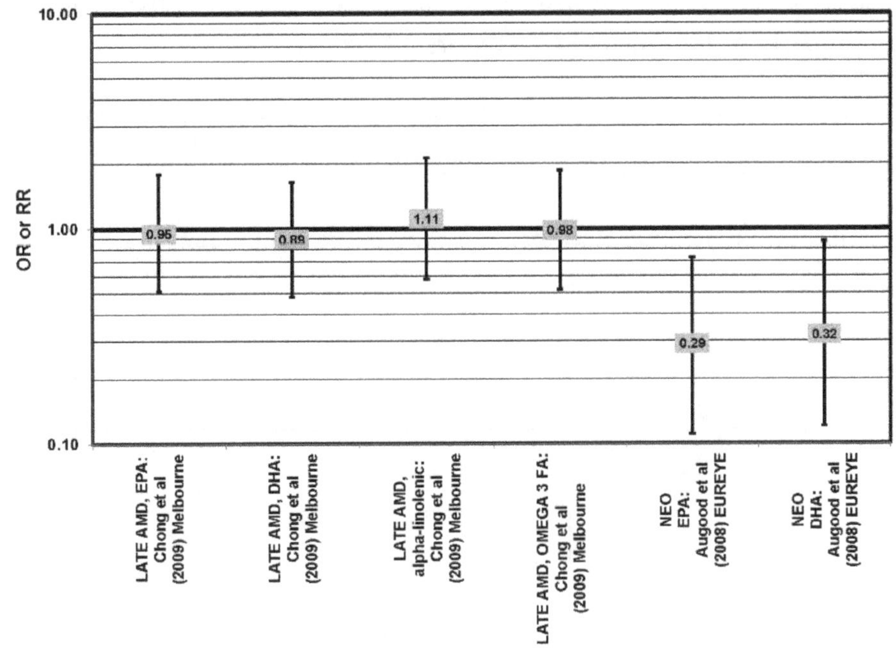

In one intervention trial, supplementation of 12 women with 800 mg DHA per day for four months significantly increased macular pigment optical density (MPOD), a surrogate marker for retina health, after two and four months of supplementation ($p < 0.001$). Surprisingly, women who also received 12 mg/day of lutein with the DHA did not experience as great an increase in MPOD at two months, but had similar density at four months [49]. The optimism that is engendered by the robust epidemiologic record is qualified somewhat by results from the Nutritional AMD Treatment 2 Study [50]. Patients were given either 840 mg/day DHA and 270 mg/day EPA or placebo for three years. For patients that showed the highest levels of EPA + DHA in red blood cell membranes, there was a 68% lower risk for chorodial neovascularization (CNV), but not for other indicators of AMD status. For the full cohort of patients, supplementation with DHA and EPA was without effect relative to placebo.

The possible connection between omega-6/omega-3 fatty acid ratio and development and progression of AMD has been investigated. Mance *et al.* divided 125 AMD patients into five groups according to the Clinical Age-Related Maculopathy Staging System and measured intake of dietary fatty acids using the validated food frequency questionnaire. A statistically significant difference was found between the omega-6/omega-3 ratio in neovascular AMD compared to all other groups, with the ratio of 11:1 found in the stage 5 group. Additionally, the stage 4 group had a statistically significant difference in the ratio compared to stages 1, 2 and 3, with the ratio in the first three groups at about 7–7.5:1 [51]. Christen *et al.* also found that the ratio of omega-6/omega-3 fatty acids was directly associated with risk for AMD in a group of 38,022 women enrolled in the Women's Health Study [43].

Despite these studies showing a beneficial role of omega-3 fatty acids in eye health, cross-sectional analysis of 4003 AREDS participants showed no association between DHA intake (OR = 0.94; 95% CI: 0.77, 1.16), EPA intake (OR = 0.96; 95% CI: 0.84, 1.15) and late AMD (OR = 0.82; 95% CI: 0.59, 1.13). There was also no association between intake of either DHA or EPA and risk for drusen (OR = 0.94; 95% CI: 0.77, 1.16) (OR = 0.96; 95% CI: 0.84, 1.15). Although those in the third quartile of EPA intake had 30% less risk for late AMD compared to those with the lowest intakes (95% CI: 0.53, 0.93), this association was lost at higher levels of EPA intake [52]. In the Melbourne cohort, there was also no association between intake of EPA, DHA or alpha-linolenic acid (another omega-3 fatty acid) and risk for early or late AMD [45] (Figures 8 and 9).

Figure 11. Odds or risk ratio for early AMD, late AMD or neovascular AMD (NEO); high *vs.* low intake of omega-6 fatty acids: retrospective and cross-sectional studies.

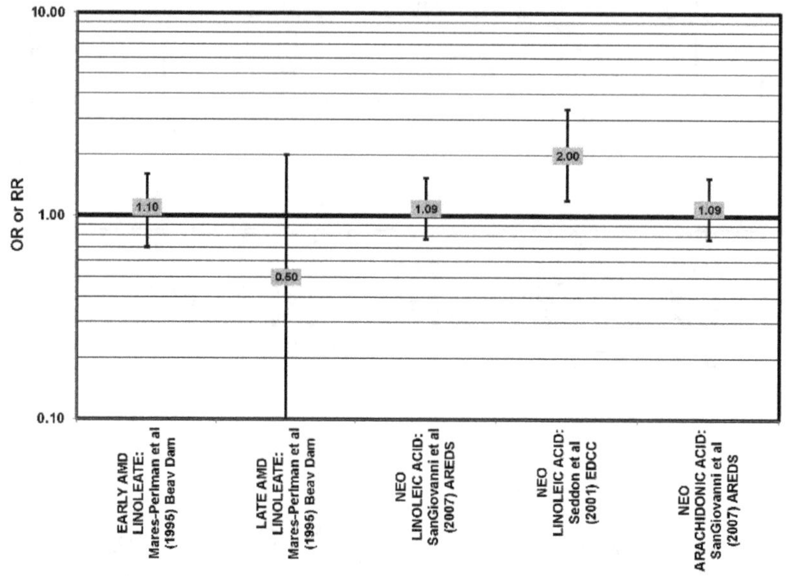

Figure 12. Odds or risk ratio for intermediate AMD, neovascular AMD (NEO) or AMD progression; high *vs.* low intake of omega-6 fatty acids: prospective studies.

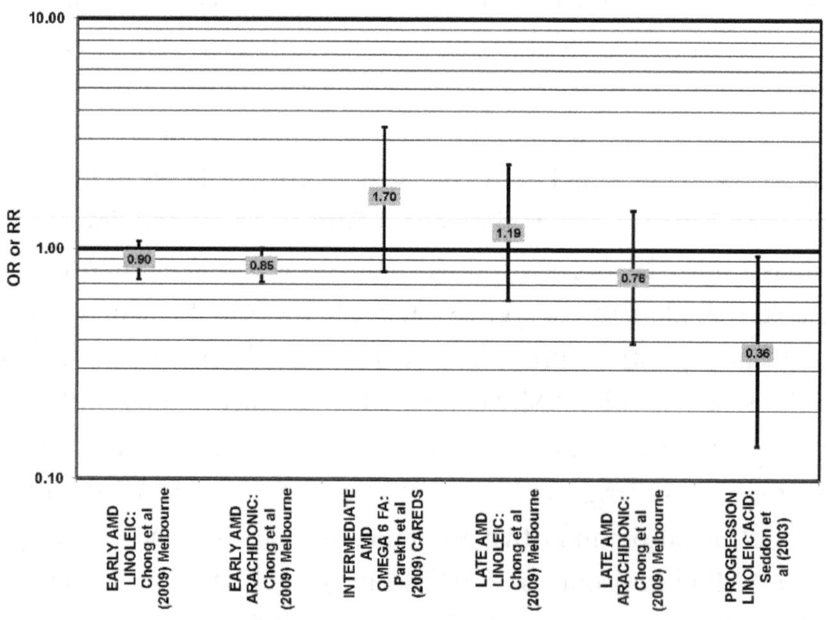

With the exception of the EDCC and NHS + HPFUS, most retrospective, cross-sectional and prospective studies found no relationship between omega-6 fatty acid intake (independent of omega-3 fatty acids) and AMD (Figures 11 and 12) [42,45,53–55]. The EDCC did indicate that high intakes of linoleic acid appeared to increase risk for neovascular AMD (OR = 2.00; 95% CI: 1.19, 3.37) [40]

(Figure 11). Additionally, the NHS + HPFUS also found that those with the highest intakes of linolenic acid had increased risk for any stage AMD [44]. The Carotenoids in Age Related Eye Disease Study (CAREDS) found that those consuming the highest amounts of omega-3 fatty acids were at higher risk for intermediate AMD [54]. An additional study found that over seven years, early AMD patients with intakes of omega-3 fatty acids in the highest quartile were at increased risk for AMD. However, this association was lost with a more rigid definition of AMD [55] (Figures 9 and 10).

4.2. Fish Intake

The effect of fish on risk for AMD is of great interest, as fish is a common dietary source of omega-3 fatty acids [56]. Cross-sectional analyses of AREDS participants indicated that consumption of at least two servings of fish per week was associated with decreased risk for neovascular AMD compared to zero servings per week (OR = 0.61; 95% CI: 0.37, 1.00; $p = 0.01$ for trend). Consumption of more than one serving of baked or broiled fish was associated with a decreased risk of neovascular AMD (OR = 0.65; 95% CI: 0.45, 0.93; $p = 0.02$, for trend) [42] (Figure 13).

Figure 13. Relationship between early indicators of AMD (DRUSEN, PIG AB), early, late or neovascular (NEO) AMD and fish intake: retrospective and cross-sectional studies.

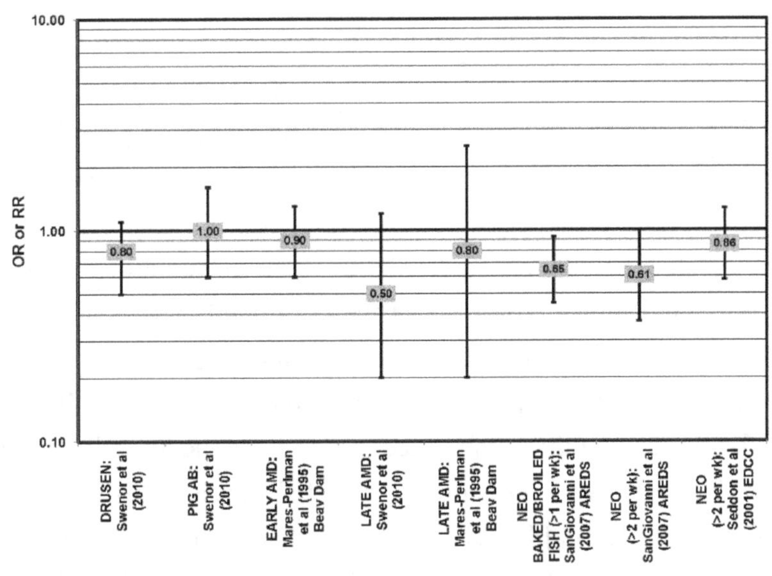

Two prospective studies analyzing the effect of fish intake on risk for AMD corroborated the observation of competition between omega-3 and omega-6 fatty acids in modulating eye health that was observed in the EDCC analysis [40]. Data from the Blue Mountains Eye Study showed that among 2454 participants with low linoleic acid (omega-6) consumption, one serving of fish/week was associated with a reduced risk of incident early AMD (OR = 0.69; 95% CI: 0.49, 0.98) ten years after baseline [46] (Figure 14). Another study reported that among those consuming at least two servings of fish/week, those consuming below the median amount of linoleic acid were at a slightly reduced risk for progression to advanced AMD compared to those consuming above the median (RR = 0.36; 95% CI: 0.14, 0.95; $p = 0.045$, for trend) (Figure 14). The beneficial associations of fish intake were not observed in those with higher intakes of linoleic acid, nor were they observed before adjusting for linoleic acid intake [57] (Figure 14). Although these observations contradict those in the quintile intake analysis of the EDCC, the prospective design of these studies increases the likelihood of a competition between omega-3 fatty acids and linoleic acid [40,46,57]. Additionally, analysis of the Women's Health Study observed that consumption of one or more servings of fish/week was associated with a 42% lower risk of AMD compared to consumption of less than one serving of fish per month [43].

Figure 14. Relationship between early indicators of AMD (DRUSEN, PIG AB), early, late or neovascular (NEO) AMD and fish intake: prospective studies.

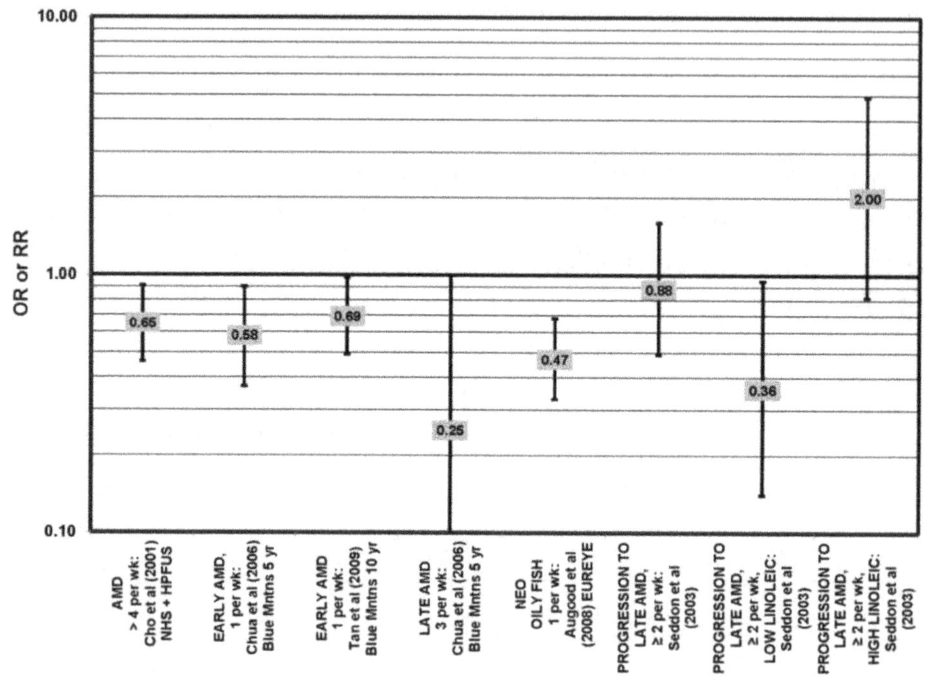

Additional prospective studies support the role of fish in reducing AMD risk, even without adjusting for omega-6 fatty acid intake. Analysis of the combined NHS + HPFUS indicated that those who consumed more than four servings of fish/wk had a reduced risk for any stage of AMD relative to those consuming less than four servings per week (RR = 0.65; 95% CI: 0.46, 0.91) [44] (Figure 14). Another study reported that consuming fish once a week reduced risk for early AMD by 42% (OR = 0.58; 95% CI: 0.37, 0.90), while consumption of fish three times a week reduced risk for late AMD by 75% (95% CI: 0.06, 1.00) [47] (Figure 14). Data from EUREYE indicated that weekly consumption of oily fish was associated with a reduced risk of neovascular AMD (OR = 0.47; 95% CI: 0.33, 0.68) [48] (Figure 12).

The EDCC, retrospective analysis of the Beaver Dam Eye Study and cross-sectional data from the Blue Mountains Eye Study did not find an association between fish intake and early or late AMD [40,53,58,59] (Figure 13).

4.3. Polyunsaturated Fat and Nut Intake

Nuts are a popular source of polyunsaturated fatty acids. In the prospective Blue Mountains Eye Study, it was found that one to two servings of nuts/week was associated with a decreased risk of early AMD (OR = 0.65; 95% CI: 0.47, 0.91) among nonsmokers with low HDL and high intake of beta-carotene [46,56] (Figure 15). All other studies, such as the EDCC, Melbourne Collaborative

Cohort, POLANUT (dietary survey study of the Pathologies Oculaires Liées à l'Age study) and cross-sectional analysis of the Blue Mountains Eye Study, did not find a significant association between these types of fatty acids and AMD risk [40,45,55,58] (Figure 16).

Figure 15. Odds or risk ratio for early AMD, intermediate AMD, progression to late AMD, and neovascular AMD (NEO); high *vs.* low intake of fat-containing foods: retrospective and prospective studies.

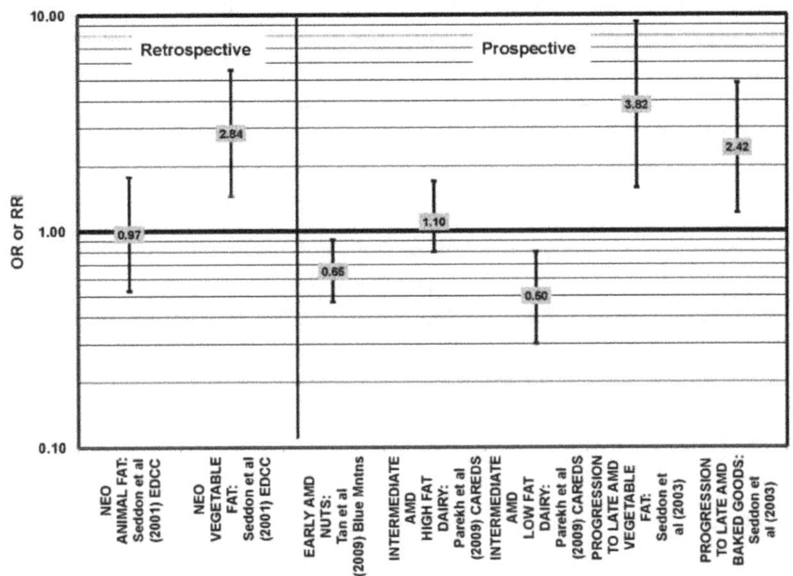

Figure 16. AMD odds or risk ratio; high *vs.* low intake of polyunsaturated fatty acids: retrospective and cross-sectional studies, prospective.

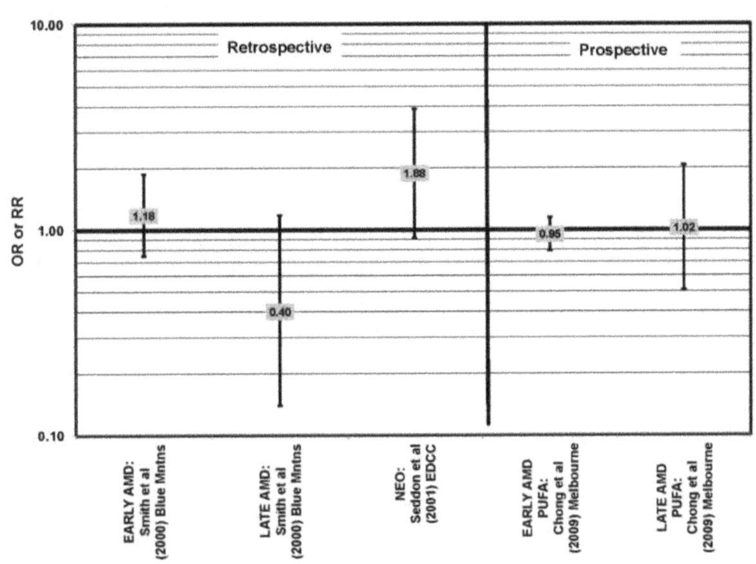

4.4. Monounsaturated Fatty Acids

Many studies, including the EDCC, Beaver Dam Eye Study, CAREDS, Melbourne Collaborative Cohort and the POLANUT study, did not find a significant association between consumption of monounsaturated fatty acids, such as oleic acid, and any stage of AMD risk [40,45,53–55,60]

(Figures 17 and 18). Cross-sectional analysis of 3654 subjects from the Blue Mountains Eye Study, and cross-sectional analysis of AREDS found a slightly harmful trend of increasing consumption of monounsaturated fatty acids and increasing risk for early and neovascular AMD (p = 0.05) and (OR = 1.80; 95% CI: 1.27, 2.56), respectively. Oleic acid, a commonly consumed monounsaturated fatty acid, was not significantly associated with disease risk in AREDS [42,53,58] (Figure 17).

Figure 17. Odds or risk ratio for early AMD, intermediate AMD, late AMD or neovascular AMD (NEO); high *vs.* low intake of monounsaturated fatty acids: retrospective, cross-sectional studies.

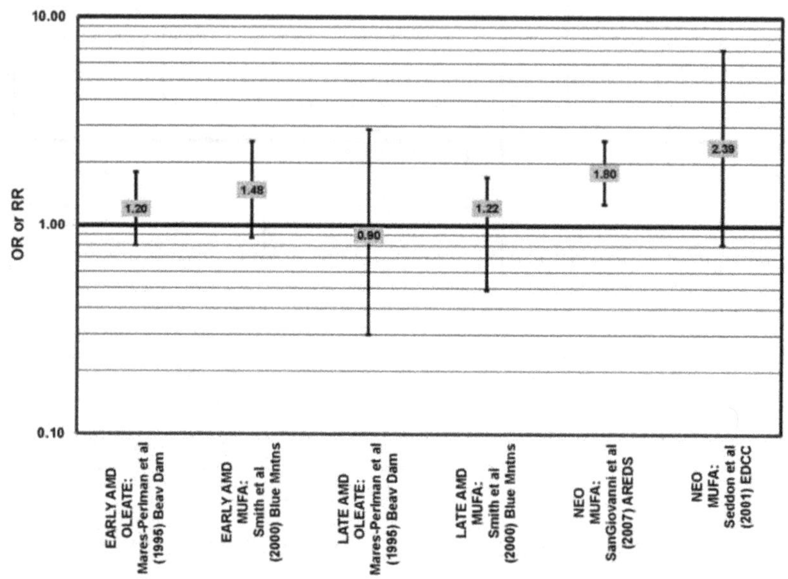

Figure 18. Odds or risk ratio for early AMD, intermediate AMD or late AMD; high *vs.* low intake of monounsaturated fatty acids: prospective studies.

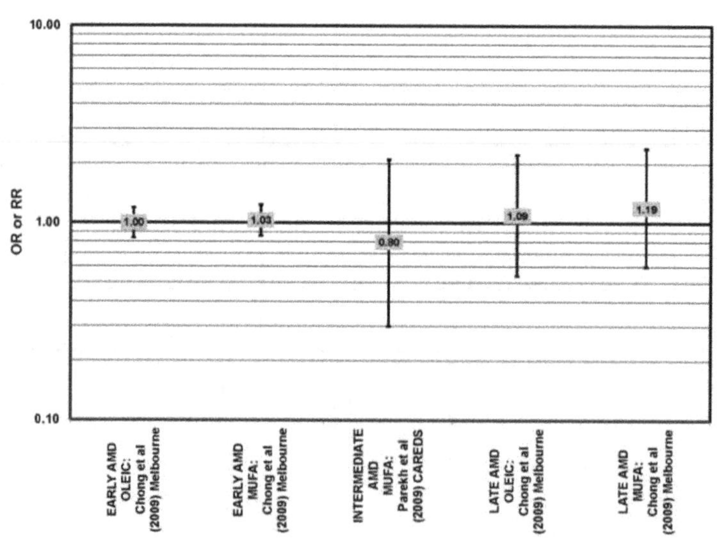

4.5. Saturated Fat

No studies have reported retinal benefits through consumption of saturated fatty acids The EDCC, CAREDS, Blue Mountain Eye Study, Melbourne cohort, POLANUT and Cardiovascular Health and

Age Related Maculopathy study did not find an association between saturated fat intake and risk for AMD [40,45,54,55,58,60] (Figures 15 and 19). However, analysis of the Beaver Dam Eye study and AREDS showed an association between high saturated fat intake and increased risk for AMD [42,53] (Figure 19).

Figure 19. Odds or risk ratio for early AMD, intermediate AMD, late AMD or neovascular AMD (NEO); high *vs.* low intake of saturated fat: retrospective, cross-sectional and prospective studies.

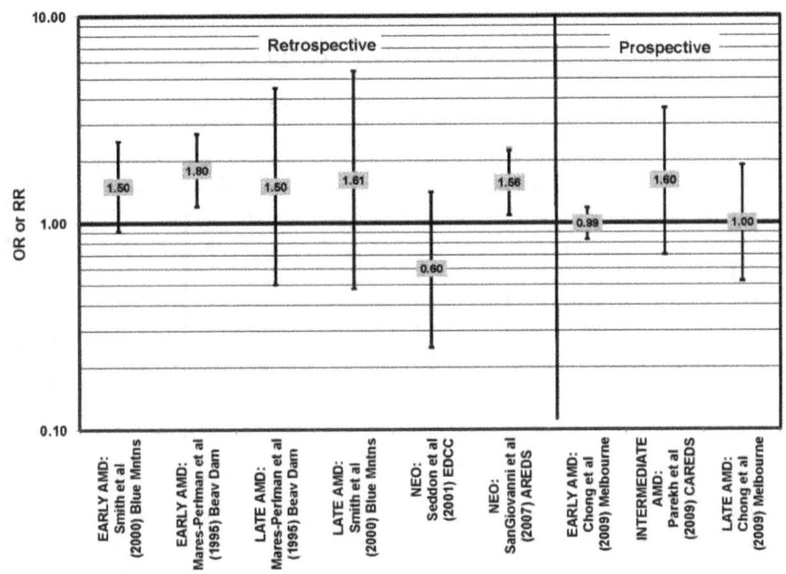

4.6. Trans Fatty Acids

The EDCC and Melbourne Collaborate Cohort analyzed the role of trans-fatty acid intake in AMD risk. Both did not find a significant relationship with early, late or neovascular AMD risk, nor with AMD progression [45,55] (Figure 20).

Figure 20. Odds or risk ratio for late AMD or neovascular AMD (NEO); high *vs.* low intake trans-fatty acids: retrospective and prospective studies.

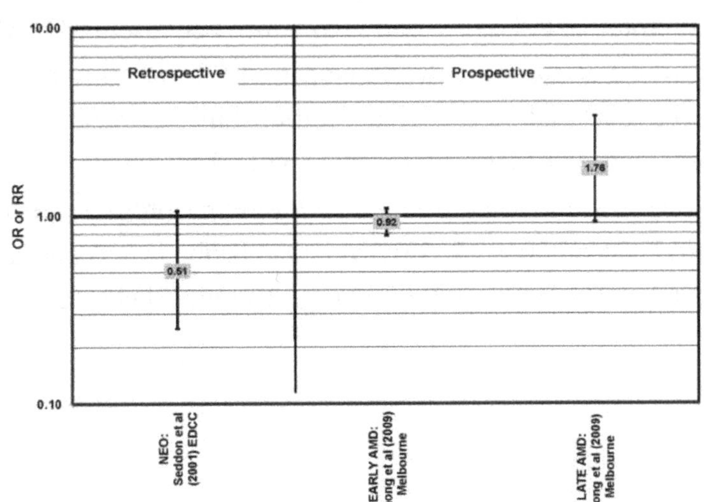

4.7. Cholesterol

Excessive cholesterol intake is related to poor cardiovascular health and elevated cholesterol levels. Similarly, no studies have found retinal benefits through high cholesterol intake. Cholesterol intake was not found to be associated with neovascular AMD risk in cross-sectional analysis of AREDS, with early AMD in the Blue Mountains Eye Study or with early or late AMD in the Melbourne cohort [40,42,45,58]. The Beaver Dam Eye and Blue Mountains Eye studies found an association of high cholesterol intake with increased risk for early AMD [53,58] (Figure 21).

Figure 21. Odds or risk ratio for early AMD, late AMD or neovascular AMD (NEO); high *vs.* low intake of dietary cholesterol: retrospective and cross-sectional studies.

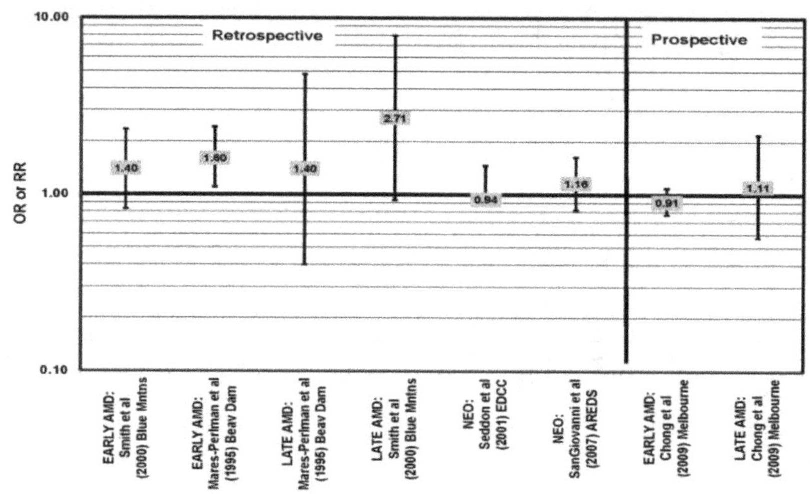

4.8. Total Fat

Only CAREDS has found a potential beneficial role of total fat intake. Women in CAREDS over the age of 75 with a high fat intake appeared to be protected from intermediate AMD (OR = 0.50; 95% CI: 0.30, 1.00) [54] (Figure 22). Retrospective analysis of the Beaver Dam Eye study and EDCC found no relationship between total fat intake and risk for neovascular AMD [40,53]. Similarly, cross-sectional analysis of the National Health and Nutrition Education Evaluation Survey (NHANES) and several prospective cohorts did not find a relationship between total fat intake and AMD risk [45,54,55,61]. It was found that those consuming the highest levels of total fat were at increased risk for any stage of AMD, as well as increased risk for AMD progression in the POLANUT study ($p = 0.007$), NHS + HPFUS (95% CI: 1.17, 2.01; $p = 0.008$, for trend) and a study of 261 dry AMD patients (RR = 2.90; 95% CI: 1.15, 7.32; $p = 0.01$, for trend) [57,60] (Figure 23).

Figure 22. AMD odds or risk ratio; high *vs.* low intake of total fat: retrospective and cross-sectional studies.

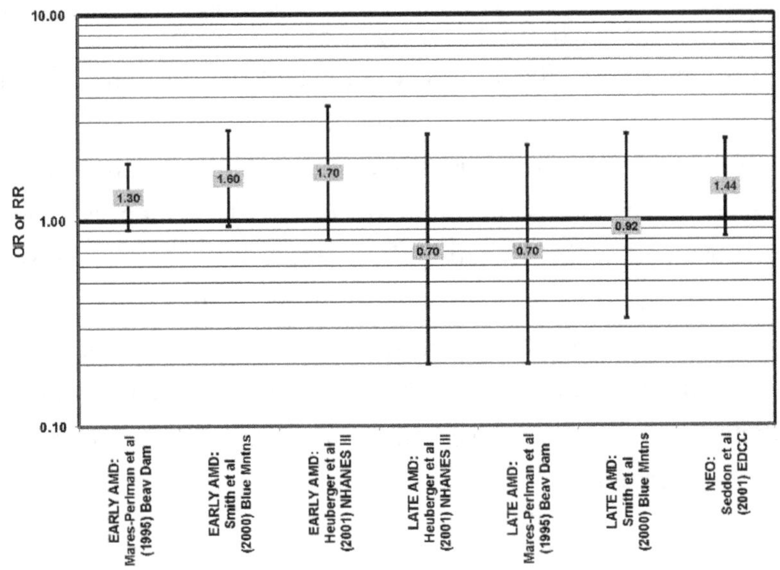

Figure 23. Odds or risk ratio for AMD, intermediate AMD or progression to late AMD; high *vs.* low intake of total fat: prospective studies.

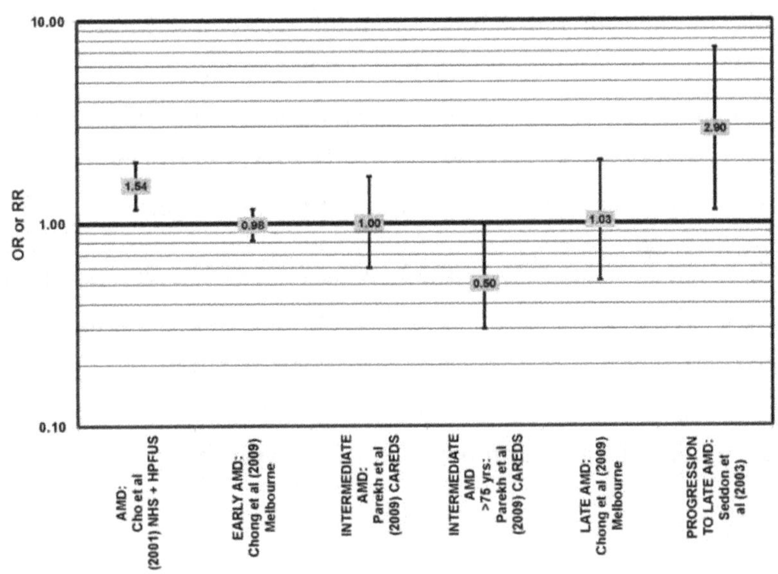

4.9. Animal versus Vegetable Fats

A few cohorts studied the associations of either animal or vegetable fats on AMD risk. The EDCC did not find an association between animal fat intake and risk for neovascular AMD, but found that compared to those consuming the lowest amounts of vegetable fat, those consuming the highest amounts had an increased risk for neovascular AMD (OR = 2.84; 95% CI: 1.45, 5.57; $p = 0.006$, for trend) [40] (Figure 15). Furthermore, a prospective study of 261 dry AMD patients found that over 4.6 years, compared to those consuming the lowest levels of vegetable fat, those consuming the highest levels were at an increased risk for progression to advanced AMD (RR = 3.82; 95% CI: 1.58, 9.28; $p = 0.003$, for trend) [57] (Figure 15).

4.10. Summary

To date, the body of observational epidemiologic data indicates that increased consumption of EPA and DHA reduces risk for neovascular and early AMD. However, such a relationship was not ascertained between consumption of omega-6 fatty acids and risk for AMD in the majority of studies that analyze this relationship. The relation of fish consumption and AMD is not as strong as the DHA and EPA components of fish individually. This suggests that the benefits of omega-3 fatty acids might be attenuated, due to interactions with other components of fish, such as omega-6 fatty acids [25]. In addition, the foods consumed with the fish and potential decreases in consumption of other food groups to compensate for increased fish are difficult to disentangle and may confound the results. The impact of monounsaturated and saturated fat consumption on AMD risk is unclear at this time. This may be due in part to different analytic approaches across studies. Further investigation into relationships between intakes of animal and vegetable fat, specifically trans-fat, as well as cholesterol, and risk for AMD may be warranted.

5. Carotenoids

5.1. Lutein and Zeaxanthin

Lutein and zeaxanthin are the only carotenoids found at appreciable levels in the macula [49,62–66] (Figures 24–34). In addition, their biophysical and biochemical capacities may play a role in the pathogenesis and progression of retinal diseases. For example, lutein and zeaxanthin have the ability to absorb blue light before it reaches the photoreceptors [67,68]. Furthermore, their concentration and potential biologic function may be modified by diet or supplement use.

The EDCC found that high intakes (OR = 0.43; 95% CI: 0.20, 0.70; $p < 0.001$), as well as blood levels (OR = 0.30; 95% CI: 0.20, 0.60; $p < 0.001$) of lutein/zeaxanthin were protective against neovascular AMD [69,70] (Figure 29). Another case control study of 72 patients and 66 controls corroborated this relationship and found that the prevalence of neovascular AMD was reduced in patients with the highest intake of lutein compared to those with the lowest (OR = 0.19; 95% CI: 0.05, 0.67) [71] (Figure 29).

Figure 24. AMD odds or risk ratio; high *vs.* low blood levels of lutein and/or zeaxanthin: retrospective and cross-sectional studies.

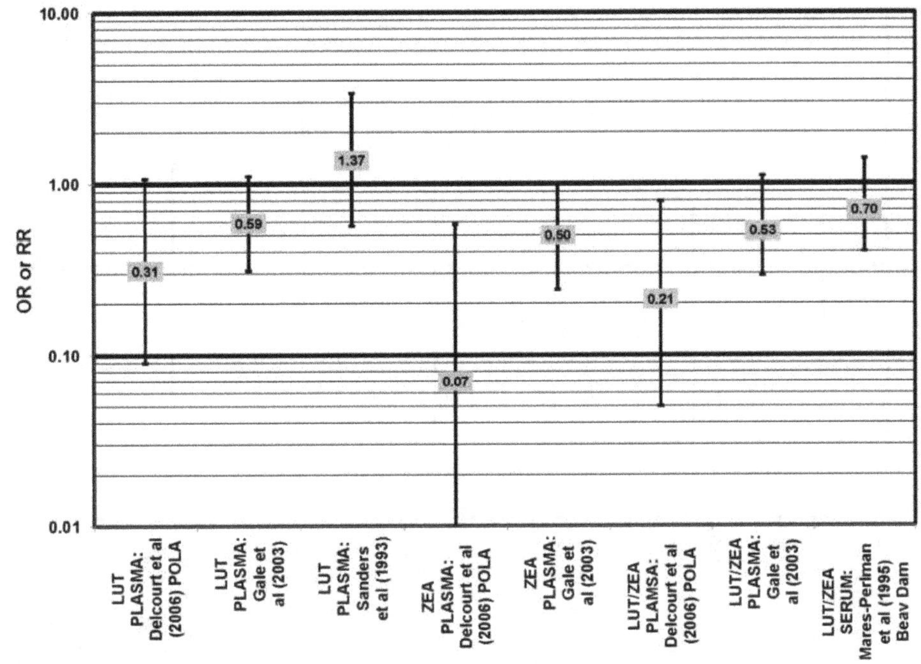

Figure 25. Odds or risk ratio for pigmentary abnormalities; high *vs.* low intake of lutein and zeaxanthin: retrospective and cross-sectional studies.

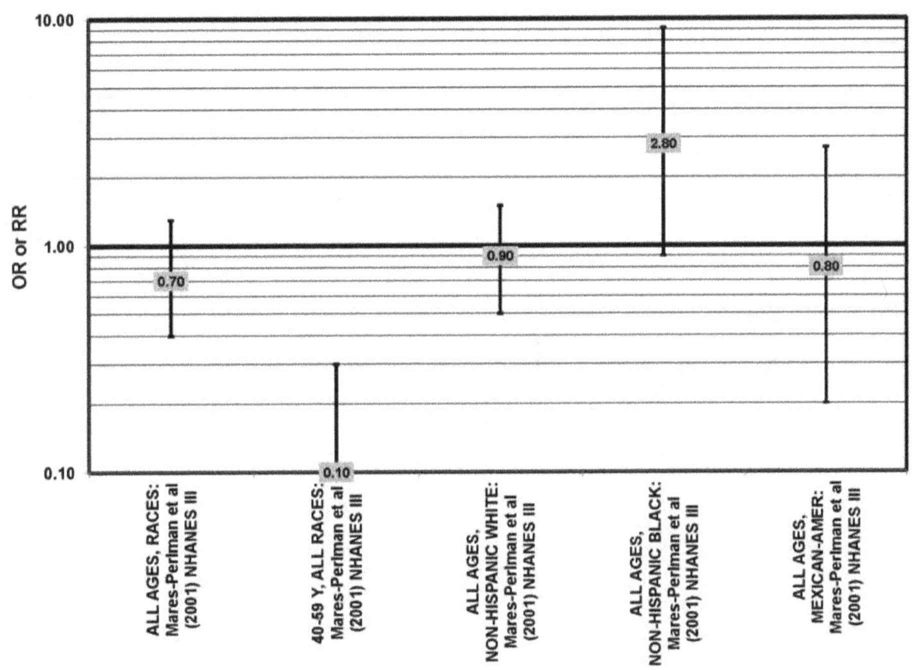

Figure 26. Odds or risk ratio for pigmentary abnormalities; high *vs.* low serum levels of lutein and zeaxanthin: retrospective and cross-sectional studies.

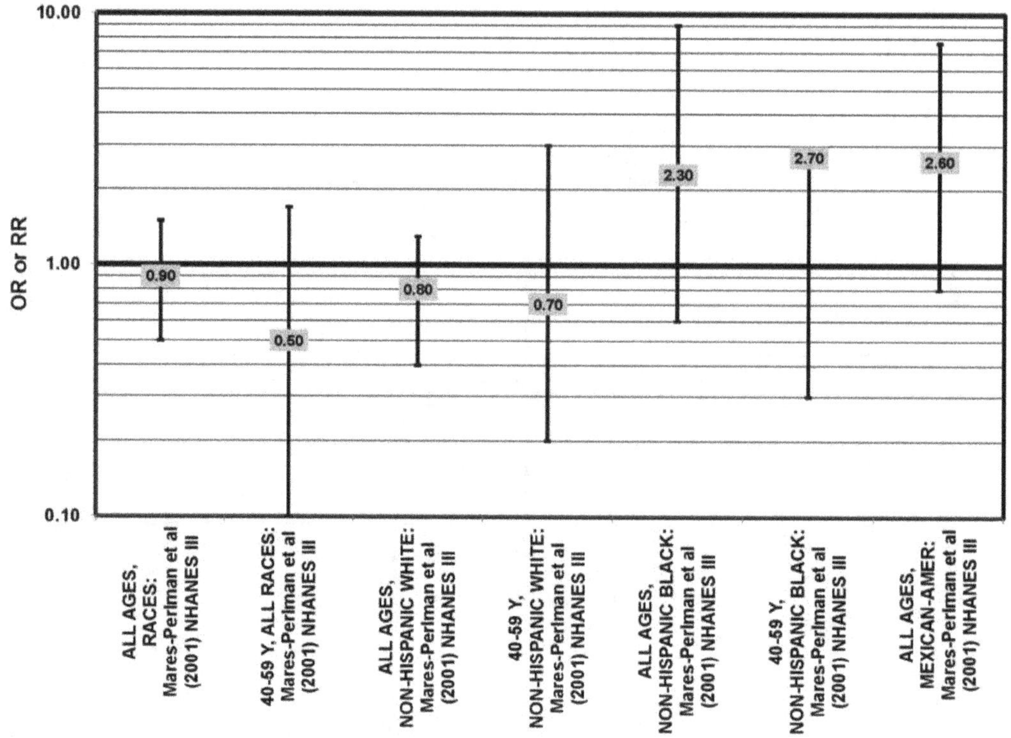

Figure 27. Odds or risk ratio for soft drusen; high *vs.* low intake of lutein and zeaxanthin:retrospective studies.

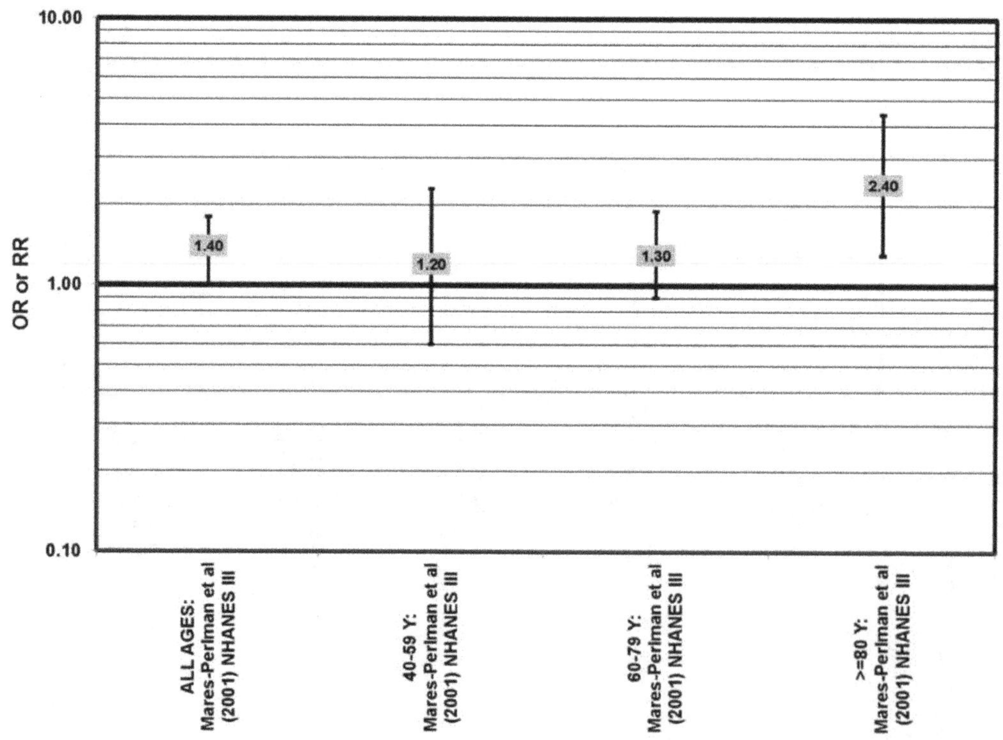

Figure 28. Odds or risk ratio for late AMD or geographic atrophy (GA); high *vs.* low intake of lutein and zeaxanthin from food: retrospective and cross-sectional studies.

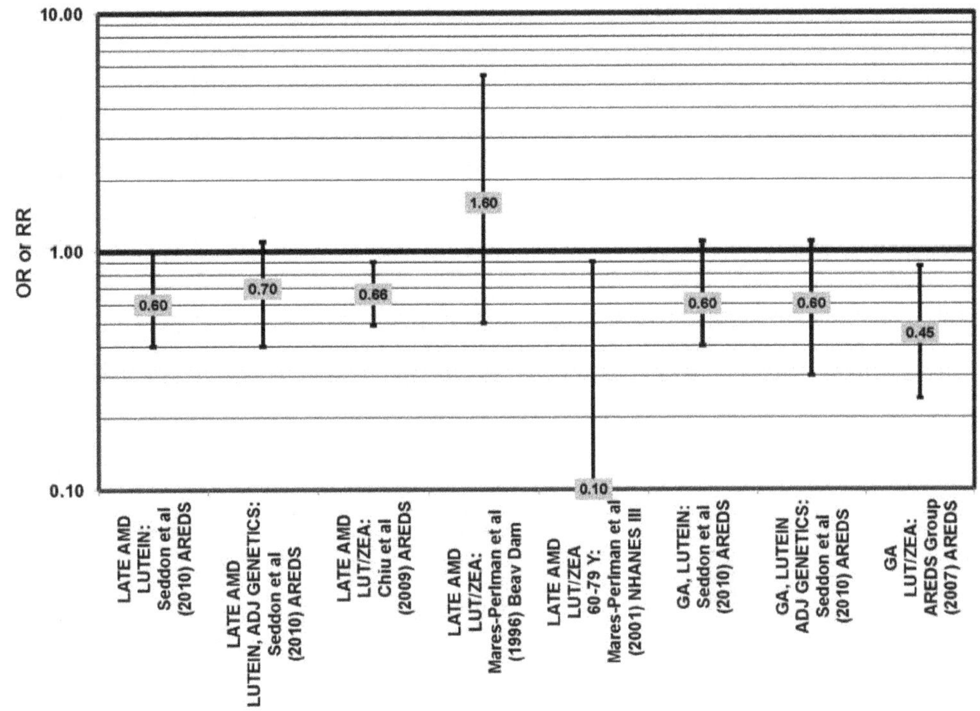

Figure 29. Odds or risk ratio for exudative or neovascular AMD; high *vs.* low intake or blood levels of lutein and/or zeaxanthin: retrospective and cross-sectional studies.

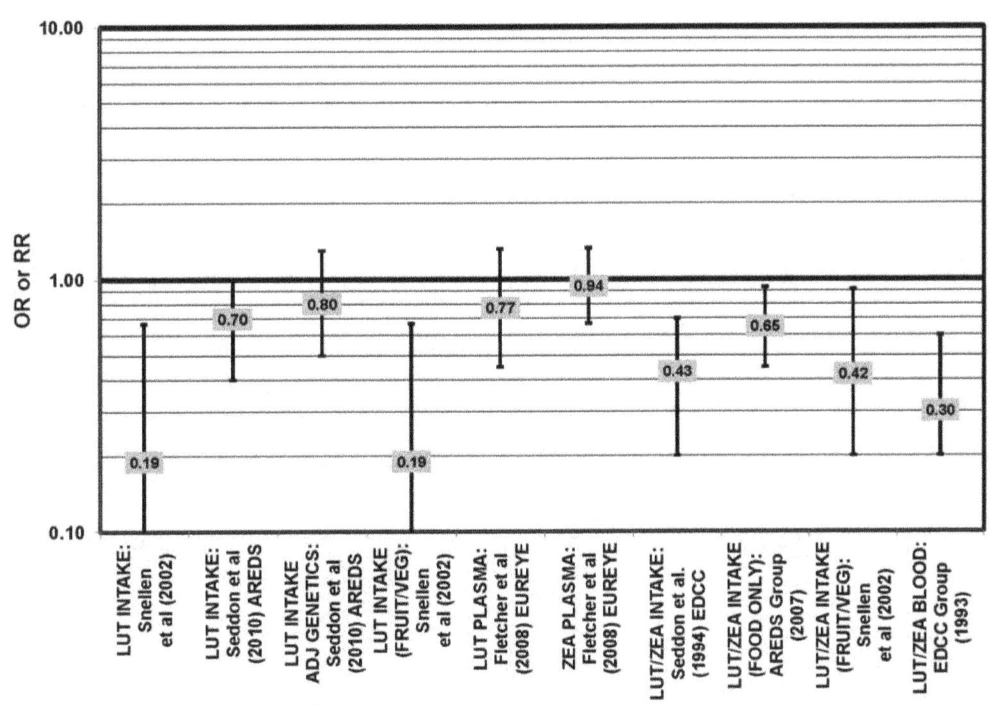

Figure 30. AMD odds or risk ratio; high *vs.* low intake of lutein and zeaxanthin: prospective studies.

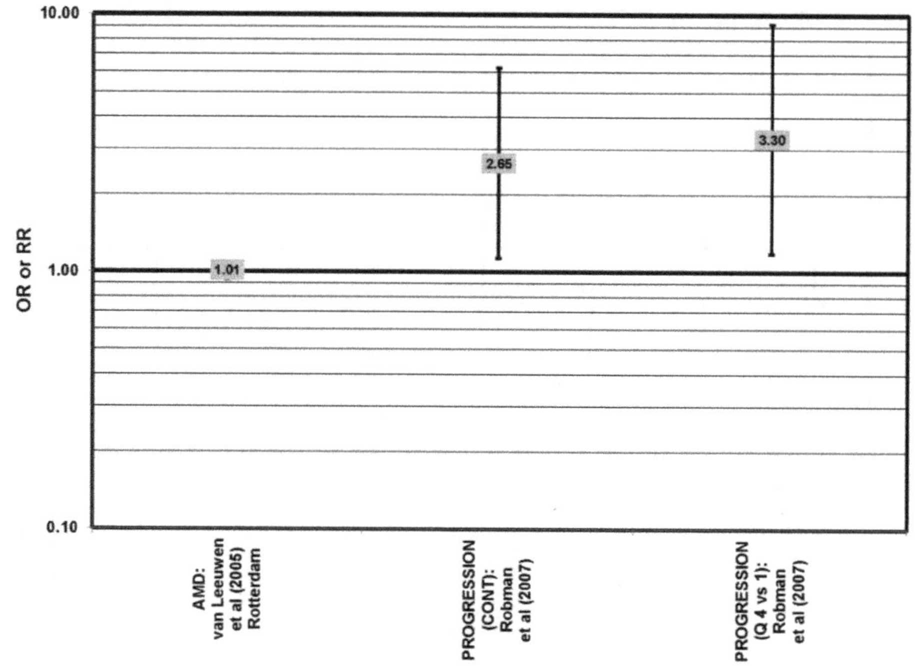

Figure 31. Late AMD odds or risk ratio; high *vs.* low intake of lutein and zeaxanthin: prospective studies.

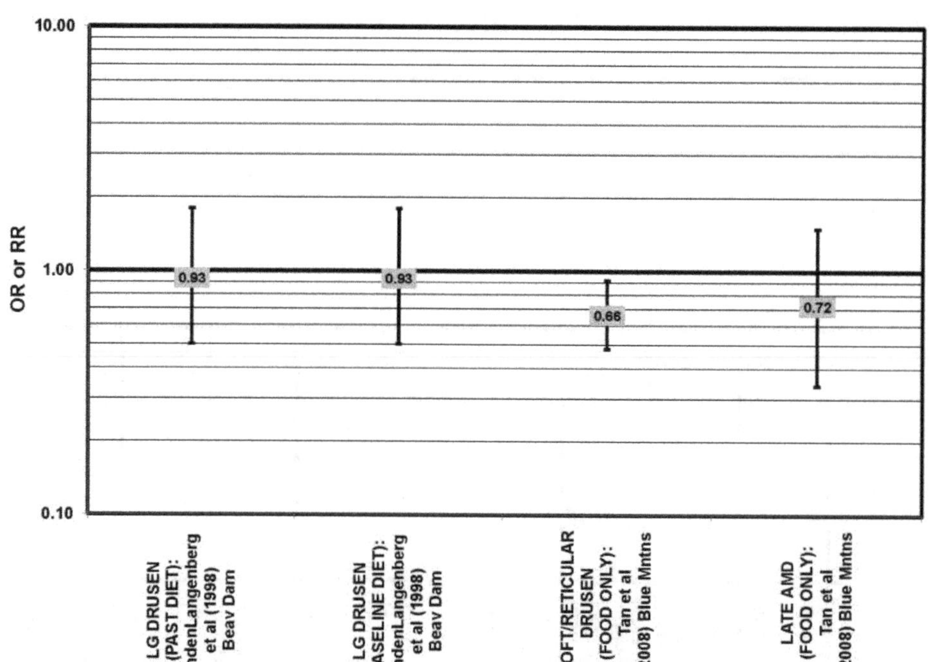

Figure 32. Neovascular AMD odds or risk ratio; high *vs.* low intake of lutein and zeaxanthin: prospective studies.

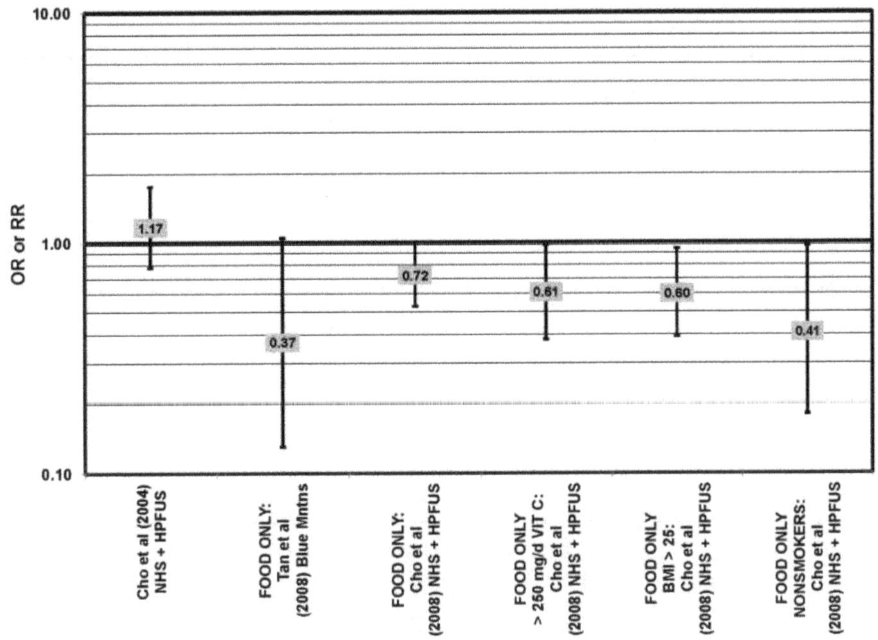

Figure 33. Odds or risk ratio for late AMD, severe AMD, geographic atrophy (GA), exudative AMD (EXUD) or neovascular AMD (NEO); high *vs.* low intake or blood levels of beta-carotene: retrospective and cross-sectional studies.

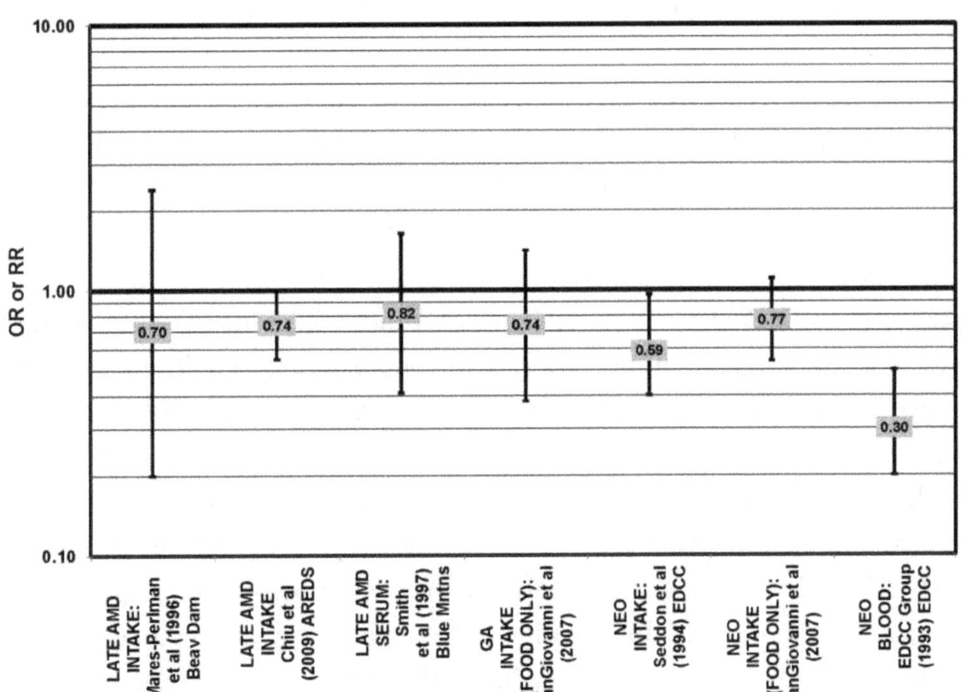

Figure 34. Odds or risk ratio for exudative AMD (EXUD) or neovascular AMD (NEO); high *vs.* low intake or blood levels of total carotenoids: retrospective and cross-sectional studies.

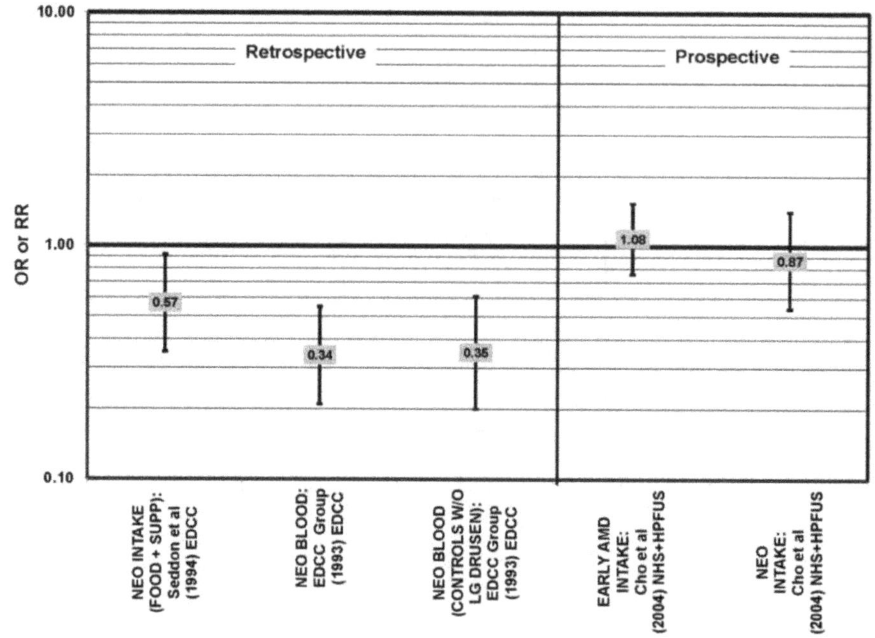

A number of cross-sectional studies support such findings. A study of 380 elderly English men and women found that those with the highest plasma levels of zeaxanthin had less risk for any stage of AMD than those with the lowest plasma levels (OR = 0.50; 95% CI: 0.24, 1.00). The associations between AMD risk and plasma lutein or plasma lutein/zeaxanthin showed the same trend, but were non-significant [72] (Figure 24). Cross-sectional analysis of the POLA (Pathologies Oculaires Liées à l'Age Study) cohort revealed that those with the highest levels of zeaxanthin (OR = 0.07; 95% CI: 0.01, 0.58) or a combination of lutein and zeaxanthin (OR = 0.21; 95% CI: 0.05, 0.79) in their blood had a reduced risk for any stage of AMD, although the amount of lutein alone in the blood (OR = 0.31; 95% CI: 0.09; 1.07) was not significantly associated with disease risk [73] (Figure 24).

Cross-sectional analysis of NHANES III revealed that those aged 40–59 who consumed the highest levels of dietary lutein and zeaxanthin had less risk for pigment abnormalities compared to those who consumed the lowest amounts (OR = 0.10; 95% CI: 0.10, 0.30) (Figure 25). However, these inverse relationships were not observed in the overall study population or among specific ethnic groups for intake or blood levels of lutein and/or zeaxanthin (Figures 25 and 26). There was no relationship between lutein/zeaxanthin blood levels and risk for soft drusen among any age group of Non-Hispanic whites in the NHANES III cohort, nor was there a relationship between lutein/zeaxanthin intake and risk for soft drusen among those aged 40–79 (Figure 27). Interestingly, 60–79-year-olds consuming the highest level of lutein/zeaxanthin did have a reduced risk for late AMD (OR = 0.10; 95% CI: 0.00, 0.90) (Figure 28). However, this inverse relationship was not observed in the overall NHANES III population [74]. Data from this cohort suggests that the associations of lutein and zeaxanthin on risk for disease are highly related to the age of those consuming these carotenoids.

Cross-sectional analysis at baseline of 4003 participants in the AREDS study indicated that those in the third quartile of consumption of lutein/zeaxanthin had 20% reduced risk for drusen compared to those in the first quartile of intake (OR = 0.80; 95% CI: 0.67, 0.97). Those in the third quartile of lutein/zeaxanthin intake also had a reduced risk for late AMD (OR = 0.66; 0.49, 0.90) (Figure 28). However, the association became non-significant in those subjects with the highest consumption of lutein/zeaxanthin for both outcomes [52].

The beneficial roles of lutein and zeaxanthin in retina health are supported in data from small intervention studies. Elderly men and women supplemented with 13.7 g/day lacto-wolfberry (a potent source of zeaxanthin) for 90 days increased serum zeaxanthin levels and antioxidant capacity in serum and also reduced pigment changes and soft drusen accumulation relative to the placebo group [75]. A small trial of 108 German men and women supplemented daily with 12 mg lutein and 1 mg zeaxanthin for six months increased MPOD compared to placebo ($p < 0.001$), a change which was maintained even after supplementation stopped [76]. Another placebo controlled trial of 49 elderly women showed that 12 mg/day of lutein supplementation significantly increased MPOD after four months [49]. In another study of 100 men and women, it was shown that increases in MPOD following lutein supplementation were dose-dependent [55,77]. In a small study of 36 subjects, a statistically significant increase in MPOD and improvements in visual acuity and contrast sensitivity were seen in subjects supplemented with 10 mg lutein, 2 mg zeaxanthin and 10 mg meso-zeaxanthin [78]. In a study of 108 early AMD patients, significant increases in MPOD were seen in those supplemented with 20 mg lutein/day and in those supplemented with 10 mg/day lutein plus 10 mg/day zeaxanthin [79]. Data from these trials should be regarded with caution, because of their short duration and limited controls and/or clinical endpoints.

The Zeaxanthin and Visual Function study was a one-year randomized double-masked placebo-controlled study to evaluate the benefits of zeaxanthin, separate from lutein, on visual function, as well as the effects of combining lutein and zeaxanthin in patients with atrophic AMD. Patients received either 8 mg zeaxanthin/day, 9 mg lutein/day ("faux placebo" group) or a combination of both carotenoids. After one year, MPOD increased in all three groups and was not different among the groups. Patients taking zeaxanthin experienced the greatest improvement in high contrast visual acuity and clearance of central scotomas, which are areas of partially diminished or entirely degenerated visual acuity surround by a normal field of vision. Patients taking lutein experienced the most improvement in low contrast acuity and glare recovery. Patients supplemented with both carotenoids saw the least improvement overall, which was attributed to a competition between the carotenoids in the retina [80]. Similarly, a majority of AMD patients given Ocuvite (supplement of 12 g lutein, 1 g zeaxanthin and antioxidants) in the Lutein Nutritional Effects Measured by Autofluorescence (LUNA) study showed elevated MPOD. However, a significant minority did not, perhaps owing to different absorption capacities between individuals.

The Carotenoids in Age-Related Maculopathy in Italians Study (CARMIS) was a randomized intervention in which patients received a combination of 10 mg lutein, 1 mg zeaxanthin, 4 mg astaxanthin and an antioxidant supplement or did not receive any supplements. After 24 months, those receiving supplements had improved and stabilized visual acuity ($p = 0.003$), as well as improved contrast sensitivity at both 12 and 24 months ($p = 0.001$), compared to the non-supplemented group [81].

The Lutein Antioxidant Supplement Trial (LAST) was a randomized, double-masked, placebo-controlled trial of 90 atrophic AMD patients who either received 10 mg lutein, 10 mg lutein with an antioxidant supplement or a maltodextrin placebo. In both groups that received lutein, there was an improvement in MPOD ($p < 0.05$), visual acuity ($p < 0.05$) and contrast sensitivity (at six, 12, 18 degrees, $p < 0.05$) after 12 months of supplementation. The group receiving lutein alone also had improvements in the Amsler grid ($p < 0.01$), a grid of horizontal and vertical lines used to monitor the central visual field and detect visual disturbances, and in glare recovery (AREDS stage II, $p = 0.02$); AREDS stage IV, $p = 0.05$) [82]. In follow-up analysis it was observed that those patients with the greatest increases in MPOD with lutein supplementation were those with the lowest baseline levels, suggesting that lutein supplementation is most beneficial for high risk patients [83]. The data also indicates a saturation of carotenoids in the macula [84].

Some studies did not find any associations of lutein and zeaxanthin on risk for AMD. Case control studies of AMD patients, including data from the Beaver Dam Eye study and AREDS, did not find any difference in blood levels of lutein/zeaxanthin between patients and controls, nor did they report any effect of plasma lutein/zeaxanthin levels on risk for AMD [85–87] (Figures 24 and 29). Cross-sectional studies reported similar findings. A study comprised of 722 elderly Japanese reported no difference in serum lutein/zeaxanthin between those with and without late AMD. Analysis of EUREYE and the Beaver Dam Eye study also found no effect of lutein/zeaxanthin intake on risk for early or late AMD [88–90] (Figures 28 and 29). Prospective studies also did not find an effect of lutein and zeaxanthin intake on AMD risk or incidence of pigment abnormalities. The Rotterdam cohort found no association between any stage of AMD and intake of lutein/zeaxanthin [91]. Data from the Blue Mountains Eye Study found no effect of lutein and zeaxanthin on risk for early AMD five years after baseline (OR = 1.00, 95% CI: 0.60. 1.60), on risk for atrophic or neovascular AMD ten years after baseline (OR = 0.66; 95% CI: 0.48, 0.92) or on risk for drusen 10 years after baseline [92,93] (Figures 34 and 35). Similarly, past or present intake of lutein did not affect the five year incidence of pigment abnormalities in the Beaver Dam Eye study [94]. Analysis of men and women in the NHS + HPFUS revealed that those with the highest intakes of lutein and zeaxanthin did not have significantly less risk for early AMD than those with the lowest intakes after adjusting for smoking status, BMI, age, energy intake, alcohol intake, fish intake and use of hormone replacement therapy, and subsequent analyses did not find an association between early or neovascular AMD and lutein/zeaxanthin intake [95,96] (Figures 30–32). There was slightly lower risk for neovascular AMD among those who consumed high levels of lutein and zeaxanthin from food (RR = 0.72; 95% CI: 0.53, 0.99), and this effect became more robust in subgroups of this population (Figure 35). Men and women who consumed >250 mg/day vitamin C (RR = 0.61; 95% CI: 0.38, 0.98) had a BMI of at least 25 (RR = 0.60; 95% CI: 0.39, 0.94) and were nonsmokers (RR = 0.41; 95% CI: 0.18, 0.97; $p = 0.07$, for trend); the highest level of lutein/zeaxanthin intake was associated with a protective effect on neovascular AMD [96] (Figure 32).

Figure 35. Odds or risk ratio for early AMD indicators (SOFT DRUSEN, LESION) or early AMD; high *vs.* low antioxidant index (AOX) intake or use of multivitamin supplements: retrospective and cross-sectional studies.

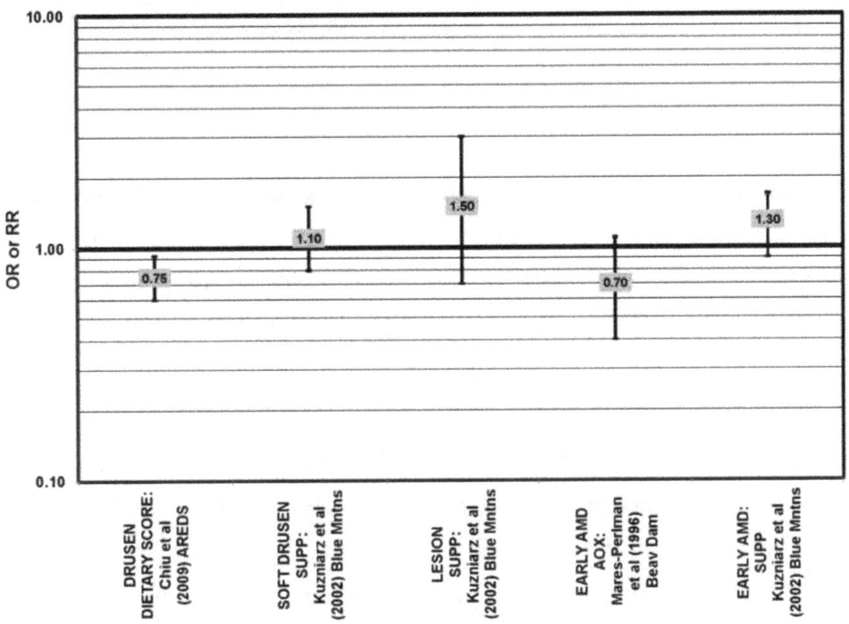

Finally, retrospective analysis of the NHANES III cohort suggested that elevated intake of these carotenoids may increase risk for drusen appearance and AMD, with the effect appearing to be driven by the most elderly participants [74]. In addition, a prospective study of 254 early AMD patients showed that lutein/zeaxanthin intake was associated with increased risk for any stage of AMD after controlling for age, smoking, family history, source study and follow-up duration [55] (Figures 27 and 30).

5.2. Beta-Carotene

Beta-carotene is another carotenoid that has been investigated in many studies for its potential ability to modulate AMD risk. The EDCC found that increased consumption (OR = 0.59; 95% CI: 0.40, 0.96; $p = 0.03$) and blood levels (OR = 0.30; 95% CI: 0.20, 0.50; $p < 0.001$ for trend) of beta-carotene reduced the risk for neovascular AMD [69,70] (Figure 33). Further support was found in a cross-sectional study of 722 elderly Japanese that reported that those with late AMD had significantly lower serum levels of beta-carotene ($p < 0.05$) [88].

The remainder of studies evaluating the role of beta-carotene did not find an effect of this carotenoid on risk for AMD. Case control studies, including the Blue Mountain Eye Study and Beaver Dam Eye Study, did not find any difference in blood beta-carotene levels between AMD patients and controls and found no association between serum beta-carotene levels and risk for AMD [85,86,97,98]. Data from cross-sectional studies, including data from NHS, Beaver Dam Eye Study and AREDS, are consistent with findings that beta-carotene has no effect on risk for pigment abnormalities, AMD or drusen, respectively [52,90,97,99]. Prospective data from the Rotterdam cohort and Baltimore Longitudinal Study of Aging show no association between beta-carotene intake or serum levels of beta-carotene, respectively, and risk for any stage of AMD. Similarly, in the Blue Mountains Eye study, there was no association between beta-carotene intake and early AMD five years after baseline or late AMD 10 years after baseline [92]. In the NHS + HPFUS, there was also no association between beta-carotene intake and neovascular AMD [95]. The Beaver Dam Eye Study found no association between past or present intake of beta-carotene and risk for pigment abnormalities [94]. The Alpha Tocopherol Beta Carotene Study (ATBC) found that beta-carotene supplementation alone had no effect on AMD risk (OR = 1.04; 95% CI: 0.74, 1.47) [91–95,100,101] (Figure 33).

5.3. Alpha-Carotene

In addition to beta-carotene, the EDCC also evaluated the effect of the isomer, alpha-carotene, on risk for AMD. In this study, higher blood levels of alpha-carotene (OR = 0.50; 95% CI: 0.30, 0.80; $p = 0.003$, for trend) were associated with decreased risk for neovascular AMD [70]. Prospective analysis of the Beaver Dam Eye Study also found that those with an elevated past intake of dietary alpha-carotene were at a reduced risk for the appearance of large drusen (OR = 0.52; 95% CI: 0.30, 1.00) [94]).

The remainder of case control and prospective studies, as well as more recent NHS data reported that alpha-carotene does not significantly affect risk for AMD. Case-control analysis of patients in the Beaver Dam Eye Study, EDCC and three additional studies did not find any association between serum levels of alpha-carotene and any stage of AMD or any difference in blood levels of alpha-carotene between AMD patients and controls [69,85,86,90,98,102].

5.4. Lycopene

Lycopene is commonly found in the American diet in tomato-based products [103]. Evidence for a potential role of lycopene in retina health was found in a small case control study, which found that AMD patients had less lycopene in their serum, LDL and HDL than in healthy controls ($p = 0.006$) [85]. Similarly, a nested case-control study of 167 patients from the Beaver Dam Eye Study found that higher lycopene blood levels were associated with decreased risk for any stage of AMD (OR = 0.45; 95% CI: 0.22, 0.91) [98].

The remaining observational, cross-sectional and prospective studies did not find a relationship between lycopene and AMD. The EDCC found no association between intake or blood levels and risk for neovascular AMD (OR = 0.80; 95% CI: 0.50, 1.30; $p = 0.4$, for trend) [69,70]. Furthermore, cross-sectional analysis of elderly Japanese found no association between serum lycopene levels and late AMD risk, and cross-sectional analysis of the Beaver Dam Eye Study found no effect of lycopene intake and risk for early or late AMD. Prospective studies, such as the Rotterdam cohort and Blue Mountains Eye study, found no association between lycopene intake and any stage AMD or early AMD, respectively (HR = 1.01; 95% CI: 0.97, 1.04) (OR = 0.80; 95% CI: 0.50, 1.40) [91,92]. Recent NHS data found no association between serum lycopene levels and risk for pigment abnormalities, and the NHS + HPFUS found no association between early or neovascular AMD and lycopene intake [95].

5.5. Cryptoxanthin

Cryptoxanthin is a carotenoid found in foods, such as avocado, basil and mango [103]. The EDCC and a cross-sectional analysis of 722 elderly Japanese found that increased blood levels of cryptoxanthin were associated with decreased risk for any stage of AMD [88]. The remaining studies did not find any associations between cryptoxanthin and AMD. A case control study did not find any difference in blood cryptoxanthin levels between patients and controls [85]. The Beaver Dam Eye study found no association between serum levels of beta-cryptoxanthin and risk for any stage of AMD [98]. The EDCC Beaver Dam Eye study, Rotterdam study, Blue Mountains Eye study and NHS + HPFUS also showed that intake of cryptoxanthin had no effect on risk for neovascular, early or late AMD [69,90–92,95].

5.6. Total Carotenoids

Total carotenoid levels have also been analyzed for their potential to confer retinal benefit. In the EDCC, increasing intake of total carotenoids was associated with decreased risk for neovascular AMD (OR = 0.57; 95% CI: 0.35, 0.92; $p = 0.02$, for trend) [69], and analysis of blood levels corroborated these relationships: OR = 0.34 (95% CI: 0.21, 0.55; $p < 0.001$, for trend) (Figure 34) [70]. Similar results were obtained when AMD cases were compared to controls without large drusen. Another smaller case-control study with 48 AMD patients found that total carotenoid plasma levels were significantly lower in patients with late AMD compared to those in the early stages of the disease ($p < 0.05$), although there was no difference in plasma levels between AMD patients and healthy controls [104]. This may imply that carotenoids play a more important role in disease progression rather than disease onset. This finding is comparable to that of another case-control study of 197 Japanese men and women that reported that eyes with early AMD and the normal eye of an AMD patient had comparable macular carotenoid levels, which were both higher than those of an eye with late AMD ($p < 0.001$). However, in this study, macular carotenoid levels of all AMD patients were also significantly lower than those of age-matched healthy subjects ($p < 0.001$), as determined by Raman spectroscopy [105].

Despite these reported beneficial effects of carotenoids on the retina, four case-control studies did not find any difference in blood levels of total carotenoids between AMD patients and healthy controls [85,86,106,107]. Furthermore, prospective analyses of the NHS + HPFUS found no association between early or neovascular AMD and total carotenoid intake [95] (Figure 34).

5.7. Summary

Taken together, these observational studies suggest that of all of the carotenoids studied, lutein and zeaxanthin may confer the most benefit to the retina. These benefits may be specific for certain types or stages of AMD. Advanced AMD shows the most consistent inverse relationships between lutein intake and risk for lesions. Data concerning the effects of lutein and zeaxanthin on outcomes, such as visual acuity and contrast sensitivity, suggest that 10 mg of lutein/day, without zeaxanthin, may confer the most retinal benefit. That said, intervention studies, such as AREDS II, will clarify the role of these carotenoids in the risk for onset and progression of specific AMD outcomes.

6. Vitamin A

Analysis of vitamin A/retinol intake and blood levels has also been examined for its role in retinal health, as many carotenoids are byproducts of vitamin A. NHANES I found that those who consumed increased amounts of fruits and vegetables rich in vitamin A had a decreased risk for any stage of AMD (OR = 0.59; 95% CI: 0.37, 0.99) [108]. Also, a prospective analysis of the Beaver Dam Eye Study found that those with an elevated past intake (OR = 0.53; 95% CI: 0.30, 1.00) or current intake (OR = 0.45; 95% CI: 0.20, 1.00) of pro-vitamin A carotenoids were at a reduced risk for the appearance of large drusen [94].

Case control analyses found that patients and healthy controls did not have different plasma levels of vitamin A and that plasma levels were not different in different stages of AMD [86,104,106,107]. Additionally, EDCC and AREDS found that intake of retinol did not modulate risk for neovascular AMD [69,99]. Cross-sectional analyses found no relationship between intake of vitamin A rich food and AMD risk in NHANES III or between intake of retinol or vitamin A and pigment abnormalities in the NHS [102,108]. Prospective analysis of the Blue Mountain Eye study found that vitamin A and retinol intake did not affect risk for AMD [92]. Additionally, prospective data from the Baltimore Longitudinal study showed no effect of plasma retinol levels and severe AMD risk, and the NHS + HPFUS found no association between early or neovascular AMD and vitamin A intake [95,100]. Analysis of four examinations from the Beaver Dam Eye Study showed that supplementation with vitamin A was associated with an increased risk for late AMD (OR = 3.05; 95% CI: 1.60, 5.82) [109]. In summary, the epidemiologic data regarding the relationship between vitamin A/retinol intake and blood levels and the risk of AMD are mixed, and no reliable trend can be reported.

7. Vitamin E

Vitamin E (alpha-tocopherol) is a lipophilic antioxidant that some studies suggest has a role in retina health and diminishing risk for AMD. A case-control study of 48 AMD patients indicated that plasma vitamin E levels were significantly lower in patients with late AMD compared to patients with early AMD or healthy age-matched controls ($p < 0.05$), and these effects remained even after adjusting for cholesterol levels. This adjustment is of interest, because vitamin E is lipid soluble and associates with cholesterol on lipoprotein particles [104]. Another case-control study of 25 elderly AMD patients found that vitamin E serum levels were significantly lower in AMD patients compared to healthy controls ($p < 0.001$). In this study, patients and controls had similar cholesterol levels [110]. A third case-control study found that comparison of serum vitamin E levels in 35 AMD patients with 66 controls showed that vitamin E was inversely associated with risk for AMD [107].

Cross-sectional analysis of the 2584 participants of the POLA study showed that after adjusting for plasma lipid levels, those with the highest levels of plasma vitamin E had a reduced risk for signs of early AMD, such as pigment changes or soft drusen (OR = 0.72; 95% CI: 0.53, 0.98; $p = 0.04$, for trend) and late AMD (OR = 0.18; 95% CI: 0.05, 0.67; $p = 0.004$, for trend) [111]. These associations remained even in populations of different ethnicity. A cross-sectional study of 722 elderly Japanese found that patients with late AMD had marginally significant lower levels of serum alpha-tocopherol than healthy controls ($p = 0.056$) [88]. Baseline analysis of 4003 participants of the AREDS cohort indicated that those consuming the highest amounts of vitamin E had a marginally reduced risk for late AMD compared to those consuming the smallest amounts (OR = 0.66; 95% CI: 0.45, 0.99; $p = 0.052$, for trend) [52].

Some prospective study data corroborate the cross-sectional data. The Baltimore Longitudinal Study of Aging indicated that among 976 men and women, those with the highest plasma tocopherol levels were at a reduced risk for any stage of AMD, even after adjusting for age, gender and nuclear opacity (OR = 0.43; 95% CI: 0.25, 0.73) [100]. In the Rotterdam prospective cohort, vitamin E intake was also associated with a slight reduction in risk for AMD (HR = 0.92; 95% CI: 0.84, 1.00) [91]. Among 498 women in the NHS, increasing amounts of vitamin E intake were associated with a decreased prevalence of pigment abnormalities, an indicator of early AMD [102].

There is also a significant amount of case control, prospective and intervention data suggesting that there is no relationship between vitamin E levels and AMD risk. A case-control study of 167 cataract patients from the Beaver Dam Eye Study revealed that there was no association between alpha-tocopherol (OR = 0.80; 95% CI: 0.40, 1.50) serum levels or gamma-tocopherol (OR = 1.30; 95% CI: 0.70, 2.40) serum levels and any stage of AMD. The EDCC and an additional study of 26 neovascular patients also found no association between serum vitamin E levels and risk for AMD [70,98,106]. Furthermore, a case-control study with 34 AMD patients found no difference in serum, LDL or HDL levels of alpha- or gamma-tocopherol between AMD patients and healthy controls [85]. Additionally, case-control studies comprised of 56–165 AMD patients found no difference in blood alpha-tocopherol levels between patients and healthy controls [86,97,112]. The EDCC found no association between vitamin E intake (OR = 1.07; 95% CI: 0.63, 1.84; p = 0.98, for trend) or supplementation (OR = 0.97; 95% CI: 0.6, 1.50, p = 0.28, for trend) and risk for neovascular AMD (OR = 1.46; 95% CI: 0.88, 2.44) [69]. Similarly, in case-control analysis of the AREDS, there was no association between vitamin E intake and risk for drusen, geographic atrophy or neovascular AMD [99].

Cross-sectional analysis of the AREDS population revealed that intake of vitamin E was not associated with risk for drusen [52]. Retrospective analysis of the Beaver Dam cohort (n = 1968) also indicated that past intake of vitamin E with or without supplementation did not have a significant effect on early or late AMD [90]. Cross-sectional analysis of 4753 elderly men and women found no increased risk for neovascular AMD in those with the lowest plasma levels of alpha-tocopherol (OR = 0.82; 95% CI: 0.47, 1.41) [89]. In prospective analysis of the Beaver Dam cohort, past intake of vitamin E was associated with a decreased risk for large drusen five years after baseline (OR = 0.40; 95% CI: 0.20, 0.90; p = 0.04 for trend), but there was no association with present vitamin E intake or past or present vitamin E supplementation, nor was there an association between past or present intake of vitamin E and risk for pigment abnormalities [94]. In the Physicians' Health Study, vitamin E supplementation was not associated with risk for any stage of AMD (RR = 0.87; 95% CI: 0.53, 1.43) [113]. Similarly, a prospective analysis of 118,428 men and women who participated in the NHS + HPFUS showed that vitamin E intake had no effect on risk for early or neovascular AMD [95].

The Women's Health Study (WHS), a randomized double-masked placebo controlled trial, gave 39,421 women either 600 IU vitamin E every other day or placebo for 10 years. After adjusting for age, aspirin intake and beta-carotene, vitamin E had no effect on risk for visually significant AMD (RR = 0.93; 95% CI: 0.72, 1.19), late AMD (RR = 1.13; 95% CI: 0.67, 1.92) or AMD with or without vision loss (RR = 0.90; 95% CI: 0.77, 1.06) [114]. The ATBC Study gave subjects either daily supplements of 50 mg vitamin E, 20 mg beta-carotene, both or placebo, and after five to eight years of intervention, alpha-tocopherol supplementation alone had no effect on risk for AMD (OR = 1.13; 95% CI: 0.81, 1.59) [101]. The Vitamin E and Age-related Cataract and Maculopathy (VECAT), a clinical trial of 1193 elderly participants, indicated that supplementation with 500 IU vitamin E for four years also had no effect on incidence of early AMD (RR = 1.05; 95% CI: 0.69, 1.61) or late AMD (RR = 1.36; 95% CI: 0.67, 2.77) [115]. Lastly, in a randomized, double masked, placebo-controlled trial of 14,236 male physicians over the age of 50, alternate day use of 400 IU of vitamin E for an average of eight years had no effect on diagnosis of AMD (HR, 1.03; 95% CI, 0.78–1.37) [116].

A 10 year follow-up of subjects from the Blue Mountains Eye study showed those with the highest intakes of vitamin E were at greater risk for late stage atrophic AMD (RR = 2.55; 95% CI: 1.14, 5.70), and there was no association between vitamin E intake and neovascular AMD (RR = 1.96; 95% CI: 0.74, 5.15) [93]. Analysis of all four examinations of the Beaver Dam Eye study reported a positive association between vitamin E supplementation and incident late AMD (OR = 1.78; 95% CI: 1.04, 3.05) [109].

While there is a large body of evidence to say there is an inverse relationship between vitamin E consumption and risk for AMD, there is also a substantial amount of evidence to say that no relationship exists. Some evidence even suggests a direct relationship with certain stages of AMD. Overall, there is not a consistent relationship from the data to date.

8. Vitamin C

Case control, observational and prospective analyses do not suggest that vitamin C plays a large role in modulating AMD risk. This includes exposure to vitamin C in blood supplements or diet, some of which monitored intake over 10 years and/or were from large cohorts [61,62,92–96,98,101,111–113,116]. Nevertheless, in a case control study of 48 Italian AMD patients, it was found that patients with late AMD had significantly lower plasma vitamin C levels than those patients with early AMD ($p < 0.05$), but there was no difference in plasma levels of vitamin C between AMD patients and healthy controls [104]. Additionally, a case control study of 56 AMD patients found significantly decreased serum vitamin C levels in AMD patients compared to controls [112]. This may be attributable to the small sample size of the study [89,111,112].

Two different cross-sectional analyses of the baseline data from AREDS (of 4519 and 4403 participants) studied the effects of a single nutrient or groups of nutrients on AMD risk, and both analyses indicated that after multivariate adjustment, vitamin C intake alone had no association with drusen formation, late AMD, geographic atrophy or neovascular AMD [52,99]. Analyses of the Beaver Dam Eye Study found that past intake of vitamin C (with or without supplements) did not have a significant effect on risk for early or late AMD [90]. Prospective analyses, including the Physician's Health Study, Rotterdam study, Baltimore Longitudinal, Blue Mountains Eye Study, Beaver Dam Eye Study and NHS + HPFUS, also indicate that vitamin C intake or blood levels are not associated with risk for AMD; respectively, [91,93,94,100,113]. In a randomized, double masked placebo controlled trial of 14,236 male physicians, daily supplementation of 500 mg vitamin C for eight years had no effect on risk for AMD (HR, 0.99; 95% CI, 0.75–1.31) [116].

Data collected at four different examinations of the Beaver Dam Eye Study found that use of vitamin C supplements was associated with increased risk for late AMD (OR = 2.47; 95% CI: 1.40, 4.80) [109]. This corroborated data from the Blue Mountains Eye Study, which found that those with the highest intakes of vitamin C had an increased risk for early AMD after five years, compared to those with the lowest intakes of vitamin C (OR = 2.30; 95% CI: 1.30, 4.00; $p = 0.002$, for trend) [92].

Overall, the body of epidemiological evidence does not inform a consistent relationship between Vitamin C and risk for AMD, and further investigation is warranted.

9. Antioxidant Combinations or Multivitamins

The case-control EDCC found no effect of multivitamin supplementation on risk for neovascular AMD (OR = 0.82; 95% CI 0.57, 1.18). There was, however, an association between antioxidant index and late AMD [69]. Participants who had the highest blood levels of selenium, vitamin C or vitamin E, had a reduced risk for neovascular AMD (OR = 0.30; 95% CI: 0.10, 0.70; $p = 0.005$, for trend) compared to those who had the lowest amounts of at least three of the nutrients [70] (Figure 36).

Figure 36. Odds or risk ratio for late AMD, exudative AMD (EXUD) or neovascular AMD (NEO); high *vs.* low antioxidant index (AOX) intake or blood levels or use of multivitamin supplements: retrospective and cross-sectional studies.

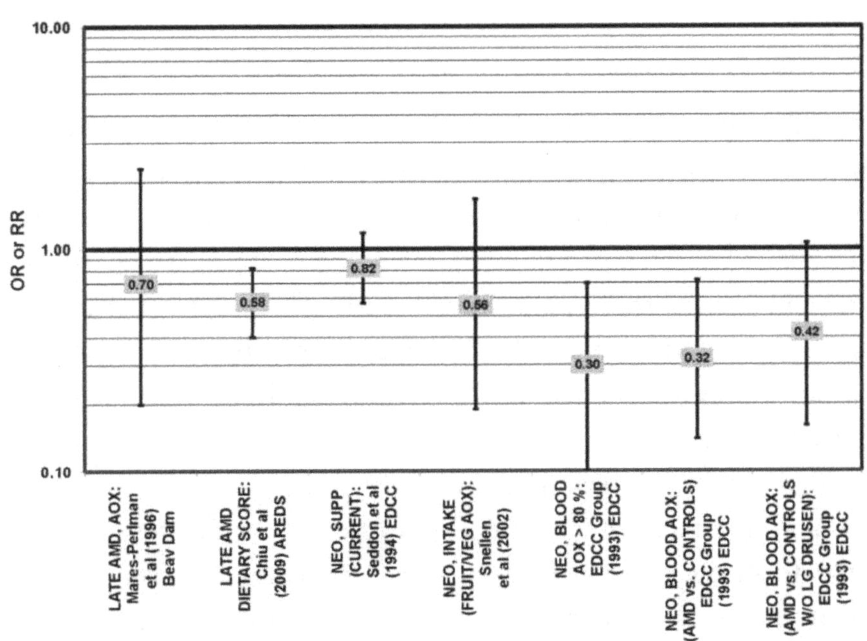

In cross-sectional analysis of 4003 participants in AREDS, a compound score, which included dietary intake of vitamin E, vitamin C, zinc, lutein/zeaxanthin, DHA, EPA and low dietary glycemic index was created to compare overall diet to the risk for AMD. Low scores indicated lowest intake of such nutrients and *vice versa.* Compared to those subjects with the lowest score, those with the highest score were at a reduced risk for drusen (OR = 0.75; 95% CI: 0.60, 0.93; $p = 0.048$, for trend) and late stage AMD (OR = 0.58; 95% CI: 0.40, 0.82; $p = 0.002$, for trend) [52] (Figures 35 and 36). Additionally, in prospective analyses, the Rotterdam study indicated that after adjusting for age, sex, BMI, smoking, blood pressure, atherosclerotic score, alcohol intake and total cholesterol, subjects that had intakes of beta-carotene, vitamin C, vitamin E and zinc above the median had reduced risk for AMD (HR = 0.65; 95% CI: 0.46, 0.92) [91] (Figure 37).

Figure 37. Odds or risk ratio for AMD, early AMD or neovascular (NEO) AMD; high *vs.* low intake of antioxidant combination or use of multivitamin supplement: prospective studies, intervention.

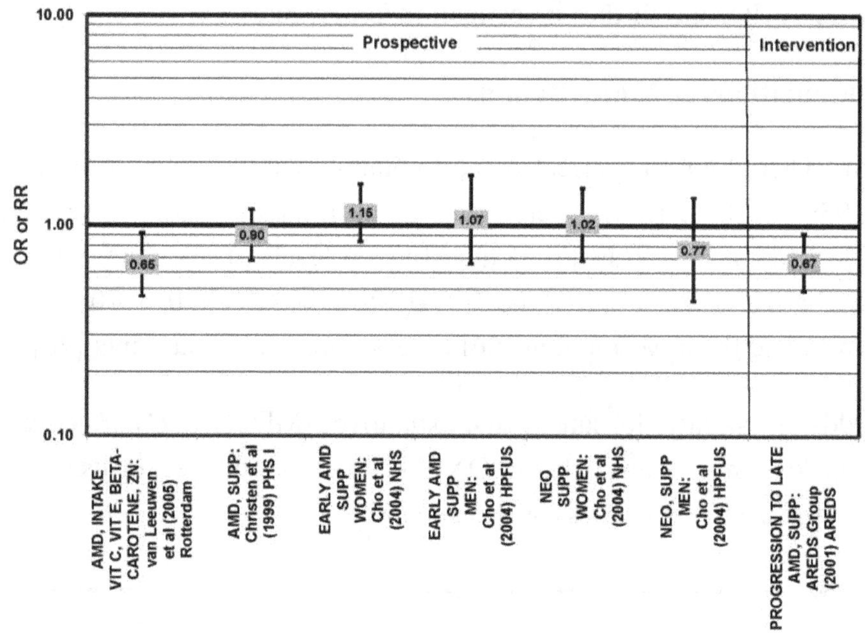

In the randomized, double masked, placebo controlled AREDS study, participants either received an antioxidant cocktail or placebo, Results indicated that supplementation with a cocktail of beta-carotene, vitamin E, vitamin C, zinc and copper reduced progression from intermediate to advanced AMD by 34% (95% CI: 0.47, 0.91) over about six years of follow-up [92,117,118] (Figure 37). Another clinical trial of 27 patients with early AMD showed that daily supplementation with 180 mg vitamin C, 30 mg vitamin E, 22.5 mg zinc, 1 mg copper, 10 mg lutein, 1 mg zeaxanthin and 4 mg astaxanthin improved function in the central retina as measured by electroretinogram ($p < 0.01$) (data not shown) [119].

In a double-masked, placebo controlled trial of dry AMD patients, it was shown that supplementation with vitamin E, zinc, magnesium, vitamin B6 and folate for 18 months maintained visual acuity, compared to placebo treatment, in which there was a decrease in visual acuity ($p = 0.03$). The antioxidant supplement group also reported greater vision stability in the areas of visual acuity and contrast sensitivity ($p = 0.05$) [120]. Another double-masked, placebo controlled trial of dry AMD patients found that supplementation with antioxidants and omega-3 fatty acids maintained visual acuity over six months, while the placebo group lost visual acuity ($p < 0.05$) [121].

The Carotenoids with Co-antioxidants in Age Related Maculopathy (CARMA) trial, a randomized, double masked placebo controlled clinical trial, gave 433 adults a daily dose of 12 mg lutein, 12 mg alpha tocopherol, 150 mg vitamin C, 20 mg zinc oxide and 0.4 mg copper gluconate. It was found that eyes in the supplemented group progressed along the AMD severity scale at a slower rate compared to the placebo group. However, there was no statistically significant difference between development of AMD in the supplemented *versus* placebo group [122]. Among the evidence that challenges a role for antioxidants and AMD is a case-control study of 72 cases and 66 controls, which could not find a significant association between antioxidant intake and AMD (OR = 0.56; 95% CI: 0.19, 1.67) [71]

(Figure 36). A cross-sectional analysis of 1968 participants of the Beaver Dam Eye Study showed that dietary antioxidants (measured with an antioxidant index) had no association with risk for early or late AMD [90] (Figures 35 and 36). A cross-sectional analysis of the baseline data from 2873 participants of the Blue Mountains Eye Study found vitamin supplements to be without effect on risk for early AMD (OR = 1.30; 95% CI: 0.90, 1.70) [123] (Figure 35). There was also no effect on risk for soft drusen (OR = 1.10; 95% CI: 0.80, 1.50) or AMD lesions (OR = 1.50; 95% CI: 0.70, 3.00) [123] (Figure 35). Further, prospective analysis of four examinations of the Beaver Dam Eye Study indicated that multivitamin supplementation had no effect on early or late AMD [109]. Among women in the NHS, as well as men in the HPFUS, there was no association between risk for early or neovascular AMD and use of a multivitamin supplement [95] (Figure 37). Finally, the Physicans Health Study reported that supplementation with a multivitamin had no effect on AMD (RR = 0.90; 95% CI: 0.68, 1.19) [113] (Figure 37).

Epidemiologic support for the value of antioxidant combinations deserves additional study. The AREDS trial indicates that multivitamin supplementing may be beneficial, and several smaller studies have corroborated such results. In addition, some studies have found that a dietary intake high in nutrients with antioxidant properties reduces risk of early AMD in individuals with high genetic risk [124]. Clearly, data from the AREDS II trial should be invaluable to determine whether or not supplementation with individual or specific combinations of nutrients provides advantage with regard to preserving retinal integrity. Furthermore, since multivitamins do not appear to be harmful to the retina, use of a supplement or eating a diet rich in fruits and vegetables may be an advisable practice, as well as consuming a diet rich in antioxidants, especially in those at high genetic risk [25,124].

10. Zinc

Zinc is essential for many physiological processes, including immunity, reproduction and neuronal development [125]. Since concentrations of zinc are very high in the retina, it has been hypothesized that zinc supplementation may aid retinal health.

There have been no case-control investigations of zinc and AMD risk. Retrospective analysis of 1968 participants of the Beaver Dam Eye study found that compared to people with the lowest amount of zinc intake from foods, those with the highest amount had a reduced risk for early AMD (OR = 0.60; 95% CI: 0.40, 1.00; $p < 0.05$). There was no association with late AMD [90] (Figure 38).

A cross-sectional study of 44 subjects indicated that while there was no difference in zinc and copper levels in the neural retina (analyzed *ex vivo*) between healthy subjects and those with AMD ($p > 0.09$), there was significantly less zinc and copper in the RPE and choroid in AMD patients compared to healthy subjects ($p = 0.002$) [126].

Prospective analysis of the Rotterdam study showed that among 4170 participants, increased consumption of zinc was associated with a reduced risk for any stage of AMD (HR = 0.91; 95% CI: 0.83, 0.98) [91] (Figure 39). Data from 1709 participants of the Beaver Dam Eye Study indicated that there was a decrease in risk for pigment abnormalities five years after baseline for those with past zinc intake (food and supplements) in the highest quintile (OR = 0.38; 95% CI: 0.20, 1.00; $p = 0.03$, for trend) [94] (Figure 39). A 10 year follow-up analysis showed that those with the highest zinc intake were at a reduced risk for any type of AMD (OR = 0.56; 95% CI: 0.32, 0.97), as well as early AMD (OR = 0.54; 95% CI: 0.32, 0.97), compared to all other participants [93] (Figure 39).

Figure 38. Odds or risk ratio for early AMD indicators, early AMD or late AMD; high *vs.* low intake of zinc: retrospective and cross-sectional studies.

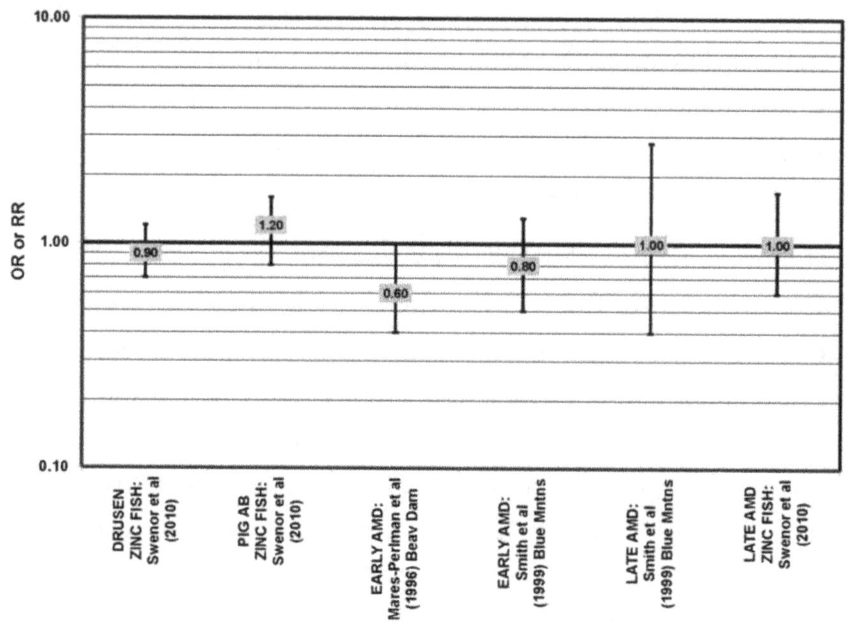

Figure 39. Odds or risk ratio for AMD, early AMD or late AMD; high *vs.* low intake (with or without supplements) of zinc: prospective and intervention studies.

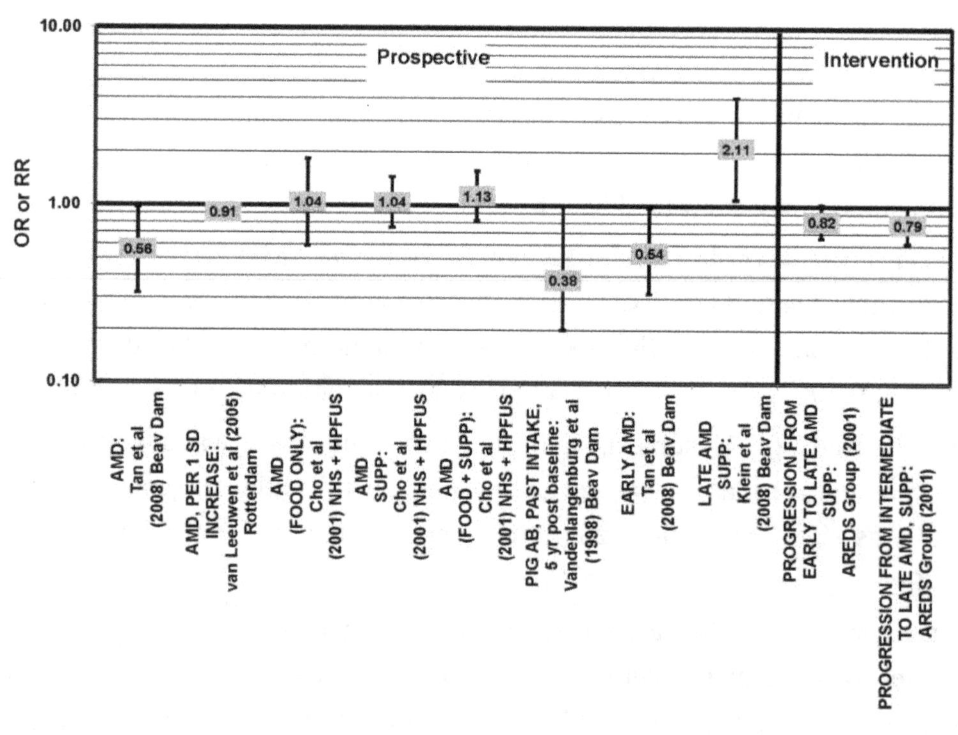

In AREDS, participants who consumed zinc were less likely to progress from intermediate to more advanced AMD than those who did not (OR = 0.79; 95% CI: 0.62, 0.99). However, there was no significant effect of zinc supplementation on progression to late AMD when the analysis included those with grade 2 AMD [117] (Figure 39). Other than the AREDS study, there have been a few clinical trials that have analyzed the effect of zinc on AMD. In a study of 90 subjects, Newsome *et al.* found that 100 mg zinc twice a day for two years reduced vision loss (one-tailed $p = 0.001$) [127]. Although this dose of zinc has been thought to induce toxicity in some patients, adverse effects related to zinc toxicity were not observed in the study population [127–129]. Another trial of 80 dry AMD patients found that supplementation with 25 mg zinc monocysteine twice a day for six months improved several indicators of retinal function, such as visual acuity, contrast sensitivity and macular flash recovery time ($p < 0.0001$) [130].

A large cross-sectional study of 2,873 participants of the Blue Mountains Eye Study found that zinc had no effect on early AMD [123]. This finding was confirmed in second analysis of slightly more subjects (3654) from the same study for early (OR = 0.80; 95% CI: 0.50, 1.30) or late AMD (OR = 1.00; 95% CI: 0.40, 2.80) [131] (Figure 38). Similarly, five years after baseline, zinc intake had no effect on early AMD incidence [92]. Swenor *et al.* found that compared to those who consumed less than 0.07 servings per week of fish with a high zinc content (for example, crab and oysters), those who consumed more than 0.07 servings per week did not have any change in risk for the appearance of drusen, pigment abnormalities or late AMD [59] (Figure 38).

A prospective study of 104,208 elderly men and women also showed that there was no association between risk for AMD and ten years of zinc intake (RR = 1.13; 95% CI: 0.82, 1.57) [132] (Figure 39). Compared to those with the lowest amount of zinc intake from food, those with the highest food intake did not have a reduced risk of AMD (RR = 1.04; 95% CI: 0.59, 1.83) [132] (Figure 39). There was also no association between AMD risk and zinc supplementation (RR = 1.04; 95% CI: 0.75, 1.45) [132] (Figure 39).

Although two trials have shown that zinc alone can improve vision, a placebo-controlled trial of 112 AMD subjects found that 200 mg zinc per day for two years had no effect on vision [133]. Analysis of the Beaver Dam Eye Study indicated that use of zinc supplements was associated with an increased risk for late AMD (OR = 2.11; 95% CI: 1.09, 4.07) [109] (Figure 39). In summary, the data to date is not robust, and we should await results from AREDS II to determine if zinc supplementation confers protection with regard to retinal function.

11. Vitamin D

There have been only a few observational studies regarding the role of vitamin D in ameliorating AMD risk [134] (Figures 40–42). Parekh *et al.* found that among 7752 participants of NHANES III, non-Hispanic whites with the highest serum levels of 1,25$(OH)_2$ vitamin D had a reduced risk for early AMD (OR = 0.64; 95% CI: 0.40, 0.90) compared to those with the lowest serum levels (Figure 40). However, there was no beneficial effect in non-Hispanic blacks or Mexican Americans (Figure 40). Combining all races, there was also a reduced risk for soft drusen in those with the highest serum levels of 1,25$(OH)_2$ vitamin D compared to those with the lowest levels (OR = 0.76; 95% CI: 0.60, 0.96) (Figure 40). There was no effect of serum levels of vitamin D on the appearance of pigment abnormalities or advanced AMD (Figure 40). Adjustments for sex and other covariates did not influence the observations [134].

Figure 40. Odds ratio for early AMD, indicators of early AMD (PIG AB, SOFT DRUSEN) or advanced AMD; high *vs.* low serum levels of vitamin D: retrospective studies.

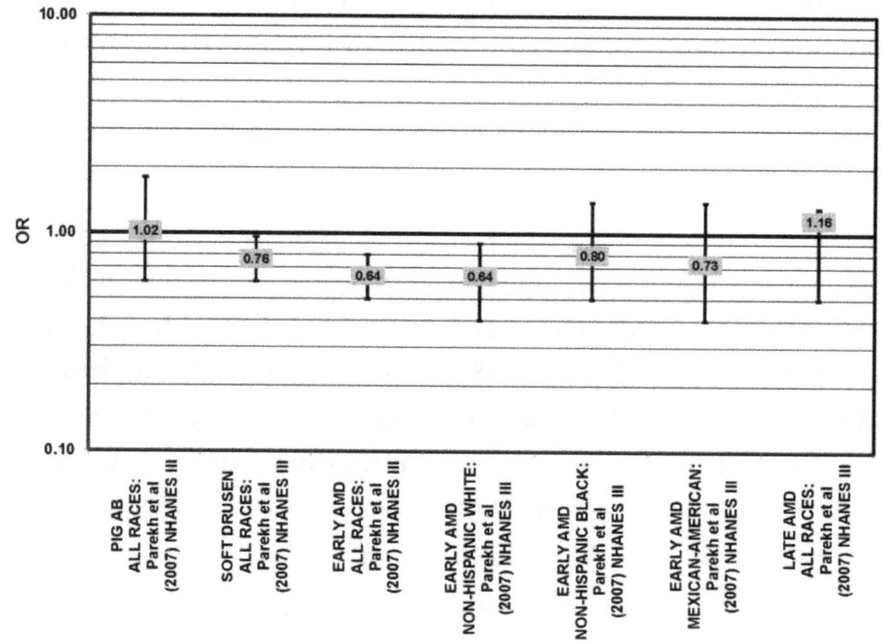

Figure 41. Odds ratio for early AMD, indicators of early AMD (PIG AB, SOFT DRUSEN) or advanced AMD; high *vs.* low intake of milk or fish in those at least 40 years of age: retrospective studies.

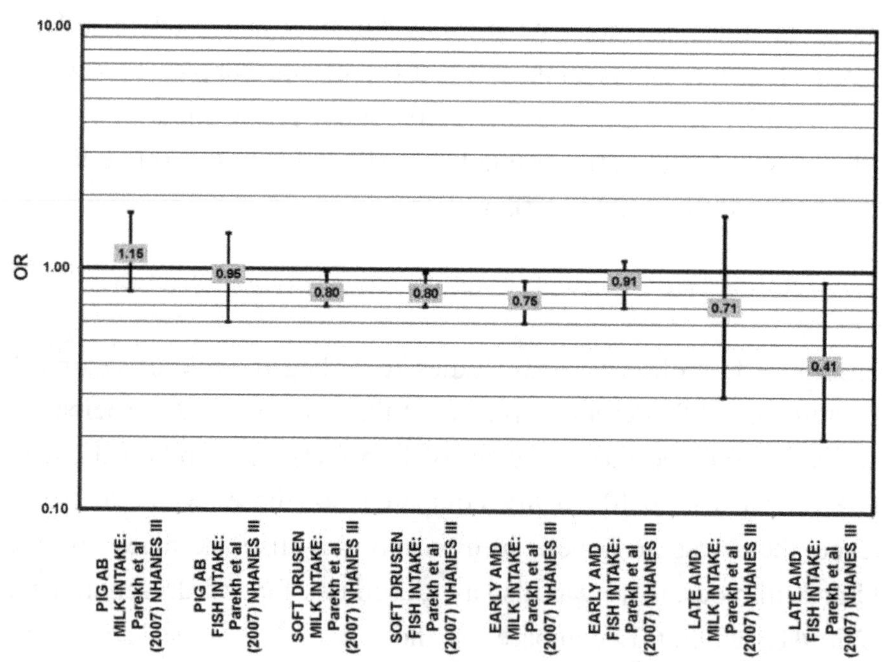

Figure 42. Odds ratio for early AMD, indicators of early AMD (SOFT DRUSEN, PIG AB) or advanced AMD upon vitamin D supplementation in in those at least 40 years of age who do not consume milk daily: retrospective studies.

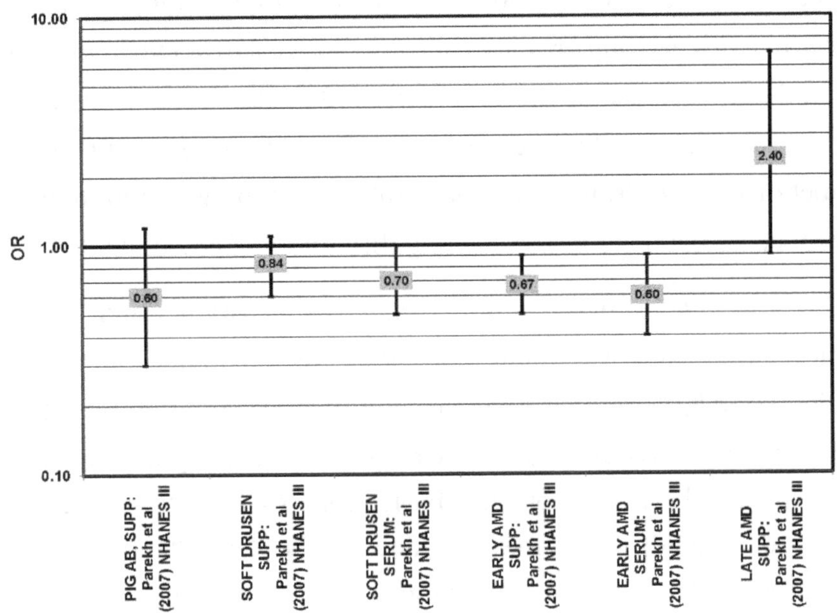

Millen *et al.* examined 1313 postmenopausal women and found a protective association of vitamin D status with the prevalence of AMD. In women younger than 75 years who had 25-hydroxyvitamin D (25[OH]D) concentrations higher than 38 nmol/L, there was a 48% decrease in the odds of early AMD. Adjustment for BMI and physical activity attenuated this observation. However, a statistically significant direct association between 25(OH) D and early AMD was observed in women aged 75 years or older (p for trend = 0.05). Additionally, significantly decreased odds of developing early AMD were observed among women in the fifth quintile for vitamin D intake [135].

Milk and fish are two of the most common sources of vitamin D in the American diet, and in exploratory analyses of the NHANES III study, it was found that among participants at least 40 years of age, those who consumed milk at least daily were at a reduced risk for early AMD (OR = 0.75; 95% CI: 0.60, 0.90) and soft drusen (OR = 0.80; 95% CI: 0.70, 0.98), compared to those who consumed it less than weekly (Figure 41). Pigment abnormalities and advanced AMD were not affected by milk consumption (Figure 41). In CAREDS, among women under age 75, those with the highest consumption of low-fat dairy products were at a reduced risk for intermediate AMD (OR = 0.50; 95% CI: 0.30, 0.80) [54] (Figure 15). Those over the age of 40 who consumed fish at least once a week were at a reduced risk for soft drusen (OR = 0.80; 95% CI: 0.70, 0.97) and advanced AMD (OR = 0.41; 95% CI: 0.20, 0.90), compared to those who consumed fish less than twice a month (Figure 41). For those in this age group that did not consume milk daily, supplementation did attenuate early AMD risk (OR = 0.67; 95% CI: 0.50, 0.90), but not risk for soft drusen, pigment abnormalities, or advanced AMD [134] (Figure 42). Although risk for early AMD did not correspond to risks associated with early AMD indicators, results of this study do leave open the possibility that vitamin D may help decrease risk for certain forms of AMD. The majority of data suggest a protective effect of Vitamin D on risk of certain forms of AMD.

12. Dietary Patterns

Diet is a potentially modifiable risk factor for AMD. As shown in the above sections, different nutritional factors may influence the development and/or progression of AMD. However, dietary components may interact with each other, either in a single food or a meal, and alteration in intake or elimination of one food may increase intake of another [136]. As shown above, associations of single nutrients and AMD are often inconsistent across studies. In addition, it is often difficult to disentangle single aspects of a diet or lifestyle from each other [137]. Examining overall diet quality in relation to AMD may better account for the relationships among different diet components [136].

A case control study of 696 men and women (437 AMD patients and 259 unrelated controls), measured dietary information using a 97-item block food frequency questionnaire, Health Habits and History Questionnaire (HHHQ)-DietSys Analysis software, Healthy Eating Index (HEI) and the Alternate Healthy Eating Index (AHEI). Those who were in the highest quartile, compared to the lowest, of diet quality using the AHEI, but not HEI, score were at significantly decreased odds of AMD (0.54, 95% CI 0.30–0.90). This may be due to the fact that the AHEI utilizes specific modifications to incorporate nutritional parameters related to chronic disease, such as emphasis on fat quality in addition to quantity [136]. In a study of 2005 women enrolled in CAREDS, diet quality was measured using a modified 2005 Healthy Eating Index score, and a six point healthy lifestyle score (HLS). Women in the highest quintile compared to the lowest for the mHEI score had 46% lower odds for early AMD (OR = 0.54; 95% CI, 0.33–0.88). Women whose diet scores were in the highest quintile, compared to the lowest, had diets significantly lower in fat (as a percent of energy) and diets higher in median servings of fish, vegetables, dairy, grains and meats or alternatives. The higher quintiles compared to the lower also had more physical activity and fewer years of smoking, lower likelihood of hypertension, lower systolic blood pressure, lower BMI and lower level of serum C-reactive protein. Furthermore, women who had a HLS score of six, which reflected the healthiest of three score components (smoking, physical activity and diet), had 71% lower odds for early AMD compared to those with scores 0–2 [137].

11. Conclusions

The proportion of the aged in many societies is growing exponentially. This imposes huge compromises to the public health budgets that must advance quality of life and avoid medical costs for these elderly citizens. Effective means to prevent progress to advanced AMD are clearly crucial toward this end. It appears that a diet that is regularly rich in fruits and vegetables, with sufficient fish, supports good retina health. Supplementation should be considered in the absence of sufficient regular dietary supplies of omega-3 fatty acids, lower glycemic index diets and several micronutrients. Overall healthy lifestyles, including diet, appear to also be beneficial for AMD. The results of the AREDS II trial will inform about the utility of nutrients, e.g., lutein, zeaxanthin, beta carotene and zinc with regard to retinal function.

Disclaimer

Any opinions, findings, conclusions, or recommendations expressed in this publication are those of the authors and do not necessarily reflect the views of the US Department of Agriculture.

References

1. Gehrs, K.M.; Anderson, D.H.; Johnson, L.V.; Hageman, G.S. Age-related macular degeneration-Emerging pathogenetic and therapeutic concepts. *Ann. Med.* **2006**, *38*, 450–471.
2. Biarnes, M.; Mones, J.; Alonso, J.; Arias, L. Update on geographic atrophy in age-related macular degeneration. *Optom. Vis. Sci.* **2011**, *88*, 881–889.
3. Klein, R.; Cruickshanks, K.J.; Nash, S.D.; Krantz, E.M.; Javier Nieto, F.; Huang, G.H.; Pankow, J.S.; Klein, B.E. The prevalence of age-related macular degeneration and associated risk factors. *Arch. Ophthalmol.* **2010**, *128*, 750–758.
4. The Bright Focus Foundation. Facts on Macular Degeneration, Macular Degeneration Research. 2012. Avaiable online: http://www.brightfocus.org/macular/about/understanding/facts.html. (accessed on 31 January 2013).
5. National Eye Institute, N.I.H. *Facts about Age-Related Macular Degeneration*; National Eye Institute: Bethesda, MD, USA, 2010.
6. Zarbin, M.A. Age-related macular degeneration: Review of pathogenesis. *Eur. J. Ophthalmol.* **1998**, *8*, 199–206.
7. Sung, C.H.; Chuang, J.Z. The cell biology of vision. *J. Cell Biol.* **2010**, *190*, 953–963.
8. Sivaprasad, S.; Bailey, T.A.; Chong, V.N. Bruch's membrane and the vascular intima: Is there a common basis for age-related changes and disease? *Clin. Exp. Ophthalmol.* **2005**, *33*, 518–523.
9. Shakib, M.; Zinn, K.M. Fine structure and function of ocular tissues. The choroid, bruch's membrane, and the retinal pigment epithelium. *Int. Ophthalmol. Clin.* **1973**, *13*, 189–204.
10. Curcio, C.A.; Millican, C.L. Basal linear deposit and large drusen are specific for early age-related maculopathy. *Arch. Ophthalmol.* **1999**, *117*, 329–339.
11. Ding, X.; Patel, M.; Chan, C.C. Molecular pathology of age-related macular degeneration. *Prog. Retin. Eye Res.* **2009**, *28*, 1–18.
12. Jager, R.D.; Mieler, W.F.; Miller, J.W. Age-related macular degeneration. *N. Engl. J. Med.* **2008**, *358*, 2606–2617.
13. Al-Hussaini, H.; Schneiders, M.; Lundh, P.; Jeffery, G. Drusen are associated with local and distant disruptions to human retinal pigment epithelium cells. *Exp. Eye Res.* **2009**, *88*, 610–612.
14. Wang, A.L.; Lukas, T.J.; Yuan, M.; Du, N.; Tso, M.O.; Neufeld, A.H. Autophagy and exosomes in the aged retinal pigment epithelium: Possible relevance to drusen formation and age-related macular degeneration. *PLoS One* **2009**, *4*, e4160.
15. Davis, M.D.; Gangnon, R.E.; Lee, L.Y.; Hubbard, L.D.; Klein, B.E.; Klein, R.; Ferris, F.L.; Bressler, S.B.; Milton, R.C. Age-Related Eye Disease Study Group. The age-related eye disease study severity scale for age-related macular degeneration: Areds report no. 17. *Arch. Ophthalmol.* **2005**, *123*, 1484–1498.

16. The Age-Related Eye Disease Study Research Group. The age-related eye disease study (areds) system for classifying cataracts from photographs: AREDS Report No. 4. *Am. J. Ophthalmol.* **2001**, *131*, 167–175.

17. Friedman, D.S.; O'Colmain, B.J.; Munoz, B.; Tomany, S.C.; McCarty, C.; de Jong, P.T.; Nemesure, B.; Mitchell, P.; Kempen, J.; Eye Diseases Prevalence Research Group. Prevalence of age-related macular degeneration in the united states. *Arch. Ophthalmol.* **2004**, *122*, 564–572.

18. Hageman, G.S.; Anderson, D.H.; Johnson, L.V.; Hancox, L.S.; Taiber, A.J.; Hardisty, L.I.; Hageman, J.L.; Stockman, H.A.; Borchardt, J.D.; Gehrs, K.M.; *et al.* A common haplotype in the complement regulatory gene factor h (hf1/cfh) predisposes individuals to age-related macular degeneration. *Proc. Natl. Acad. Sci. USA* **2005**, *102*, 7227–7232.

19. Edwards, A.O.; Ritter, R., III; Abel, K.J.; Manning, A.; Panhuysen, C.; Farrer, L.A. Complement factor h polymorphism and age-related macular degeneration. *Science* **2005**, *308*, 421–424.

20. Haines, J.L.; Hauser, M.A.; Schmidt, S.; Scott, W.K.; Olson, L.M.; Gallins, P.; Spencer, K.L.; Kwan, S.Y.; Noureddine, M.; Gilbert, J.R.; *et al.* Complement factor h variant increases the risk of age-related macular degeneration. *Science* **2005**, *308*, 419–421.

21. Klein, R.J.; Zeiss, C.; Chew, E.Y.; Tsai, J.Y.; Sackler, R.S.; Haynes, C.; Henning, A.K.; SanGiovanni, J.P.; Mane, S.M.; Mayne, S.T.; *et al.* Complement factor h polymorphism in age-related macular degeneration. *Science* **2005**, *308*, 385–389.

22. Gorin, M.B. Genetic insights into age-related macular degeneration: Controversies addressing risk, causality, and therapeutics. *Mol. Aspects Med.* **2012**, *33*, 467–486.

23. Peeters, A.; Magliano, D.J.; Stevens, J.; Duncan, B.B.; Klein, R.; Wong, T.Y. Changes in abdominal obesity and age-related macular degeneration: The atherosclerosis risk in communities study. *Arch. Ophthalmol.* **2008**, *126*, 1554–1560.

24. Smiddy, W.E.; Fine, S.L. Prognosis of patients with bilateral macular drusen. *Ophthalmology* **1984**, *91*, 271–277.

25. Weikel, K.A.; Chiu, C.J.; Taylor, A. Nutritional modulation of age-related macular degeneration. *Mol. Aspects Med.* **2012**, *33*, 318–375.

26. Jenkins, D.J.; Wolever, T.M.; Taylor, R.H.; Barker, H.; Fielden, H.; Baldwin, J.M.; Bowling, A.C.; Newman, H.C.; Jenkins, A.L.; Goff, D.V. Glycemic index of foods: A physiological basis for carbohydrate exchange. *Am. J. Clin. Nutr.* **1981**, *34*, 362–366.

27. Chiu, C.J.; Taylor, A. Dietary hyperglycemia, glycemic index and metabolic retinal diseases. *Prog. Retin. Eye Res.* **2011**, *30*, 18–53.

28. Chiu, C.-J.; Liu, S.; Willett, W.C.; Wolever, T.M.S.; Brand-Miller, J.C.; Barclay, A.C.; Taylor, A. Informing food choices and health outcomes by use of the dietary glycemic index. *Nutr. Rev.* **2011**, *69*, 231–242.

29. Chiu, C.J.; Milton, R.C.; Gensler, G.; Taylor, A. Association between dietary glycemic index and age-related macular degeneration in nondiabetic participants in the age-related eye disease study. *Am. J. Clin. Nutr.* **2007**, *86*, 180–188.

30. Chiu, C.J.; Hubbard, L.D.; Armstrong, J.; Rogers, G.; Jacques, P.F.; Chylack, L.T., Jr.; Hankinson, S.E.; Willett, W.C.; Taylor, A. Dietary glycemic index and carbohydrate in relation to early age-related macular degeneration. *Am. J. Clin. Nutr.* **2006**, *83*, 880–886.

31. Chiu, C.J.; Milton, R.C.; Klein, R.; Gensler, G.; Taylor, A. Dietary carbohydrate and the progression of age-related macular degeneration: A prospective study from the age-related eye disease study. *Am. J. Clin. Nutr.* **2007**, *86*, 1210–1218.

32. Chiu, C.J.; Klein, R.; Milton, R.C.; Gensler, G.; Taylor, A. Does eating particular diets alter risk of age-related macular degeneration in users of the age-related eye disease study supplements? *Br. J. Ophthalmol.* **2009**, *93*, 1241–1246.

33. Kaushik, S.; Wang, J.J.; Flood, V.; Tan, J.S.; Barclay, A.W.; Wong, T.Y.; Brand-Miller, J.; Mitchell, P. Dietary glycemic index and the risk of age-related macular degeneration. *Am. J. Clin. Nutr.* **2008**, *88*, 1104–1110.

34. Weikel, K.A.; Fitzgerald, P.; Shang, F.; Caceres, M.A.; Bian, Q.; Handa, J.T.; Stitt, A.W.; Taylor, A. Natural history of age-related retinal lesions that precede amd in mice fed high or low glycemic index diets. *Investig. Ophthalmol. Vis. Sci.* **2012**, *53*, 622–632.

35. Uchiki, T.; Weikel, K.A.; Jiao, W.; Shang, F.; Caceres, A.; Pawlak, D.B.; Handa, J.T.; Brownlee, M.; Nagaraj, R.; Taylor, A. Glycation-altered proteolysis as a pathobiologic mechanism that links dietary glycemic index, aging, and age-related disease (in non diabetics). *Aging Cell* **2012**, *11*, 1–13.

36. Ludwig, D.S. The glycemic index: Physiological mechanisms relating to obesity, diabetes, and cardiovascular disease. *JAMA* **2002**, *287*, 2414–2423.

37. Brand-Miller, J.C.; Holt, S.H.; Pawlak, D.B.; McMillan, J. Glycemic index and obesity. *Am. J. Clin. Nutr.* **2002**, *76*, 281S–285S.

38. Schweigert, F.J.; Reimann, J. Micronutrients and their relevance for the eye—Function of lutein, zeaxanthin and omega-3 fatty acids. *Klin. Monbl. Augenheilkd.* **2011**, *228*, 537–543.

39. Pilkington, S.M.; Watson, R.E.; Nicolaou, A.; Rhodes, L.E. Omega-3 polyunsaturated fatty acids: Photoprotective macronutrients. *Exp. Dermatol.* **2011**, *20*, 537–543.

40. Seddon, J.M.; Rosner, B.; Sperduto, R.D.; Yannuzzi, L.; Haller, J.A.; Blair, N.P.; Willett, W. Dietary fat and risk for advanced age-related macular degeneration. *Arch. Ophthalmol.* **2001**, *119*, 1191–1199.

41. Seddon, J.M.; George, S.; Rosner, B. Cigarette smoking, fish consumption, omega-3 fatty acid intake, and associations with age-related macular degeneration: The us twin study of age-related macular degeneration. *Arch. Ophthalmol.* **2006**, *124*, 995–1001.

42. SanGiovanni, J.P.; Chew, E.Y.; Clemons, T.E.; Davis, M.D.; Ferris, F.L., III; Gensler, G.R.; Kurinij, N.; Lindblad, A.S.; Milton, R.C.; Seddon, J.M.; *et al.* The relationship of dietary lipid intake and age-related macular degeneration in a case-control study: Areds report no. 20. *Arch. Ophthalmol.* **2007**, *125*, 671–679.

43. Christen, W.G.; Schaumberg, D.A.; Glynn, R.J.; Buring, J.E. Dietary omega-3 fatty acid and fish intake and incident age-related macular degeneration in women. *Arch. Ophthalmol.* **2011**, *129*, 921–929.

44. Cho, E.; Hung, S.; Willett, W.C.; Spiegelman, D.; Rimm, E.B.; Seddon, J.M.; Colditz, G.A.; Hankinson, S.E. Prospective study of dietary fat and the risk of age-related macular degeneration. *Am. J. Clin. Nutr.* **2001**, *73*, 209–218.

45. Chong, E.W.; Robman, L.D.; Simpson, J.A.; Hodge, A.M.; Aung, K.Z.; Dolphin, T.K.; English, D.R.; Giles, G.G.; Guymer, R.H. Fat consumption and its association with age-related macular degeneration. *Arch. Ophthalmol.* **2009**, *127*, 674–680.
46. Tan, J.S.; Wang, J.J.; Flood, V.; Mitchell, P. Dietary fatty acids and the 10-year incidence of age-related macular degeneration: The blue mountains eye study. *Arch. Ophthalmol.* **2009**, *127*, 656–665.
47. Chua, B.; Flood, V.; Rochtchina, E.; Wang, J.J.; Smith, W.; Mitchell, P. Dietary fatty acids and the 5-year incidence of age-related maculopathy. *Arch. Ophthalmol.* **2006**, *124*, 981–986.
48. Augood, C.; Chakravarthy, U.; Young, I.; Vioque, J.; de Jong, P.T.; Bentham, G.; Rahu, M.; Seland, J.; Soubrane, G.; Tomazzoli, L.; *et al.* Oily fish consumption, dietary docosahexaenoic acid and eicosapentaenoic acid intakes, and associations with neovascular age-related macular degeneration. *Am. J. Clin. Nutr.* **2008**, *88*, 398–406.
49. Johnson, E.J.; Chung, H.Y.; Caldarella, S.M.; Snodderly, D.M. The influence of supplemental lutein and docosahexaenoic acid on serum, lipoproteins, and macular pigmentation. *Am. J. Clin. Nutr.* **2008**, *87*, 1521–1529.
50. Souied, E.H.; Delcourt, C.; Querques, G.; Bassols, A.; Merle, B.; Zourdani, A.; Smith, T.; Benlian, P. Oral docosahexaenoic acid in the prevention of exudative age-related macular degeneration: The nutritional amd treatment 2 study. *Ophthalmology* **2013**, *7*, 7–9.
51. Mance, T.C.; Kovacevic, D.; Alpeza-Dunato, Z.; Stroligo, M.N.; Brumini, G. The role of omega6 to omega3 ratio in development and progression of age-related macular degeneration. *Coll. Antropol.* **2011**, *2*, 307–310.
52. Chiu, C.J.; Milton, R.C.; Klein, R.; Gensler, G.; Taylor, A. Dietary compound score and risk of age-related macular degeneration in the age-related eye disease study. *Ophthalmology* **2009**, *116*, 939–946.
53. Mares-Perlman, J.A.; Brady, W.E.; Klein, R.; VandenLangenberg, G.M.; Klein, B.E.; Palta, M. Dietary fat and age-related maculopathy. *Arch. Ophthalmol.* **1995**, *113*, 743–748.
54. Parekh, N.; Voland, R.P.; Moeller, S.M.; Blodi, B.A.; Ritenbaugh, C.; Chappell, R.J.; Wallace, R.B.; Mares, J.A. Association between dietary fat intake and age-related macular degeneration in the carotenoids in age-related eye disease study (careds): An ancillary study of the women's health initiative. *Arch. Ophthalmol.* **2009**, *127*, 1483–1493.
55. Robman, L.; Vu, H.; Hodge, A.; Tikellis, G.; Dimitrov, P.; McCarty, C.; Guymer, R. Dietary lutein, zeaxanthin, and fats and the progression of age-related macular degeneration. *Can. J. Ophthalmol.* **2007**, *42*, 720–726.
56. Meyer, B.J.; Mann, N.J.; Lewis, J.L.; Milligan, G.C.; Sinclair, A.J.; Howe, P.R. Dietary intakes and food sources of omega-6 and omega-3 polyunsaturated fatty acids. *Lipids* **2003**, *38*, 391–398.
57. Seddon, J.M.; Cote, J.; Rosner, B. Progression of age-related macular degeneration: Association with dietary fat, transunsaturated fat, nuts, and fish intake. *Arch. Ophthalmol.* **2003**, *121*, 1728–1737.
58. Smith, W.; Mitchell, P.; Leeder, S.R. Dietary fat and fish intake and age-related maculopathy. *Arch. Ophthalmol.* **2000**, *118*, 401–404.
59. Swenor, B.K.; Bressler, S.; Caulfield, L.; West, S.K. The impact of fish and shellfish consumption on age-related macular degeneration. *Ophthalmology* **2010**, *117*, 2395–2401.

60. Delcourt, C.; Carriere, I.; Cristol, J.P.; Lacroux, A.; Gerber, M. Dietary fat and the risk of age-related maculopathy: The polanut study. *Eur. J. Clin. Nutr.* **2007**, *61*, 1341–1344.

61. Heuberger, R.A.; Mares-Perlman, J.A.; Klein, R.; Klein, B.E.; Millen, A.E.; Palta, M. Relationship of dietary fat to age-related maculopathy in the third national health and nutrition examination survey. *Arch. Ophthalmol.* **2001**, *119*, 1833–1838.

62. Granado, F.; Olmedilla, B.; Blanco, I. Nutritional and clinical relevance of lutein in human health. *Br. J. Nutr.* **2003**, *90*, 487–502.

63. Dictzcl, M.; Zcimcr, M.; Heimes, B.; Claes, B.; Pauleikhoff, D.; Hense, H.W. Determinants of macular pigment optical density and its relation to age-related maculopathy: Results from the muenster aging and retina study (mars). *Investig. Ophthalmol. Vis. Sci.* **2011**, *52*, 3452–3457.

64. Schalch, W.; Cohn, W.; Barker, F.M.; Kopcke, W.; Mellerio, J.; Bird, A.C.; Robson, A.G.; Fitzke, F.F.; van Kuijk, F.J. Xanthophyll accumulation in the human retina during supplementation with lutein or zeaxanthin—The luxea (lutein xanthophyll eye accumulation) study. *Arch. Biochem. Biophys.* **2007**, *458*, 128–135.

65. Landrum, J.T.; Bone, R.A.; Joa, H.; Kilburn, M.D.; Moore, L.L.; Sprague, K.E. A one year study of the macular pigment: The effect of 140 days of a lutein supplement. *Exp. Eye Res.* **1997**, *65*, 57–62.

66. Hammond, B.R., Jr.; Johnson, E.J.; Russell, R.M.; Krinsky, N.I.; Yeum, K.-J.; Edwards, R.B.; Snodderly, D.M. Dietary modification of human macular pigment density. *Investig. Ophthalmol. Vis. Sci.* **1997**, *38*, 1795–1801.

67. Ma, L.; Dou, H.-L.; Wu, Y.-Q.; Huang, Y.-M.; Huang, Y.-B.; Xu, X.-R.; Zou, Z.-Y.; Lin, X.-M. Lutein and zeaxanthin intake and the risk of age-related macular degeneration: A systematic review and meta-analysis. *Br. J. Nutr.* **2012**, *107*, 350–359.

68. SanGiovanni, J.P.; Neuringer, M. The putative role of lutein and zeaxanthin as protective agents against age-related macular degeneration: Promise of molecular genetics for guiding mechanistic and translational research in the field. *Am. J. Clin. Nutr.* **2012**, *96*, 10.

69. Seddon, J.M.; Ajani, U.A.; Sperduto, R.D.; Hiller, R.; Blair, N.; Burton, T.C.; Farber, M.D.; Gragoudas, E.S.; Haller, J.; Miller, D.T.; *et al.* Dietary carotenoids, vitamins a, c, and e, and advanced age-related macular degeneration. Eye disease case-control study group. *JAMA* **1994**, *272*, 1413–1420.

70. Eye Disease Case-Control Study Group. Antioxidant status and neovascular age-related macular degeneration. *Arch. Ophthalmol.* **1993**, *111*, 104–109.

71. Snellen, E.L.; Verbeek, A.L.; van den Hoogen, G.W.; Cruysberg, J.R.; Hoyng, C.B. Neovascular age-related macular degeneration and its relationship to antioxidant intake. *Acta Ophthalmol. Scand.* **2002**, *80*, 368–371.

72. Gale, C.R.; Hall, N.F.; Phillips, D.I.W.; Martyn, C.N. Lutein and zeaxanthin status and risk of age-related macular degeneration. *Investig. Ophthalmol. Vis. Sci.* **2003**, *44*, 2461–2465.

73. Delcourt, C.; Carriere, I.; Delage, M.; Barberger-Gateau, P.; Schalch, W. Plasma lutein and zeaxanthin and other carotenoids as modifiable risk factors for age-related maculopathy and cataract: The pola study. *Investig. Ophthalmol. Vis. Sci.* **2006**, *47*, 2329–2335.

74. Mares-Perlman, J.A.; Fisher, A.I.; Klein, R.; Palta, M.; Block, G.; Millen, A.E.; Wright, J.D. Lutein and zeaxanthin in the diet and serum and their relation to age-related maculopathy in the third national health and nutrition examination survey. *Am. J. Epidemiol.* **2001**, *153*, 424–432.
75. Bucheli, P.; Vidal, K.; Shen, L.; Gu, Z.; Zhang, C.; Miller, L.E.; Wang, J. Goji berry effects on macular characteristics and plasma antioxidant levels. *Optom. Vis. Sci.* **2011**, *88*, 257–262.
76. Zeimer, M.; Hense, H.W.; Heimes, B.; Austermann, U.; Fobker, M.; Pauleikhoff, D. The macular pigment: Short- and intermediate-term changes of macular pigment optical density following supplementation with lutein and zeaxanthin and co-antioxidants. The luna study. *Ophthalmologe* **2009**, *106*, 29–36.
77. Bone, R.A.; Landrum, J.T. Dose-dependent response of serum lutein and macular pigment optical density to supplementation with lutein esters. *Arch. Biochem. Biophys.* **2010**, *504*, 50–55.
78. Loughman, J.; Nolan, J.M.; Howard, A.N.; Connolly, E.; Meagher, K.; Beatty, S. The impact of macular pigment augmentation on visual performance using different carotenoid formulations. *Investig. Ophthalmol. Vis. Sci.* **2012**, *53*, 7871–7880.
79. Ma, L.; Yan, S.F.; Huang, Y.M.; Lu, X.R.; Qian, F.; Pang, H.L.; Xu, X.R.; Zou, Z.Y.; Dong, P.C.; Xiao, X.; *et al.* Effect of lutein and zeaxanthin on macular pigment and visual function in patients with early age-related macular degeneration. *Ophthalmology* **2012**, *119*, 2290–2297.
80. Richer, S.P.; Stiles, W.; Graham-Hoffman, K.; Levin, M.; Ruskin, D.; Wrobel, J.; Park, D.W.; Thomas, C. Randomized, double-blind, placebo-controlled study of zeaxanthin and visual function in patients with atrophic age-related macular degeneration: The zeaxanthin and visual function study (zvf) fda ind #78, 973. *Optometry* **2011**, *82*, 667–680.
81. Piermarocchi, S.; Saviano, S.; Parisi, V.; Tedeschi, M.; Panozzo, G.; Scarpa, G.; Boschi, G.; Lo Giudice, G. Carotenoids in age-related maculopathy italian study (CARMIS): Two-year results of a randomized study. *Eur. J. Ophthalmol.* **2012**, *22*, 216–225.
82. Richer, S.; Stiles, W.; Statkute, L.; Pulido, J.; Frankowski, J.; Rudy, D.; Pei, K.; Tsipursky, M.; Nyland, J. Double-masked, placebo-controlled, randomized trial of lutein and antioxidant supplementation in the intervention of atrophic age-related macular degeneration: The veterans last study (lutein antioxidant supplementation trial). *Optometry* **2004**, *75*, 216–230.
83. Richer, S.; Devenport, J.; Lang, J.C. Last ii: Differential temporal responses of macular pigment optical density in patients with atrophic age-related macular degeneration to dietary supplementation with xanthophylls. *Optometry* **2007**, *78*, 213–219.
84. Trieschmann, M.; Beatty, S.; Nolan, J.M.; Hense, H.W.; Heimes, B.; Austermann, U.; Fobker, M.; Pauleikhoff, D. Changes in macular pigment optical density and serum concentrations of its constituent carotenoids following supplemental lutein and zeaxanthin: The luna study. *Exp. Eye Res.* **2007**, *84*, 718–728.
85. Cardinault, N.; Abalain, J.H.; Sairafi, B.; Coudray, C.; Grolier, P.; Rambeau, M.; Carre, J.L.; Mazur, A.; Rock, E. Lycopene but not lutein nor zeaxanthin decreases in serum and lipoproteins in age-related macular degeneration patients. *Clin. Chim. Acta* **2005**, *357*, 34–42.
86. Sanders, T.A.B.; Haines, A.P.; Wormald, R.; Wright, L.A.; Obeid, O. Essential fatty acids, plasma cholesterol, and fat-soluble vitamins in subjects with age-related maculopathy and matched control subjects. *Am. J. Clin. Nutr.* **1993**, *57*, 428–433.

87. Seddon, J.M.; Reynolds, R.; Rosner, B. Associations of smoking, body mass index, dietary lutein, and the lipc gene variant rs10468017 with advanced age-related macular degeneration. *Mol. Vis.* **2010**, *16*, 2412–2424.
88. Michikawa, T.; Ishida, S.; Nishiwaki, Y.; Kikuchi, Y.; Tsuboi, T.; Hosoda, K.; Ishigami, A.; Iwasawa, S.; Nakano, M.; Takebayashi, T. Serum antioxidants and age-related macular degeneration among older japanese. *Asia Pac. J. Clin. Nutr.* **2009**, *18*, 1–7.
89. Fletcher, A.E.; Bentham, G.C.; Agnew, M.; Young, I.S.; Augood, C.; Chakravarthy, U.; de Jong, P.T.; Rahu, M.; Seland, J.; Soubrane, G.; *et al.* Sunlight exposure, antioxidants, and age-related macular degeneration. *Arch. Ophthalmol.* **2008**, *126*, 1396–1403.
90. Mares-Perlman, J.; Klein, R.; Klein, B.E.K.; Greger, J.L.; Brady, W.E.; Palta, M.; Ritter, L.L. Association of zinc and antioxidant nutrients with age-related maculopathy. *Arch. Ophthalmol.* **1996**, *114*, 991–997.
91. Van Leeuwen, R.; Boekhoorn, S.; Vingerling, J.R.; Witteman, J.C.; Klaver, C.C.; Hofman, A.; de Jong, P.T. Dietary intake of antioxidants and risk of age-related macular degeneration. *JAMA* **2005**, *294*, 3101–3107.
92. Flood, V.; Smith, W.; Wang, J.J.; Manzi, F.; Webb, K.; Mitchell, P. Dietary antioxidant intake and incidence of early age-related maculopathy: The blue mountains eye study. *Ophthalmology* **2002**, *109*, 2272–2278.
93. Tan, J.S.; Wang, J.J.; Flood, V.; Rochtchina, E.; Smith, W.; Mitchell, P. Dietary antioxidants and the long-term incidence of age-related macular degeneration: The blue mountains eye study. *Ophthalmology* **2008**, *115*, 334–341.
94. VandenLangenberg, G.M.; Mares-Perlman, J.A.; Klein, R.; Klein, B.E.; Brady, W.E.; Palta, M. Associations between antioxidant and zinc intake and the 5-year incidence of early age-related maculopathy in the beaver dam eye study. *Am. J. Epidemiol.* **1998**, *148*, 204–214.
95. Cho, E.; Seddon, J.M.; Rosner, B.; Willett, W.C.; Hankinson, S.E. Prospective study of intake of fruits, vegetables, vitamins, and carotenoids and risk of age-related maculopathy. *Arch. Ophthalmol.* **2004**, *122*, 883–892.
96. Cho, E.; Hankinson, S.E.; Rosner, B.; Willett, W.C.; Colditz, G.A. Prospective study of lutein/zeaxanthin intake and risk of age-related macular degeneration. *Am. J. Clin. Nutr.* **2008**, *87*, 1837–1843.
97. Smith, W.; Mitchell, P.; Rochester, C. Serum beta carotene, alpha tocopherol, and age-related maculopathy: The blue mountains eye study. *Am. J. Ophthalmol.* **1997**, *124*, 838–840.
98. Mares-Perlman, J.A.; Brady, W.E.; Klein, R.; Klein, B.E.; Bowen, P.; Stacewicz-Sapuntzakis, M.; Palta, M. Serum antioxidants and age-related macular degeneration in a population-based case-control study. *Arch. Ophthalmol.* **1995**, *113*, 1518–1523.
99. San Giovanni, J.P.; Chew, E.Y.; Clemons, T.E.; Ferris, F.L., III; Gensler, G.; Lindblad, A.S.; Milton, R.C.; Seddon, J.M.; Sperduto, R.D. The relationship of dietary carotenoid and vitamin a, e, and c intake with age-related macular degeneration in a case-control study: Areds report no. 22. *Arch. Ophthalmol.* **2007**, *125*, 1225–1232.
100. West, S.; Vitale, S.; Hallfrisch, J.; Munoz, B.; Muller, D.; Bressler, S.; Bressler, N.M. Are antioxidants or supplements protective for age-related macular degeneration? *Arch. Ophthalmol.* **1994**, *112*, 222–227.

101. Teikari, J.M.; Laatikainen, L.; Virtamo, J.; Haukka, J.; Rautalahti, M.; Liesto, K.; Albanes, D.; Taylor, P.; Heinonen, O.P. Six-year supplementation with alpha-tocopherol and beta-carotene and age-related maculopathy. *Acta Ophthalmol. Scand.* **1998**, *76*, 224–229.
102. Morris, M.S.; Jacques, P.F.; Chylack, L.T.; Hankinson, S.E.; Willett, W.C.; Hubbard, L.D.; Taylor, A. Intake of zinc and antioxidant micronutrients and early age-related maculopathy lesions. *Ophthalmic Epidemiol.* **2007**, *14*, 288–298.
103. Maiani, G.; Caston, M.J.; Catasta, G.; Toti, E.; Cambrodon, I.G.; Bysted, A.; Granado-Lorencio, F.; Olmedilla-Alonso, B.; Knuthsen, P.; Valoti, M.; *et al.* Carotenoids: Actual knowledge on food sources, intakes, stability and bioavailability and their protective role in humans. *Mol. Nutr. Food Res.* **2009**, *53*, S194–S218.
104. Simonelli, F.; Zarrilli, F.; Mazzeo, S.; Verde, V.; Romano, N.; Savoia, M.; Testa, F.; Vitale, D.F.; Rinaldi, M.; Sacchetti, L. Serum oxidative and antioxidant parameters in a group of italian patients with age-related maculopathy. *Clin. Chim. Acta* **2002**, *320*, 111–115.
105. Obana, A.; Hiramitsu, T.; Gohto, Y.; Ohira, A.; Mizuno, S.; Hirano, T.; Bernstein, P.S.; Fujii, H.; Iseki, K.; Tanito, M.; *et al.* Macular carotenoid levels of normal subjects and age-related maculopathy patients in a japanese population. *Ophthalmology* **2008**, *115*, 147–157.
106. Blumenkranz, M.S.; Russell, S.R.; Robey, M.G.; Kott-Blumenkranz, R.; Penneys, N. Risk factors in age-related maculopathy complicated by choroidal neovascularization. *Ophthalmology* **1986**, *93*, 552–558.
107. Ishihara, N.; Yuzawa, M.; Tamakoshi, A. Antioxidants and angiogenetic factor associated with age-related macular degeneration (exudative type). *Nippon Ganka Gakkai Zasshi* **1997**, *101*, 248–251.
108. Goldberg, J.; Flowerdew, G.; Smith, E.; Brody, J.A.; Tso, M.O.M. Factors associated with age-related macular degeneration. *Am. J. Epidemiol.* **1988**, *128*, 700–710.
109. Klein, B.E.; Knudtson, M.D.; Lee, K.E.; Reinke, J.O.; Danforth, L.G.; Wealti, A.M.; Moore, E.; Klein, R. Supplements and age-related eye conditions the beaver dam eye study. *Ophthalmology* **2008**, *115*, 1203–1208.
110. Belda, J.I.; Roma, J.; Vilela, C.; Puertas, F.J.; Diaz-Llopis, M.; Bosch-Morell, F.; Romero, F.J. Serum vitamin e levels negatively correlate with severity of age-related macular degeneration. *Mech. Ageing Dev.* **1999**, *107*, 159–164.
111. Delcourt, C.; Cristol, J.P.; Tessier, F.; Leger, C.L.; Descomps, B.; Papoz, L. Age-related macular degeneration and antioxidant status in the pola study. Pola study group. Pathologies oculaires liees a l'age. *Arch. Ophthalmol.* **1999**, *117*, 1384–1390.
112. Shen, X.L.; Jia, J.H.; Zhao, P.; Fan, R.; Pan, X.Y.; Yang, H.M.; Liu, L. Changes in blood oxidative and antioxidant parameters in a group of chinese patients with age-related macular degeneration. *J. Nutr. Health Aging* **2012**, *16*, 201–204.
113. Christen, W.G.; Ajani, U.A.; Glynn, R.J.; Manson, J.E.; Schaumberg, D.A.; Chew, E.C.; Buring, J.E.; Hennekens, C.H. Prospective cohort study of antioxidant vitamin supplement use and the risk of age-related maculopathy. *Am. J. Epidemiol.* **1999**, *149*, 476–484.
114. Christen, W.G.; Glynn, R.J.; Sesso, H.D.; Kurth, T.; MacFadyen, J.; Bubes, V.; Buring, J.E.; Manson, J.E.; Gaziano, J.M. Age-related cataract in a randomized trial of vitamins e and c in men. *Arch. Ophthalmol.* **2010**, *128*, 1397–1405.

115. Taylor, H.R.; Tikellis, G.; Robman, L.D.; McCarty, C.A.; McNeil, J.J. Vitamin e supplementation and macular degeneration: Randomised controlled trial. *BMJ* **2002**, *325*, 11.
116. Christen, W.G.; Glynn, R.J.; Sesso, H.D.; Kurth, T.; Macfadyen, J.; Bubes, V.; Buring, J.E.; Manson, J.E.; Gaziano, J.M. Vitamins e and c and medical record-confirmed age-related macular degeneration in a randomized trial of male physicians. *Ophthalmology* **2012**, *119*, 1642–1649.
117. Age-Related Eye Disease Study Research Group. A randomized, placebo-controlled, clinical trial of high-dose supplementation with vitamins c and e and beta carotene for age-related cataract and vision loss: Areds report no. 9. *Arch. Ophthalmol.* **2001**, *119*, 1439–1452.
118. Chew, E.Y.; Lindblad, A.S.; Clemons, T. Summary results and recommendations from the age-related eye disease study. *Arch. Ophthalmol.* **2009**, *127*, 1678–1679.
119. Parisi, V.; Tedeschi, M.; Gallinaro, G.; Varano, M.; Saviano, S.; Piermarocchi, S. Carotenoids and antioxidants in age-related maculopathy italian study: Multifocal electroretinogram modifications after 1 year. *Ophthalmology* **2008**, *115*, 324–333.
120. Richer, S. Multicenter ophthalmic and nutritional age-related macular degeneration study—Part 2: Antioxidant intervention and conclusions. *J. Am. Optom. Assoc.* **1996**, *67*, 30–49.
121. Cangemi, F.E. Tozal study: An open case control study of an oral antioxidant and omega-3 supplement for dry amd. *BMC Ophthalmol.* **2007**, *7*, 3.
122. Beatty, S.; Chakravarthy, U.; Nolan, J.M.; Muldrew, K.A.; Woodside, J.V.; Denny, F.; Stevenson, M.R. Secondary outcomes in a clinical trial of carotenoids with coantioxidants *versus* placebo in early age-related macular degeneration. *Ophthalmology* **2012**, *120*, 600–606.
123. Kuzniarz, M.; Mitchell, P.; Flood, V.M.; Wang, J.J. Use of vitamin and zinc supplements and age-related maculopathy: The blue mountains eye study. *Ophthalmic Epidemiol.* **2002**, *9*, 283–295.
124. Ho, L.; van Leeuwen, R.; Witteman, J.C.; van Duijn, C.M.; Uitterlinden, A.G.; Hofman, A.; de Jong, P.T.; Vingerling, J.R.; Klaver, C.C. Reducing the genetic risk of age-related macular degeneration with dietary antioxidants, zinc, and omega-3 fatty acids: The rotterdam study. *Arch. Ophthalmol.* **2011**, *129*, 758–766.
125. King, J.C. Zinc: An essential but elusive nutrient. *Am. J. Clin. Nutr.* **2011**, *94*, 679S–684S.
126. Erie, J.C.; Good, J.A.; Butz, J.A.; Pulido, J.S. Reduced zinc and copper in the retinal pigment epithelium and choroid in age-related macular degeneration. *Am. J. Ophthalmol.* **2009**, *147*, 276–282.
127. Newsome, D.A.; Swartz, M.; Leone, N.C.; Elston, R.C.; Miller, E. Oral zinc in macular degeneration. *Arch. Ophthalmol.* **1988**, *106*, 192–198.
128. Yuzbasiyan-Gurkan, V.; Brewer, G.J. The therapeutic use of zinc in macular degeneration. *Arch. Ophthalmol.* **1989**, *107*, 1723–1724.
129. Trempe, C.L. Zinc and macular degeneration. *Arch. Ophthalmol.* **1992**, *110*, 1517.
130. Newsome, D.A. A randomized, prospective, placebo-controlled clinical trial of a novel zinc-monocysteine compound in age-related macular degeneration. *Curr. Eye Res.* **2008**, *33*, 591–598.
131. Smith, W.; Mitchell, P.; Webb, K.; Leeder, S.R. Dietary antioxidants and age-related maculopathy: The blue mountains eye study. *Ophthalmology* **1999**, *106*, 761–767.

132. Cho, E.; Stampfer, M.J.; Seddon, J.M.; Hung, S.; Spiegelman, D.; Rimm, E.B.; Willett, W.C.; Hankinson, S.E. Prospective study of zinc intake and the risk of age-related macular degeneration. *Ann. Epidemiol.* **2001**, *11*, 328–336.

133. Stur, M.; Tittl, M.; Reitner, A.; Meisinger, V. Oral zinc and the second eye in age-related macular degeneration. *Investig. Ophthalmol. Vis. Sci.* **1996**, *37*, 1225–1235.

134. Parekh, N.; Chappell, R.J.; Millen, A.E.; Albert, D.M.; Mares, J.A. Association between vitamin d and age-related macular degeneration in the third national health and nutrition examination survey, 1988 through 1994. *Arch. Ophthalmol.* **2007**, *125*, 661–669.

135. Millen, A.E.; Voland, R.; Sondel, S.A.; Parekh, N.; Horst, R.L.; Wallace, R.B.; Hageman, G.S.; Chappell, R.; Blodi, B.A.; Klein, M.L.; *et al.* Vitamin d status and early age-related macular degeneration in postmenopausal women. *Arch. Ophthalmol.* **2011**, *129*, 481–489.

136. Montgomery, M.P.; Kamel, F.; Pericak-Vance, M.A.; Haines, J.L.; Postel, E.A.; Agarwal, A.; Richards, M.; Scott, W.K.; Schmidt, S. Overall diet quality and age-related macular degeneration. *Ophthalmic Epidemiol.* **2010**, *17*, 58–65.

137. Mares, J.A.; Voland, R.P.; Sondel, S.A.; Millen, A.E.; Larowe, T.; Moeller, S.M.; Klein, M.L.; Blodi, B.A.; Chappell, R.J.; Tinker, L.; *et al.* Healthy lifestyles related to subsequent prevalence of age-related macular degeneration. *Arch. Ophthalmol.* **2011**, *129*, 470–480.

7

Effects of Lutein and Docosahexaenoic Acid Supplementation on Macular Pigment Optical Density

Alfredo García-Layana *, Sergio Recalde, Angel Salinas Alamán and Patricia Fernández Robredo

Ophthalmology Department, Clinica Universidad de Navarra, C/Pio XII 36, 31080, Pamplona, Spain; E-Mails: srecalde@unav.es (S.R.); asalinas@unav.es (A.S.A.); pfrobredo@unav.es (P.F.R.)

* Author to whom correspondence should be addressed; E-Mail: aglayana@unav.es;

Abstract: We studied the macular pigment ocular density (MPOD) in patients with early age macular degeneration (AMD) before and 1 year after nutritional supplementation with lutein and docosahexaenoic acid (DHA). Forty-four patients with AMD were randomly divided into two groups that received placebo ($n = 21$) or a nutritional supplement ($n = 23$, 12 mg of lutein and 280 mg of DHA daily). Heterochromatic flicker photometry was used to determine the MPOD. At baseline, the MPOD in AMD patients with placebo was 0.286 ± 0.017 meanwhile in AMD patients with supplementation it was 0.291 ± 0.016. One year later, the mean MPOD had increased by 0.059 in the placebo group and by 0.162 in patients receiving lutein and DHA. This difference between groups was significant ($p < 0.05$). Lutein and DHA supplementation is effective in increasing the MPOD and may aid in prevention of age related macular degeneration.

Keywords: lutein; docosahexaenoic acid; age-related macular degeneration; macular pigment density

---

1. Introduction

Understanding the pathogenesis of age-related macular degeneration (AMD), the most common cause of visual disability in elderly patients in developed countries, is advancing rapidly, but is still unclear [1,2]. Epidemiologic reports have suggested that diets rich in vitamins C and E, zinc, lutein, zeaxanthin, and docosahexaenoic acid (DHA) are associated with the greatest reduction in the risk of development of early and advanced AMD [3,4]. Higher dietary intake of lutein and zeaxanthin was associated independently with a decreased likelihood of having AMD [5] and dietary omega-3 long-chain polyunsaturated fatty acid intake is associated with a decreased risk of progression from bilateral drusen to advanced AMD [6]. Lutein, zeaxanthin and meso-zeaxanthin are xanthophylls (carotenoids that contain one or more polar functional groups) that selectively accumulate in the retina and are particularly dense in the foveal region, or macula, where they are the main components of the macular pigment (MP) [7]. In addition, lutein is the precursor of meso-zeaxanthin, a major component of MP [8]. They are known to function as antioxidants [9] and blue-light filters and thereby may protect the macular retina and retinal pigment epithelium from light-initiated oxidative damage [10]. Oxidative stress is high in the eye because of repeated exposure to light and the high rate of oxidative metabolism in the retina. In addition, the LAST [11] and LUNA [12] studies have evaluated the beneficial effect of lutein supplementation in patients with AMD.

DHA is a fatty acid found in the retina, with a high concentration in the rod outer segment [13,14]. Because photoreceptor outer segments are constantly being renewed, a constant supply of DHA may be required for proper retinal function. Marginal depletion may impair retinal function and influence the development of AMD [15]. Moreover, in two prospective follow-up studies it was reported that DHA intake was inversely related to the risk of AMD [3,16]. Of note is the observation that supplemental DHA increases HDL and HDL subfractions in serum [17–19]. Given that the carotenoids transport is made by lipids (HDL) [20,21], DHA supplementation could increase its transport to the retina and subsequently cause a MP ocular density (MPOD) increase. Therefore, DHA may, in part, decrease risk of AMD via increased transport of lutein into the macula. MPOD has been evaluated as a predictor of the retinal response to nutritional intervention with lutein in patients with AMD with the hope of retarding visual loss, disease progression, or both [22].

Although the formulation in the AREDS, which prevents development of advanced AMD, was comprised of vitamins C and E, beta-carotene, and zinc, currents trends in AMD nutritional prevention also are based on the use of lutein and long-chain polyunsaturated fatty acids like DHA [23].

Few data have been reported on the effect of the combined supplementation in MPOD [15]. Johnson *et al.* [15] reported that although lutein supplementation increases MPOD in nonsmoking elderly women without AMD, when lutein and DHA were administered together, the increase in MPOD was not significant. This study investigates the influence of lutein and DHA supplementation on MPOD and vision performance.

2. Experimental Section

2.1. Sample Size and Inclusion Criteria

For reasons aforementioned, we conducted a small prospective study to determine the basal MPOD in 44 patients with early AMD (stage II-III AREDS classification corresponding to small/intermediate drusen and large drusen with/without pigment changes). All subjects underwent a screening examination that included a medical history and a physical examination. Volunteers with any history of lactose intolerance, liver, kidney, or pancreatic disease, anemia, insulin-dependent diabetes, hyperlipoproteinemia or alcoholism were excluded from the study. Other exclusion criteria included current use of antihistamine drugs, steroids or nonsteroidal anti-inflammatory drugs and use of any nutrient supplement for previous 2 months or carotenoid supplements for the previous 6 months. The present project has been performed following the Declaration of Helsinki, was approved by the Ethics Committee of the Clinica Universidad de Navarra and all participants received and signed an informed consent for the study. Randomization was done by coin toss by the same ophthalmologist who enrolled them in the study.

2.2. Nutritional Supplementation

The patients with AMD were distributed randomly in two groups; one group (placebo group) were asked to take two placebo tablets daily for one year ($n = 21$), and the other group (intervention group) were asked to take two tablets daily of a supplemental complex with lutein and DHA ($n = 23$). The two intervention tablets contained a total daily dosage of 12 mg of lutein, 0.6 mg of zeaxanthin, and 280 mg of DHA. The placebo (containing sugar) and intervention tablets presented with the same look, smell, taste, packaging, and were manufactured by the same laboratory (Laboratorios Thea, Barcelona, Spain). Patients as well as ophthalmologists were blinded as to which group were taking the placebo tablets and which group were taking the intervention tablets until the end of the study.

2.3. Macular Pigment Ocular Density (MPOD) Measurement

The instrument used was the Eye Maculometer® (modified version: [24], School of Biosciences, University of Westminster, London, UK) to provide central fixation for both the foveal and parafoveal condition. This device is based on Heterochromatic Flicker Photometry (HFP) and uses Light Emitting Diodes (LED) as the near monochromatic light source, similarly to other published studies for the assessment of MPOD [22,24–27]. The Eye Maculometer® described in 1998 had only one test field and required eccentric fixation for the parafoveal measurement. This field was imaged on the fovea by direct fixation by the subject or on a patch of retina 5 degrees from the fovea by getting the subject to fixate on a small red light placed to one side of the single test field. Many subjects found this eccentric fixation was not easy to maintain. Consequently, the Eye Maculometer® was modified to provide central fixation for both the foveal and parafoveal condition. This improved device was the used in our study [24].

2.4. Visual Parameters

Visual function was tested before and after supplementation by measuring the best-corrected visual acuity with the ETDRS chart (Vectorvision, Greenville, Ohio, USA), and by contrast sensitivity with Pelli-Robson charts (Clement Clarke International, Edinburgh Way, Harlow, Essex, UK). Macular thickness was measured by Stratus optical coherence tomography (Carl Zeiss Meditec, Jena, Germany).

2.5. Statistical Analysis

Values are reported as the mean ± standard error of the mean (SEM). Statistical significance was evaluated by T student or U Mann-Whitney tests to analyze the differences between the placebo group and the nutritional supplementation group. Statistical significance was accepted at the 95% confidence level ($p < 0.05$) and analysis was performed by using the computer program SPSS (version 15.0, SPSS Inc., Chicago, IL, USA).

3. Results

3.1. Participant Characteristics

Of 69 participants screened for this study, 44 were AMD patients that were assigned randomly to receive treatment or placebo. Of the 44 participants, 26 (59.0%) were women and 18 (41.0%) were men. Mean age ± Standard Error of Mean (S.E.M.) was 67.8 ± 9.2 years for AMD patients with placebo and 69.2 ± 7.8 years for AMD patients with supplementation. Mean body mass index ± S.E.M. was 24.8 ± 1.4 kg/m^2 for placebo group and 25.2 ± 1.5 kg/m^2 for supplementation group. There were not statistical differences between both groups in any of these demographic parameters (Table 1).

Table 1. General Parameters and basal macular pigment ocular density (MPOD) in age macular degeneration (AMD) patients with placebo and supplementation with lutein and docosahexaenoic acid (DHA).

	Placebo group ($n = 21$)	Intervention group ($n = 23$)
Men/women	8/13	10/13
Age (years)	67.8 (9.2)	69.2 (7.8)
BMI (kg/m^2)	24.8 (1.4)	25.2 (1.5)
MPOD [a]	0.286 (0.017)	0.291 (0.016)

BMI = body mass index. Age, BMI, and MPOD measurements are expressed as the mean ± S.E.M. [a]$p < 0.01$.

3.2. Macular Pigment Optical Density (MPOD)

The baseline MPOD in the intervention group was (0.291 ± 0.016 unit) and was not statistically different from that of the placebo group (0.286 ± 0.017 unit) ($p > 0.05$, Table 1 and Figure 1A). Additionally, there was no significant difference between MPOD in the AREDS categories 2 and 3 ($p > 0.05$, Figure 1B).

Figure 1. (**A**) MPOD in AMD patients with placebo and AMD patients with supplementation. (**B**) MPOD separately for the Age Related Eye Disease study (AREDS) categories 2 and 3. Data are presented as means ± S.E.M.

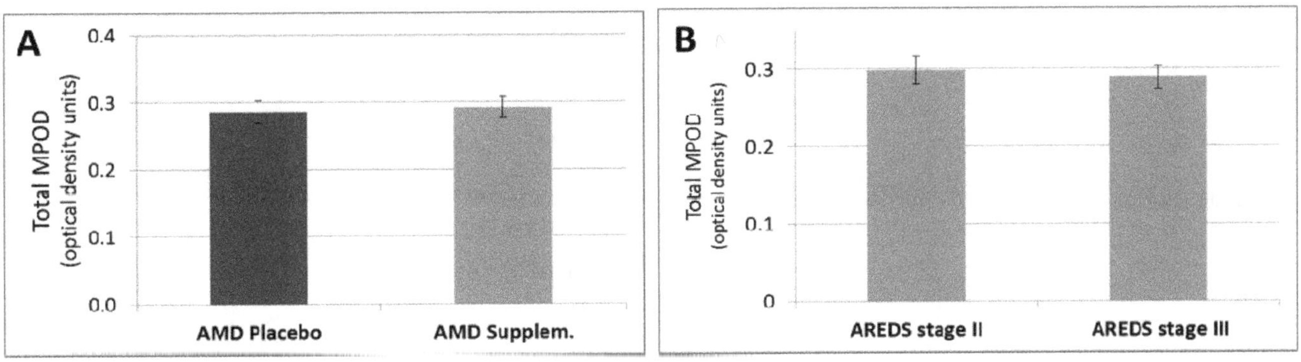

When we compared the MPOD values in patients with AMD after 1 year of follow-up, we found a significant increase in the supplementation group (0.453 ± 0.028 unit) compared to the placebo group (0.345 ± 0.026 unit) ($p < 0.01$, Table 2 and Figure 2A). Moreover, total MPOD increased very significantly after nutritional supplementation for 1 year ($p < 0.01$; Figure 2B). However, the VA, contrast sensitivity, and macular thickness did not change after 1 year of supplementation (Table 2). In addition, the increase (0.059 units) in MPOD in the group taking placebo after 1 year compared to baseline was not statistically significant. When we evaluated the non-responders to supplementation, *i.e.*, patients with less than a 5% increase in the total MPOD, four of 23 were non-responders among the patients with AMD who received nutritional supplement (17.4%).

Table 2. Ophthalmic parameters in patients with early AMD who received placebo or supplementation with lutein and DHA.

Parameters	Period	*Placebo Group (n = 21)*	*Intervention Group (n = 23)*	*P Value*
MPOD	*Baseline*	0.286 (0.017)	0.291 (0.016)	
	1 year after	0.345 (0.026)	0.453 (0.028)	$p < 0.01$
ETDRS (letters)	*Baseline*	78.3 (6.2)	76.4 (8.7)	
	1 year after	75.9 (5.8)	74.3 (9.2)	ns
Contrast sensitivity score (letters)	*Baseline*	26 (5)	25(5)	
	1 year after	26 (6)	26 (5)	ns
OCT macular thickness (μm)	*Baseline*	246 (20.7)	248 (32.5)	
	1 year after	249 (29.8)	246 (43.2)	ns

BCVA = best-corrected visual acuity; OCT = optical coherence tomography. All values are expressed as the mean (±S.E.M.). The Best Corrected Visual Acuity tested with the Early Treatment Diabetic Retinopathy Study charts and contrast sensitivity are expressed in number of letters (ETDRS). $p < 0.01$.

Figure 2. (**A**) MPOD in AMD placebo group and AMD supplemented group at time 0 (basal) and one year after treatment. (**B**) The MPOD change (1 year–0 month) in AMD placebo group and AMD supplemented group. Data are presented as means ± S.E.M. ** $p < 0.01$.

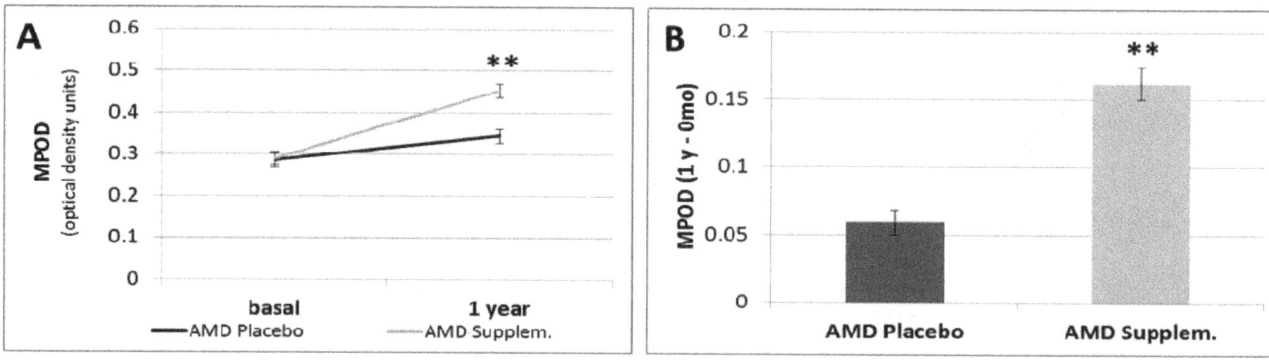

4. Discussion

This study investigates the influence of lutein and DHA supplementation on MPOD and vision performance. We found a significant increase in the MPOD levels in patients with AMD treated for 1 year with nutritional supplementation compared with the patients with AMD who received placebo, indicating that supplemental pills with lutein and DHA can significantly improve MP and increase retinal antioxidant protection in patients with this retinal disease. These results also agree with other similar studies and reaffirmed the hypothesis that the lutein and zeaxanthin macular concentrations constitute a modifiable nutritional risk factor [28]. However, visual function did not improve after supplementation, a result also reported previously [29]. Of note is that the increase in MPOD in the group taking placebo was not statistically significant. Our hypothesis is that those patients suffered the "placebo effect" and their behavior on dietetics could have changed. Probably, they were more motivated and took better care of themselves.

Our results differed from those of Johnson *et al.* [15] who found that the MPOD did not differ significantly when lutein and DHA were administered together. However, there are several differences between both populations that may explain that difference. Firstly, the population in the study of Johnson *et al.* was comprised of only women, and the current study included both genders. Secondly and probably more important, the population in the study of Johnson were patients without AMD and our supplementation was given to patients with AMD, who may have a better response to that supplementation, because those individuals with the lowest MPOD values were in the greatest need of supplementation and the most likely to benefit [15].

Additionally, the percentages of non-responders to lutein and DHA supplementation in our study were even lower than those observed by other authors in AMD patients (17.4% and 21.4%) [15]. In contrast, several recent studies in normal subjects [25] and healthy subjects with atypical spatial profile of MP (lack of a typical central peak) [27] showed a low rate of non-responders (<5%) because of the rapid increase in MP by the meso-zeaxanthin supplementation. They suggested that family history of AMD and smoking cigarettes may inhibit meso-zeaxanthin generation from lutein at the macula [25,27]. This hypothesis could explain the high rate of non-responder in our older AMD population supplemented with lutein given that it is well documented that atypical spatial profiles are more common in older subjects like AMD patients [26]. Moreover, it is possible that the non-responders in supplementation studies are individuals who lack the ability to convert lutein into meso-zeaxanthin. However, recent data has shown that when meso-zeaxanthin is provided in a supplement, it has a rapid and dramatic effect on serum carotenoid levels [27,30]. Thus, in our non-responders meso-zeaxanthin supplementation could be more effective than lutein.

Our device is based on the subjective HFP method, however several limitation need to be taken into account. For example: The inability to customise the flicker and the fact that this works in an independent mode as opposed to the yoked mode. However, we have found similar results than other authors using objective techniques [28]. Moreover, another limitation was the small sample size and the use of a subjective technique such as HFP. Therefore, the results obtained herein should be interpreted with full appreciation of their sample size and the device. This fact could result in a likelihood of chance findings in either direction. Thus, it would be necessary to complete the study with more information with respect to diet, smoking, exercise, plasma lutein levels, *etc.*

5. Conclusions

In conclusion, the daily intake of a nutritional complex containing 12 mg of lutein, 0.6 mg of zeaxanthin, and 280 mg of DHA had a beneficial effect on the MPOD levels in patients with AMD. However further clinical trials like AREDS 2 [31] are required to investigate the optimum dosage levels of all vitamins, micronutrients, and carotenoids that will protect the retina against degenerative diseases such as AMD.

Acknowledgements

Authors want to thank to all patients that collaborated in the present project. Funding: “The present work was partially funded by a Thea Laboratoires’ Grant and partially supported by RETICS (RD07/0062) from ISCIII, Ministerio de Ciencia e Innovación, Spain”.

References

1. Klaver, C.C.; Wolfs, R.C.; Vingerling, J.R.; Hofman, A.; de Jong, P.T. Age-specific prevalence and causes of blindness and visual impairment in an older population: The Rotterdam Study. *Arch. Ophthalmol.* **1998**, *116*, 653–658.
2. Klein, R.; Wang, Q.; Klein, B.E.; Moss, S.E.; Meuer, S.M. The relationship of age-related maculopathy, cataract, and glaucoma to visual acuity. *Invest. Ophthalmol. Vis. Sci.* **1995**, *36*, 182–191.
3. Cho, E.; Hung, S.; Willett, W.C.; Spiegelman, D.; Rimm, E.B.; Seddon, J.M.; Colditz, G.A.; Hankinson, S.E. Prospective study of dietary fat and the risk of age-related macular degeneration. *Am. J. Clin. Nutr.* **2001**, *73*, 209–218.
4. Landrum, J.T.; Bone, R.A. Lutein, zeaxanthin, and the macular pigment. *Arch. Biochem. Biophys.* **2001**, *385*, 28–40.

5. SanGiovanni, J.P.; Chew, E.Y.; Clemons, T.E.; Ferris, F.L., III; Gensler, G.; Lindblad, A.S.; Milton, R.C.; Seddon, J.M.; Sperduto, R.D. The relationship of dietary carotenoid and vitamin A, E, and C intake with age-related macular degeneration in a case-control study: AREDS Report No. 22. *Arch. Ophthalmol.* **2007**, *125*, 1225–1232.
6. SanGiovanni, J.P.; Chew, E.Y.; Agron, E.; Clemons, T.E.; Ferris, F.L., III; Gensler, G.; Lindblad, A.S.; Milton, R.C.; Seddon, J.M.; Klein, R.; *et al.* The relationship of dietary omega-3 long-chain polyunsaturated fatty acid intake with incident age-related macular degeneration: AREDS report no. 23. *Arch. Ophthalmol.* **2008**, *126*, 1274–1279.
7. Snodderly, D.M. Evidence for protection against age-related macular degeneration by carotenoids and antioxidant vitamins. *Am. J. Clin. Nutr.* **1995**, *62*, 1448S–1461S.
8. Johnson, E.J.; Neuringer, M.; Russell, R.M.; Schalch, W.; Snodderly, D.M. Nutritional manipulation of primate retinas, III: Effects of lutein or zeaxanthin supplementation on adipose tissue and retina of xanthophyll-free monkeys. *Invest. Ophthalmol. Vis. Sci.* **2005**, *46*, 692–702.
9. Schalch, W. Carotenoids in the retina—a review of their possible role in preventing or limiting damage caused by light and oxygen. *EXS* **1992**, *62*, 280–298.
10. Hammond, B.R., Jr.; Wooten, B.R.; Snodderly, D.M. Preservation of visual sensitivity of older subjects: Association with macular pigment density. *Invest. Ophthalmol. Vis. Sci.* **1998**, *39*, 397–406.
11. Richer, S.; Stiles, W.; Statkute, L.; Pulido, J.; Frankowski, J.; Rudy, D.; Pei, K.; Tsipursky, M.; Nyland, J. Double-masked, placebo-controlled, randomized trial of lutein and antioxidant supplementation in the intervention of atrophic age-related macular degeneration: The Veterans LAST study (Lutein Antioxidant Supplementation Trial). *Optometry* **2004**, *75*, 216–230.
12. Trieschmann, M.; Beatty, S.; Nolan, J.M.; Hense, H.W.; Heimes, B.; Austermann, U.; Fobker, M.; Pauleikhoff, D. Changes in macular pigment optical density and serum concentrations of its constituent carotenoids following supplemental lutein and zeaxanthin: The LUNA study. *Exp. Eye Res.* **2007**, *84*, 718–728.
13. Bazan, N.G.; Reddy, T.S.; Bazan, H.E.; Birkle, D.L. Metabolism of arachidonic and docosahexaenoic acids in the retina. *Prog. Lipid Res.* **1986**, *25*, 595–606.
14. Fliesler, S.J.; Anderson, R.E. Chemistry and metabolism of lipids in the vertebrate retina. *Prog. Lipid Res.* **1983**, *22*, 79–131.
15. Johnson, E.J.; Chung, H.Y.; Caldarella, S.M.; Snodderly, D.M. The influence of supplemental lutein and docosahexaenoic acid on serum, lipoproteins, and macular pigmentation. *Am. J. Clin. Nutr.* **2008**, *87*, 1521–1529.
16. Seddon, J.M.; Cote, J.; Rosner, B. Progression of age-related macular degeneration: association with dietary fat, transunsaturated fat, nuts, and fish intake. *Arch. Ophthalmol.* **2003**, *121*, 1728–1737.
17. Foulon, T.; Richard, M.J.; Payen, N.; Bourrain, J.L.; Beani, J.C.; Laporte, F.; Hadjian, A. Effects of fish oil fatty acids on plasma lipids and lipoproteins and oxidant-antioxidant imbalance in healthy subjects. *Scand. J. Clin. Lab. Invest.* **1999**, *59*, 239–248.
18. Nelson, G.J.; Schmidt, P.C.; Bartolini, G.L.; Kelley, D.S.; Kyle, D. The effect of dietary docosahexaenoic acid on plasma lipoproteins and tissue fatty acid composition in humans. *Lipids* **1997**, *32*, 1137–1146.

19. Thomas, T.R.; Smith, B.K.; Donahue, O.M.; Altena, T.S.; James-Kracke, M.; Sun, G.Y. Effects of omega-3 fatty acid supplementation and exercise on low-density lipoprotein and high-density lipoprotein subfractions. *Metabolism* **2004**, *53*, 749–754.
20. Cardinault, N.; Abalain, J.H.; Sairafi, B.; Coudray, C.; Grolier, P.; Rambeau, M.; Carre, J.L.; Mazur, A.; Rock, E. Lycopene but not lutein nor zeaxanthin decreases in serum and lipoproteins in age-related macular degeneration patients. *Clin. Chim. Acta* **2005**, *357*, 34–42.
21. Parker, R.S. Absorption, metabolism, and transport of carotenoids. *FASEB J.* **1996**, *10*, 542–551.
22. Stringham, J.M.; Hammond, B.R.; Nolan, J.M.; Wooten, B.R.; Mammen, A.; Smollon, W.; Snodderly, D.M. The utility of using customized heterochromatic flicker photometry (cHFP) to measure macular pigment in patients with age-related macular degeneration. *Exp. Eye Res.* **2008**, *87*, 445–453.
23. Coleman, H.; Chew, E. Nutritional supplementation in age related macular degeneration. *Curr. Opin. Ophthalmol.* **2007**, *18*, 220–223.
24. Mellerio, J.; Ahmadi-Lari, S.; van Kuijk, F.; Pauleikhoff, D.; Bird, A.; Marshall, J. A portable instrument for measuring macular pigment with central fixation. *Curr. Eye Res.* **2002**, *25*, 37–47.
25. Connolly, E.E.; Beatty, S.; Loughman, J.; Howard, A.N.; Louw, M.S.; Nolan, J.M. Supplementation with all three macular carotenoids: response, stability, and safety. *Invest. Ophthalmol. Vis. Sci.* **2011**, *52*, 9207–9217.
26. Kirby, M.L.; Beatty, S.; Loane, E.; Akkali, M.C.; Connolly, E.E.; Stack, J.; Nolan, J.M. A central dip in the macular pigment spatial profile is associated with age and smoking. *Invest. Ophthalmol. Vis. Sci.* **2010**, *51*, 6722–6728.
27. Nolan, J.M.; Akkali, M.C.; Loughman, J.; Howard, A.N.; Beatty, S. Macular carotenoid supplementation in subjects with atypical spatial profiles of macular pigment. *Exp. Eye Res.* **2012**, *101*, 9–15.
28. Kaya, S.; Weigert, G.; Pemp, B.; Sacu, S.; Werkmeister, R.M.; Dragostinoff, N.; Garhofer, G.; Schmidt-Erfurth, U.; Schmetterer, L. Comparison of macular pigment in patients with age-related macular degeneration and healthy control subjects—a study using spectral fundus reflectance. *Acta Ophthalmol.* **2012**, *90*, e399–e403.
29. Bartlett, H.E.; Eperjesi, F. Effect of lutein and antioxidant dietary supplementation on contrast sensitivity in age-related macular disease: A randomized controlled trial. *Eur J. Clin. Nutr.* **2007**, *61*, 1121–1127.
30. Meagher, K.A.; Thurnham, D.I.; Beatty, S.; Howard, A.N.; Connolly, E.; Cummins, W.; Nolan, J.M. Serum response to supplemental macular carotenoids in subjects with and without age-related macular degeneration. *Br. J. Nutr.* **2012**, *5*, 1–12.
31. Age-Related Eye Disease Study 2. Available online: http://www.areds2.org/ (accessed on 6 February 2013).

8

Eye Nutrition in Context: Mechanisms, Implementation and Future Directions

Barbara Demmig-Adams * and Robert B. Adams

Department of Ecology & Evolutionary Biology, University of Colorado, Boulder, CO 80309-0334, USA; E-Mail: Robert.Adams@colorado.edu

* Author to whom correspondence should be addressed;
E-Mail: Barbara.Demmig-Adams@colorado.edu

Abstract: Carotenoid-based visual cues and roles of carotenoids in human vision are reviewed, with an emphasis on protection by zeaxanthin and lutein against vision loss, and dietary sources of zeaxanthin and lutein are summarized. In addition, attention is given to synergistic interactions of zeaxanthin and lutein with other dietary factors affecting human vision (such as antioxidant vitamins, phenolics, and poly-unsaturated fatty acids) and the emerging mechanisms of these interactions. Emphasis is given to lipid oxidation products serving as messengers with functions in gene regulation. Lastly, the photo-physics of light collection and photoprotection in photosynthesis and vision are compared and their common principles identified as possible targets of future research.

Keywords: antioxidants; carotenoids; gene regulation; light collection; lipid peroxidation; lutein; photo-damage; photoprotection; programmed cell death; zeaxanthin

1. Introduction

Carotenoids possess functions as diverse as their colors (for a review, see [1]). Carotenoid function as visual cues is matched by roles in (1) visual detection of these cues and (2) protection of the vision process against overly bright light. Many animals are able to detect visual signals carrying important information content about their environment via the light-absorbing rhodopsin, formed from the carotenoid (β-carotene) cleavage product vitamin A combined with the opsin protein. On the other hand, the carotenoids zeaxanthin and lutein provide essential protection of the eye in humans and many other animals. Moreover, carotenoids are involved in the regulation of life-and-death processes at the cellular level via modulation of signaling networks that control cell division and programmed cell death [2]. The present overview places carotenoids into the context of (1) familiar organisms and objects colored by carotenoids, (2) their roles in human vision, with an emphasis on protection by zeaxanthin and lutein against vision loss, (3) various dietary sources of zeaxanthin and lutein, (4) synergistic interactions of zeaxanthin and lutein with other dietary factors affecting human vision and the emerging mechanisms of these interactions, and (5) a comparison of the photo-physics of light collection and photoprotection in photosynthesis and vision and their common principles that might be rewarding targets of future research.

2. Colors and Nomenclature of Carotenoids

The flamingo's pink plumage, the yellow of egg yolks and daffodils, the orange of peppers, and yellow-orange autumn foliage are colors conferred by carotenoids (see [1]). It is plants and photosynthetic microbes that synthesize most carotenoids; non-photosynthetic consumers, like humans and other animals, rely strictly on acquiring essential carotenoids with their food and are unable to synthesize these *de novo* (although some conversions are known to occur).

Carotenoids are typically named after organisms in which they occur in high concentrations and/or from which they were first isolated and identified. For example, *carot*ene colors the carrot and *zea*xanthin levels are high in the corn plant (scientific name: *Zea mays*). The names of the two major groups of carotenoids, carotenes (carotenoids without oxygen atoms in the molecular structure) and xanthophylls (carotenoids containing oxygen atoms) further relate to their features: *-ene* (as in carot*ene*) for the presence of many carbon-carbon double bonds (from the chemical nomenclature of *-ene* for molecules with carbon-carbon double bonds) and *xantho-phyll* (Greek for "yellow-leaf") in reference to the high level of these carotenoids in yellow autumn leaves. Zeaxanthin has a structural isomer, lutein; even though these two xanthophylls differ merely in the placement of a single C=C double bond, they possess discernible biological functions.

3. Carotenoids in the Functioning and Protection of the Human Eye

The dietary carotenoid β-carotene is provitamin A that, after being cleaved, yields two molecules of vitamin A as the chromophore (light-absorbing) component of rhodopsin. In addition, vitamin A serves as a modulator of genes serving in the immune response [1]. Chronic severe vitamin A deficiency therefore causes not only blindness, but also often death from infectious disease.

In addition to serving as precursors of constituents of the human eye, carotenoids are thought to protect the vision process, improve visual acuity and shape discrimination, and be involved in the prevention of cataracts and age-related blindness (age-related macular degeneration or AMD) (for reviews, see [3,4]). Rather than carotenes, it is zeaxanthin and lutein—two carotene-derived xanthophylls synthesized by plants and algae—that are chiefly involved in protection of the vision process.

Dietary zeaxanthin and lutein—neither of which, as stated above, can be synthesized by humans—apparently confer *multiple* beneficial effects to human health. Epidemiological studies have identified strong inverse trends between zeaxanthin and/or lutein consumption and human diseases, including age-related eye disease, various cancers, and other conditions [5–7]. The underlying mechanisms for these protective effects have yet to be fully elucidated (see Section 5 below). Plants and photosynthetic microbes synthesize zeaxanthin and lutein for their own protection against damage by intense sunlight—and the same two xanthophylls, when consumed with the human diet, apparently also protect the human eye from damage by intense light [5].

In the human eye, zeaxanthin and lutein (as well as some meso-zeaxanthin, formed from lutein) are the predominant carotenoids in the yellow spot (*macula lutea*) of the retinal macula, with higher ratios of zeaxanthin to lutein in those areas receiving the highest light exposure [8,9]. Both xanthophylls are accumulated in the blood stream (from the intestinal tract), and then further accumulated in the retina (from the blood stream). Along with this overall accumulation of xanthophylls in the eye, the ratio of zeaxanthin to lutein increases at each step (from the intestinal tract to the blood plasma to the eye), indicating a particular importance of zeaxanthin in the retina (for reviews, see [3,4,6]). Individuals suffering from age-related eye disease (such as AMD) possess lesser xanthophyll densities throughout their retinas, and there is an inverse correlation between dietary zeaxanthin and lutein intake and the risk for AMD as well as cataracts [6].

It has been suggested that the yellow zeaxanthin and lutein pigments act by providing an absorbing shield against the most harmful blue portion of sunlight and perhaps also against UV light [10], but evidence for additional or alternative functions is mounting [2,4,10]. Zeaxanthin and lutein act synergistically with the antioxidant vitamin E (and likely other antixodants), as well as with certain (omega-3) poly-unsaturated fatty acids, in photoreceptor protection (for details, see Section 4 below).

A breakthrough in the understanding of the function of retinal zeaxanthin in protecting the eye was made by the discovery that dietary zeaxanthin *prevents* programmed cell death of retinal photoreceptor cells in an intact animal model [11,12]. Because of the latter finding, one might wonder whether dietary zeaxanthin would increase cancer risk by inhibiting programmed cell death of cancer cells. However, this concern is unfounded since dietary zeaxanthin has, in fact, been associated with a lower cancer risk (see, e.g., [13]). Consumption of dietary zeaxanthin is therefore not only correlated with improved eye health but also with a lower cancer risk. While the mechanism of cancer prevention by carotenoids is presently unknown, it may involve an actual *stimulation* of programmed cell death of various cancer cells [14–16], including cancer of the eye [17]. The xanthophylls zeaxanthin and lutein share this remarkable ability, *i.e.*, to simultaneously *protect needed* cells and apparently *destroy unwanted* cells, with several other classes of dietary compounds like some phenolics and omega-3 fatty acids ([2]; see also Section 5 below). In addition to their protective effects against vision loss, zeaxanthin and lutein apparently also serve in improving vision overall. Consistent with its preferential concentration in the central region of the retina (in the fovea), a dietary supplement of zeaxanthin (8 mg daily) specifically enhanced high-contrast visual acuity and shape discrimination, while a dietary supplement of lutein (9 mg daily), consistent with its preferential distribution in the non-central regions of the retina, enhanced low-contrast visual acuity and glare recovery [3].

While zeaxanthin and lutein levels in the human retina are correlated with dietary intake of these xanthophylls, genetic factors also play a role [4,18]. Individuals with a darker iris color (with greater levels of melanin pigment) possess higher retinal levels of zeaxanthin and lutein [19]. It will be important to assess whether these differences represent a genetic difference in the ability to enrich zeaxanthin and/or lutein from the diet among individuals and populations, or whether a darker iris may prevent xanthophyll destruction by intense light.

4. Dietary Sources of Zeaxanthin & Lutein

There is evidence that the human consumer should avoid excessive supplementation with carotenoids [20,21]. For example, daily supplementation with excessive amounts of β-carotene for several years actually increased the risk of Finnish male smokers for lung cancer. In addition, blue-green algal (cyanobacterial) supplements (with high levels of a class of highly oxygenated xanthophylls called ketocarotenoids) caused crystalline ketocarotenoid deposits in the human eye [22]. Currently available blue-green algal supplements thus need to be viewed with caution, due to potential adverse effects of ketocarotenoid accumulation.

4.1. Carotenoid and Vitamin Supplements

There are additional reasons why the human consumer should avoid high-dose supplements. A comprehensive review [21] of a large number of clinical studies examining the effect of antioxidant and/or carotenoid supplements on chronic diseases demonstrated opposite effects dependent on dosage. Supplements doses similar to, or up to a few times higher than, the US daily recommended allowance (RDA) typically had positive effects (reducing disease risk), while higher doses had no effect on disease risk, and extremely high doses, above ten times the RDA, had negative effects (increasing disease risk) [21]. Some studies have reported benefits of lutein and zeaxanthin supplements (10–20 mg daily; [23,24]) for AMD patients, while other studies reported no benefits of 6 mg lutein combined with vitamins and minerals [25]. More research is needed to further explore effects of different doses of supplementation for patients already diagnosed with eye disease.

On the other hand, prevention of eye disease prior to onset may be well served by regular consumption of xanthophylls and other dietary factors as part of a whole diet based on foods containing multiple, synergistically acting ingredients. The underlying mechanisms why whole foods rich in, e.g., antioxidants and carotenoids protect against disease, while high-dose antioxidant supplements can have the opposite effects, are currently not fully understood. However, it appears that reactive oxygen species and cellular signaling networks are involved. Reactive oxygen species, which are removed by antioxidants and carotenoids, actually exert essential positive effects at low levels (they are the signals triggering up-regulation of the body's own internal antioxidant defenses), while being able to cause tissue damage at unchecked high levels (see, e.g., [26–28]). Section 5 below addresses cellular signaling networks that may be involved.

4.2. Yellow Foods

Eggs, yellow corn, and yellow peppers are probably the richest dietary sources of zeaxanthin and lutein in the United States. These food sources receive all of their yellow-to-orange color from their zeaxanthin and lutein content. In contrast, green leafy plant foods typically contain high levels of lutein, but very little zeaxanthin. This difference is due to the fact that green leaves form zeaxanthin under full sunlight and remove zeaxanthin when no longer exposed to full sunlight (for additional details, see section on "leafy greens and other plant sources" below). In contrast to green leaves, certain non-photosynthetic parts of plants, like the ear of corn, accumulate *constant high* levels of zeaxanthin. Yellow corn is a food naturally high in zeaxanthin and lutein, and all of its yellow color stems directly from these two pigments (see [29] for analysis of various corn products). White corn, on the other hand, does not provide these xanthophylls. Lines of corn with even higher levels of zeaxanthin and lutein might be identified from locally adapted varieties, or could be produced by further breeding and/or engineering.

Chicken eggs are another food with high levels of both zeaxanthin and lutein. However, chickens are no more capable of synthesizing their own xanthophylls than humans, and the coloration (and zeaxanthin and lutein content) of their eggs strictly depends on the chickens' feed. As long as a xanthophyll-rich food source is available (from alfalfa, corn, or other sources containing zeaxanthin and lutein), chickens deposit zeaxanthin and lutein into their eggs; and egg color varies with carotenoid content. Furthermore, just as different strains of corn have different levels of zeaxanthin and lutein, some chicken breeds deposit more zeaxanthin and lutein into their eggs than others [30].

4.3. Leafy Greens and Other Plant Sources

Just as is the case for animals, plants and algae also use carotenoids for *both light collection AND photoprotection* against the destructive effects of intense light. The xanthophylls zeaxanthin and lutein stand out as primary agents of photoprotection in plants. Zeaxanthin facilitates the safe removal of potentially damaging excessive excitation energy [5,31,32]; zeaxanthin's close isomer lutein plays a minor role in the same process of the dissipation of excessive excitation [33]. In addition, zeaxanthin also provides plant photoprotection by direct inhibition of the oxidation of lipids of the photosynthetic membrane (lipid peroxidation; [34,35]; see also Section 5 below).

How much zeaxanthin versus lutein can be obtained from leafy green plant foods varies greatly, as stated above. While the green parts of plants after harvest typically contain high levels of lutein, they retain mere traces of zeaxanthin. This is because plants carefully modulate the level of zeaxanthin in response to the amount of light they absorb. Leaves only produce zeaxanthin (via de-epoxidation of another xanthophyll, violaxanthin, that consists of a zeaxanthin molecule with two epoxide groups added) when exposed to high light; whenever direct high light exposure ends, zeaxanthin is quickly re-converted (re-epoxidized) to its direct xanthophyll precursor (violaxanthin). This fine control of zeaxanthin levels is important for the plant to (1) maintain its ability to safely dissipate potentially destructive excessive light one minute (via zeaxanthin as a dissipater of excess light) and (2) to quickly return to efficiently using sunlight for sugar production the next, by converting the dissipater zeaxanthin back to its direct, non-dissipating xanthophyll precursor [31,36,37].

Human consumption of zeaxanthin is highly desirable because zeaxanthin needs to be preferentially accumulated and incorporated into the parts of the mammalian retina exposed to high irradiance ([8]; see also above). For this reason, an arrest of the back-conversion of zeaxanthin to its precursor in green leaves may be a desirable trait to incorporate into crops that provide green leafy foods. Such a retention of zeaxanthin can be accomplished, e.g., by knocking out or silencing the enzyme/gene (zeaxanthin epoxidase) responsible for zeaxanthin conversion to its xanthophyll precursor and/or by overexpressing enzymes in earlier portions of the carotenoid biosynthetic pathway. Over-expression of the enzyme catalyzing synthesis of zeaxanthin from β-carotene in the plant model species *Arabidopsis* led to elevated zeaxanthin accumulation [38].

Additional mutants unable to convert zeaxanthin to its xanthophyll precursor, and thus accumulating high levels of zeaxanthin, have been produced in model plants and algae [39] and these traits can be transferred to crop plants. However, since constantly elevated zeaxanthin levels may diminish the green leaf's ability to efficiently collect sunlight during the parts of the day when light levels are low and limiting to photosynthesis, e.g., early morning and late afternoon, the effect of continuous zeaxanthin retention in leaves on the productivity of crop plants needs to be further examined. Due to the need of leaves to photosynthesize efficiently for maximal biomass production, overexpression of zeaxanthin in fruit, rather than leaves, is attractive. Tomato fruit with increased zeaxanthin content has recently been engineered via two manipulations (overexpression of lycopene-cyclase and of β-carotene hydroxylase; [40]). Zeaxanthin-rich potato has also been produced [41] as well as zeaxanthin-accumulating *E. coli* [42]. While foods engineered to contain high zeaxanthin levels should aid in augmenting dietary zeaxanthin supply for human populations at risk for zeaxanthin deficiency, attention should be given to avoiding excessive consumption of such fortified foods.

5. Xanthophylls in the Context of Other Dietary Modulators

Reviews of lifestyle- and diet-associated risk factors for age-related macular degeneration indicate that, in addition to zeaxanthin and lutein, omega-3 fatty acids, antioxidant vitamins C and E, antioxidant minerals, and other dietary factors lower the risk for AMD [43]. These factors act synergistically (via the emerging mechanisms reviewed below) in modulating key signaling networks.

5.1. Foods Contain Multiple Gene Regulators Acting in Synergy

The essential role of food components—such as vitamins—in human physiology has long been recognized. However, it is only now being realized that a multitude of additional dietary factors have profound effects on human health and the risk for disease, and may thus deserve vitamin status as well (see [5]). Many of these dietary factors possess the remarkable ability to alter expression of regulatory genes that modulate human metabolism. Most of these dietary factors are synthesized by plants or algae and are referred to as phytochemicals (from *phyto* = plant), phytonutrients, or nutraceuticals. These dietary factors modulate expression of central human genes (master control genes) that regulate processes of fundamental importance, such as cell proliferation, programmed cell death, and the immune response (see, e.g., [5,44,45]). These key processes, and any imbalances in their regulation, play a major role in all major human diseases including cancer, autoimmune diseases, and pro-inflammatory diseases (such as age-related blindness, heart disease, diabetes, and others; [46]). Macular degeneration involves excessive programmed cell death as well as inflammation. While the original literature on programmed cell death distinguishes between "programmed cell death" and "apoptosis" as a particular form of cell death, both of these processes are referred to as programmed cell death in the present review for simplicity's sake.

Dietary factors may be able to *stop* programmed cell death of vital cells and *promote* programmed cell death of unwanted cells. Such a potential to both *trigger programmed cell death of unwanted cells* while *aiding in the survival of needed cells* is not only demonstrated by zeaxanthin and lutein, but also by poly-unsaturated omega-3 fatty acids (in fish that consume omega-3 fat-producing cold-water algae; [47]), and plant compounds (phenolics) with multiple functional (phenol) groups conferring exceptionally strong antioxidant qualities to the molecule [44,48]. This potential makes these food-derived compounds highly desirable nutraceuticals.

Studies with human cancer cell lines indicate that lutein is able to induce programmed cell death of human breast cancer cells [14,15] and leukemia cells [16]. Similarly, zeaxanthin is able to promote programmed cell death of eye cancer (neuroblastoma) cells [17]. Lutein furthermore induced programmed cell death in mouse tumor cells, but decreased programmed cell death in cancer-fighting immune cells of tumor-bearing mice [14].

5.2. Gene Regulators Produced by Lipid Peroxidation

In both plants and animals, membrane lipids are actively oxidized by enzymes (e.g., lipoxygenases) that function as part of cellular signaling networks and actively respond to oxidative challenges. Lipoxygenases produce messengers that regulate programmed cell death, the immune response, and other vital processes. Lipoxygenases in both plants and animals produce multiple lipid-derived messengers (in plants collectively termed “oxylipins”, such as jasmonic acid, and in animals collectedly termed “eicosanoids”, such as prostaglandins, leukotrienes, and thromboxanes). Each messenger family typically includes members with *opposite* regulatory functions, *i.e.*, that either *promote* or *inhibit* programmed cell death ([49,50]; see Figure 1). For example, *inhibition* of lipoxygenases *prevented programmed cell death of neurons* and was discussed as a new target for the treatment of Alzheimer’s disease [51], whereas *inhibition* of lipoxygenases in leukemia cells *actively induced programmed cell death* [52]. As further detailed in the legend of Figure 1, lipoxygenases are activated by oxidants (e.g., reactive oxygen species, ROS) and are inhibited by various antioxidants. Reactive oxygen species thus activate both enzymatic and non-specific, non-enzymatic lipid peroxidation, and multiple products of both enzymatic and non-enzymatic lipid peroxidation serve as gene regulators. Likewise, antioxidants inhibit both enzymatic and non-enzymatic lipid peroxidation.

While it had been known for some time that the lipid-soluble vitamin E is able to suppress (both non-enzymatic and enzymatic) lipid peroxidation, it is now emerging that zeaxanthin and other dietary factors interact synergistically with vitamin E (see below). Suppression of lipid-peroxidation-derived modulators of programmed cell death (and/or other vital cellular processes) is an attractive mechanism for these dietary modulators’ ability to protect vital cells, while eliminating unwanted cells. This fine-tuned modulation of vital metabolic functions emphasizes the critical importance of a *balanced* dose of these dietary regulators.

Experimentation with isolated biological membranes showed that lipid-soluble antioxidants (like zeaxanthin and vitamin E) synergistically protect against oxidation of unsaturated fatty acids (that are highly susceptible to oxidation; see Figure 1). While massive oxidation of membrane lipids eventually leads to membrane damage, a more physiologically relevant effect is the rapid formation of small amounts of oxidized lipid derivatives serving as messengers that modulate the expression of genes involved in programmed cell death and other vital functions (Figure 1).

Figure 1. Schematic depiction of (1) the oxidation (by reactive oxygen species, ROS) of membrane lipids to lipid peroxides (L-OO•) that are further converted to messengers, e.g., stimulating photoreceptor cell death as well as (2) the effect of lifestyle/environmental/dietary factors on ROS and/or lipid peroxide levels. Moderate exercise generates moderate amounts of ROS serving to trigger full formation of endogenous antioxidant defenses (in the form of antioxidant enzymes requiring dietary minerals as their cofactors). Smoking, exposure to pollutants, and excessive alcohol consumption all strongly increase ROS levels. Dietary zeaxanthin (Zea), lutein (Lut), vitamins E (Vit. E) and C (Vit. C), and phenolics, as well as endogenous antioxidant enzymes, serve in synergy to lower the levels of ROS (via ROS detoxification) as well as recycle lipid peroxides (via re-reduction). Stimulation by ROS, and inhibition by various antioxidants, applies equally to non-enzymatic and enzymatic (via lipoxygenase, LOX) lipid peroxidation. Lipoxygenases contain a catalytic iron center that is active in lipid peroxidation only after oxidation (by ROS) to (active) LOX-Fe^{3+} [53], and can be inactivated by antioxidants to (inactive) LOX-Fe^{2+} [54]. Products of both enzymatic and non-enzymatic lipid peroxidation serve as gene regulators.

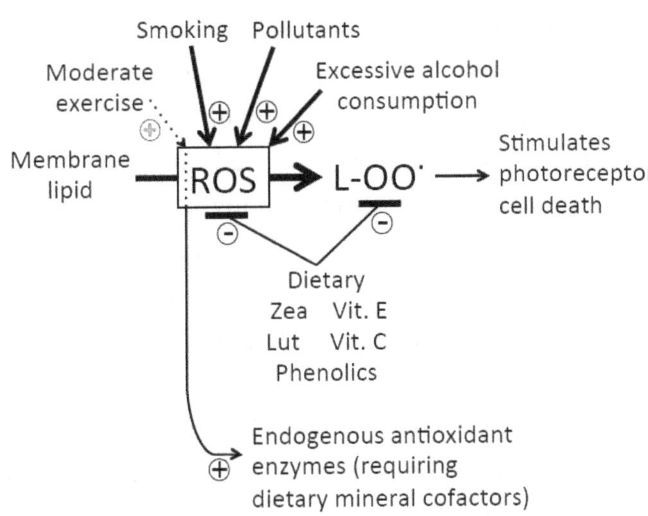

Zeaxanthin *inhibits* the oxidation of membrane lipids (lipid peroxidation; Figure 1) in plants [34,35] as well as in humans (e.g., in epithelial cells of the eye's lens; [55]). Zeaxanthin also protects lipids against peroxidation *in vitro*, and zeaxanthin's ability to provide this protection is enhanced by addition of vitamin E, with zeaxanthin having the more potent, primary effect [56,57]. While zeaxanthin and vitamin E act synergistically to suppress lipid peroxidation in biological membranes, vitamin C aids in the recycling of vitamin E at the membrane/cytosol interface, and various phenolics (with strong antioxidant effects) can do the same. Furthermore, antioxidant minerals, such as zinc, copper, and selenium, are essential cofactors of the body's internal antioxidant enzymes that also serve in the cellular antioxidant network (Figure 1). Others have drawn similar conclusions and recommended supplements consisting of cocktails of the factors above (specifically, vitamins A, B, C, E, β-carotene, zeaxanthin, lutein, selenium, zinc, and the herb *Gingko biloba*; [58]).

Dietary antioxidants must work in conjunction with the body's own internal antioxidant enzymes (Figure 1). Antioxidant enzymes require mineral cofactors from the diet, and interact with dietary xanthophylls, vitamins, and phenolics to suppress unchecked accumulation of reactive oxygen species. However, it is small amounts of reactive oxygen species (produced, e.g., via moderate physical exercise) that serve as the vitally important trigger for synthesis of the body's own antioxidant enzymes (Figure 1; [27]). It was recently been proposed that, "reactive oxygen species (ROS) and chronic oxidative changes in membrane lipids and proteins found in many chronic diseases are not the result of accidental damage. Instead, these changes are the result of a highly evolved, stereotyped, and protein-catalyzed 'oxidative shielding' response that all eukaryotes adopt when placed in a chemically or microbially hostile environment" [28]. The requirement of small amounts of ROS for induction of endogenous antioxidant defenses is the likely reason for the adverse effects of high-dose antioxidant supplements that presumably abolish the beneficial effects of ROS [21].

5.3. Poly-Unsaturated Fatty Acids

Exposure to reactive oxygen (readily formed in highly oxygenated tissues, such as the human eye) leads to preferential peroxidation of poly-unsaturated fatty acids. Poly-unsaturated fatty acids are linked to eye disease (as well as multiple other chronic diseases) in both positive and negative ways. Dietary poly-unsaturated fatty acids fall into two major groups, *i.e.*, omega-6 (mainly linoleic acid and arachidonic acid) and omega-3 fatty acids, mainly alpha-linolenic acid, *e*icosa*p*entaenoic *a*cid (EPA) and *d*ocosa*h*exaenoic *a*cid (DHA). A balanced ratio of dietary omega-6 to omega-3 fats (below 10:1 and perhaps as low as 2:1) is needed to support human health (including the health of the human eye), while the modern western diet provides a highly unbalanced ratio of about 10–20:1 [59]. Such a high, unbalanced ratio of omega-6 to omega-3 fatty acids is thought to promote programmed cell death and inflammation in some tissues, thereby increasing the risk of (1) chronic pro-inflammatory disease, like eye disease [43], diabetes, and heart disease [60,61], and a host of neuropsychiatric and neurodevelopmental disorders ([62,63]; see also [64]), as well as promoting (2) excessive cell proliferation (cancer) of other tissues [65,66].

How do poly-unsaturated fatty acids interact with vital cellular signaling networks? Both groups of fatty acids are essential (they cannot be synthesized in the human body), and form the precursors of lipid peroxidation-based regulators of gene expression discussed above. Both omega-6 and omega-3 poly-unsaturated fatty acids become incorporated into membrane lipids, where they represent the lipids most highly susceptible to either non-enzymatic or enzymatic oxidation (the unsaturated bonds of fatty acids are easily oxidized).

Oxidatively modified derivatives of omega-6 and omega-3 fatty acids typically serve as antagonists of each other in the regulation of gene expression, such that a balanced, relatively low ratio of omega-6 to omega-3 is required to prevent programmed cell death, e.g., in the eye. The omega-3 fatty acid DHA is concentrated in photoreceptor cells, and a major recent review concluded that, "DHA is necessary for vision, photoprotection, and corneal nerve regeneration" [67]. Furthermore, omega-3 supplementation has been demonstrated to prevent programmed cell death of tear gland cells [68]. Preferential lutein and zeaxanthin accumulation in membrane domains rich in poly-unsaturated fatty acids has been suggested to prevent lipid peroxidation [69]. Figure 1 focuses on stimulation by ROS, and inhibition by antioxidants, of the production of photoreceptor-death-stimulating messengers presumably derived from omega-6 fatty acids. Future research is needed to fully elucidate the effects of messengers derived from omega-3 fatty acids, and what relative and absolute concentrations of omega-6 and omega-3-derived messengers are needed to protect photoreceptors and other cells.

Current dietary recommendations are to keep the sum of all poly-unsaturated fats consumed in the human diet between 15% and 20%–30% of total fat consumption, with most of the remainder coming from mono-unsaturated fats like oleic acid found in many plant foods. While most currently used sunflower, corn, soybean, or cottonseed oils are excessively high in omega-6 fatty acids, utilization of high-oleic varieties of these oil-seed crops that either naturally contain, and/or have been genetically engineered to contain, much reduced levels of omega-6 linoleic acid should have many health benefits [70–74].

5.4. Dietary and Lifestyle Factors Increasing Disease Risk

High levels of saturated fats and/or trans fats and a high glycemic load (high and frequent consumption of carbohydrates that rapidly break down into simple sugars) as well as smoking, excess alcohol consumption, and physical inactivity promote the production of pro-inflammatory messengers and/or unchecked high levels of reactive oxygen species, and increase the risk for chronic, pro-inflammatory disease (see, e.g., [75]). Again, regular exercise (and consumption of the required mineral cofactors) is required to fully induce the body's own internal complement of antioxidant enzymes, and high doses of antioxidant supplements have the potential to remove the necessary small ROS levels and thereby interfere with this induction of defenses [21,27,28].

In conclusion, a prudent course of action for improving vision and lowering the risk of eye disease (as well as a host of other diseases) at this time is to consume a whole-food-based diet rich in zeaxanthin, lutein, various phenolics, antioxidant vitamins and minerals, with a balanced ratio of omega-3 to omega-6 fatty acids, and to avoid high-caloric, high-glycemic, saturated-, *trans*-, and omega-6-fat-rich foods as well as smoking, excess alcohol, and physical inactivity. A "healthy lifestyle with a diet containing food rich in antioxidants, especially lutein and zeaxanthin, and (omega-3) fatty acids" has been recommended to prevent or slow progression of AMD and cataracts [73]. A multi-vitamin-multi-mineral supplement (each around the RDA level) with a combination of vitamins C and E, β-carotene, and zinc with copper has been recommended for AMD but not cataracts [76]. Optimal doses of supplements have yet to be determined, but high-dose xanthophyll and/or antioxidant vitamin supplements are unlikely to be beneficial (cf. also [77]).

6. Relating the Mechanisms of Photoprotection to the Photochemistry of Photosynthesis and Human Vision

Continuing comparison of parallels between light absorption, light processing, and protection against excessive excitation in photosynthesis and human vision may be rewarding (Figure 2). Research on the photoprotection of photosynthesis has focused, e.g., on interaction of the light-absorbing chlorophylls with xanthophylls in the light-collecting system, with a lesser focus on lipid peroxidation-based messengers and signaling networks (Figure 2). On the other hand, research on human vision has identified synergies among factors involved in signaling networks, while the photo-physics of excited states of rhodopsin derivatives and their possible interaction with xanthophylls have not been fully elucidated (Figure 2). Possible practical applications based on insight into the photo-physics of visions will be addressed below.

Figure 2. Comparison of photosynthesis and vision with respect to the principal steps in the series of reactions from light absorption, by various chromophores, to transfer of excitation energy to singlet oxygen ($^1O_2$*) resulting in lipid peroxidation and formation of lipid-derived gene regulators. Light absorption occurs in chlorophyll (Chl)-antenna-protein complexes in photosynthesis, and in retinal-opsin-complexes in vision. Triplet excited chlorophyll (^{3}Chl*) is known to act as the photosensitizer in photosynthesis, passing excitation energy to oxygen, thus forming singlet oxygen. The nature of the photosensitizer in vision (X) is currently under debate. In contrast to protein-bound Chl, opsin-bound retinal does not produce singlet oxygen. However, there is current debate that, once released from opsin, all-*trans* retinal absorbs another photon and may give rise to singlet oxygen formation (see, e.g., [78]). The boxes around the different phases of the reaction series serve to indicate where research focus has previously been placed.

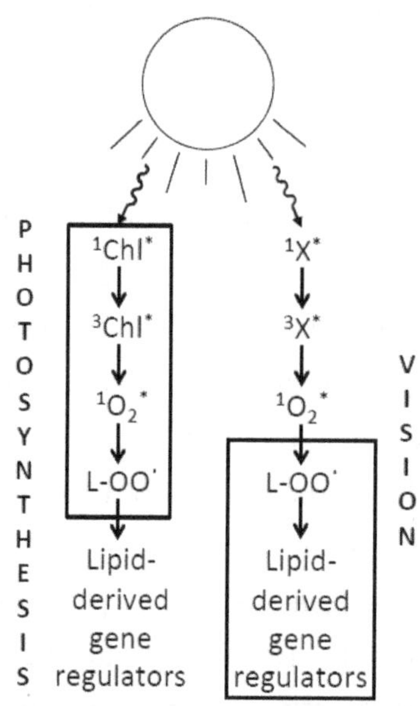

The parallels between photosynthesis and human vision are remarkable—as would be expected from an evolutionary viewpoint considering not only the homology of these systems, but also common dictates from natural selection and adaptive advantage. Both systems must be able to collect photons of light (as carriers of information in vision, or carriers of energy in photosynthesis) via light-absorbing pigments or chromophores (retinal or chlorophyll), which is achieved by the chromophore's binding to a protein (opsin or chlorophyll-binding proteins, respectively). Figure 2 summarizes some of the parallels between human vision and photosynthesis.

Chromophore-binding proteins, such as the chlorophyll-binding proteins of photosynthesis, typically help increase the lifetime of a chromophore's excited state (produced by absorption of a photon of light) long enough to allow highly efficient transfer of excitation energy (e.g., into an electron transport chain in the case of photosynthesis). Increasing the chromophore's lifetime, however, comes at a cost under high light levels; if the chromophore's excited state builds up just for fractions of a second, a conversion (via intersystem crossing) occurs to a slightly lower (triplet) excited state of the chromophore able to pass on excitation energy to oxygen, thereby forming potentially highly destructive reactive oxygen species. Chromophores thus typically act as facilitators of photo-damage, or photosensitizers, although in the vision process, it is not opsin-bound retinal, but forms of retinal (all-*trans*-retinal or its derivatives) released from opsin that absorb another photon and may act as the singlet-oxygen-producing photosensitizer ([78–87]).

The accumulation of light-absorbing pigment protein complexes typically responds to long-term light availability. Plants accumulate more chlorophyll when grown in low light, and thereby become more susceptible to over-excitation and inactivation of photochemistry under high light exposure, than plants grown in high light [32]. Similarly, animals raised in low light environments accumulated more rhodopsin, and were more susceptible to high-light-induced vision loss (for an overview, see [78]). Based on these findings and the current understanding of the mechanisms of photo-damage, it is possible that long-term light environment may affect the risk for human eye disease. Future research should assess whether predominant exposure to very low light environments in typical home and office settings may increase the risk for eye disease compared to regular exposure to modest levels of natural sunlight outdoors, e.g., in mornings and afternoons or on overcast days (with typical light intensities around only 10 μmol photons $m^{-2}{\cdot}s^{-1}$ for indoors fluorescent lighting versus around 300 and up to 2000 μmol photons $m^{-2}{\cdot}s^{-1}$ for natural sunlight outdoors during overcast skies and full midday sunlight on clear days, respectively; B. Demmig-Adams, [79]).

It has been discussed that the human eye, just like photosynthesis, must maintain "a delicate balance between maximizing the absorption of photon for vision and retinal image quality while simultaneously minimizing the risk of photo-damage when exposed to bright light" [80]. Rhodopsin presence has been proposed to be required for photo-damage in the retina ([81]; see also [82,83]), and, as pointed out above, there has been recent discussion that all-*trans*-retinal, once released from rhodopsin during the vision cycle, or specific derivatives of all-*trans*-retinal, may accumulate in the retina and act as photosensitizer(s) ("X" in Figure 2; [78,81–88]). Lutein and zeaxanthin have been suggested to confer photoprotection against such an action [84]. It is currently unknown whether or not, or how, xanthophylls may facilitate de-excitation of any excited states of chromophores in human vision. In contrast, detailed information has been accumulated on chromophore de-excitation, and an involvement of xanthophylls, in photosynthesis (see below).

A chromophore's first excited state is typically a singlet-excited state (e.g., $^{1}Chl^{*}$; Figure 2) electronically unable to pass excitation energy to oxygen in its ground (triplet) state. However, the chromophore's state reached after conversion via intersystem crossing is a triplet state (e.g., $^{3}Chl^{*}$; Figure 2) that reacts readily with oxygen, resulting in the formation of highly reactive singlet-excited oxygen. Under high light exposure, a light-absorbing system like chlorophyll-binding proteins is thus extremely vulnerable to destruction by singlet oxygen. Multiple mechanisms have evolved to provide protection by safe de-excitation of "unwanted", excessive excited states at every step of the above cascade, *i.e.*, (1) de-excitation of the chlorophyll's singlet-excited state, (2) de-excitation of its triplet state, (3) de-excitation of singlet-excited oxygen, and, finally, (4) mechanisms that re-reduce oxidized lipids.

In photosynthesis, zeaxanthin (and to a lesser extent lutein) facilitate de-excitation of excessive singlet-excited chlorophyll [31,37]; efficient de-excitation of triplet-excited chlorophyll in light-harvesting complexes can also be catalyzed by lutein and zeaxanthin [89,90]. Singlet-excited oxygen ($^1O_2$*) can be de-excited by vitamin E and various carotenoids (see [91]). Remarkably, a mixture of zeaxanthin, lutein, and a lutein derivative in the concentrations found in the human retina was shown to be more effective at singlet oxygen de-excitation than each xanthophyll alone [92]. Finally, zeaxanthin can apparently directly inhibit lipid peroxidation (L-OO$^\bullet$) in plants [34,35] and may serve in a similar function in the human eye through the synergistic interaction with vitamin E described above.

The underlying photo-physical mechanism of de-excitation of singlet-excited chlorophyll facilitated by zeaxanthin has received much attention, and evidence has been provided (for reviews, see [32,93,94]) for several different mechanisms that may yet turn out to all contribute, *i.e.*, (1) direct transfer of excitation energy from singlet-excited chlorophyll to zeaxanthin (and perhaps lutein), followed by conversion of the excitation energy to harmless heat [95]; (2) reversible charge transfer between singlet-excited chlorophyll and zeaxanthin (transfer of an electron from chlorophyll to zeaxanthin and back) resulting in loss of the excitation energy as harmless heat [96]; (3) a zeaxanthin-induced change in the chlorophyll-binding light-harvesting proteins from a conformation that lengthens the lifetime of ^{1}Chl* to a conformation allowing efficient return of ^{1}Chl* directly to ground-state chlorophyll while releasing excitation energy as harmless heat [93,94]. Zeaxanthin's close structural isomer, lutein, differs in the energy levels of its excited states as well as in its exact structure (and perhaps its interaction with membranes and proteins).

The evolutionary conservation of xanthophyll association with light-absorbing systems in widely different organisms is as remarkable as the multitude of mechanisms of xanthophyll-facilitated photoprotection. More research is needed to elucidate whether different organisms employ different ones of these multiple mechanisms—or whether the whole suite of mechanisms may be conserved across species and light-processing systems.

Acknowledgments

We wish to thank Christopher M. Cohu for preparing the figures for this review.

References

1. Demmig-Adams, B.; Rixham, C.S.; Adams, W.W., III. Carotenoids. In *McGraw-Hill Encyclopedia of Science & Technology*, 11th ed.; McGraw-Hill: New York, NY, USA, 2012; pp. 549–555.
2. Demmig-Adams, B.; Adams, W.W., III. Overview of diet-gene interaction and the example of xanthophylls. *Adv. Exp. Med. Biol.* **2010**, *698*, 17–26.
3. Richer, S.B.; Stiles, W.; Graham-Hoffman, K.; Levin, M.; Ruskin, D.; Wrobel, J.; Park, D.W.; Thomas, C. Randomized, double-blind, placebo-controlled study of zeaxanthin and visual function in patients with atrophic age-related macular degeneration. The zeaxanthin and visual function study (ZVF) FDA IND #78, 973. *Optometry* **2011**, *82*, 667–680.

4. SanGiovanni, J.P.; Neuringer, M. The putative role of lutein and zeaxanthin as protective agents against age-related macular degeneration: Promise of molecular genetics for guiding mechanistic and translational research in the field. *Am. J. Clin. Nutr.* **2012**, *96*, 1223S–1233S.
5. Demmig-Adams, B.; Adams, W.W., III. Antioxidants in photosynthesis and human nutrition. *Science* **2002**, *298*, 2149–2153.
6. Mares-Perlman, J.A.; Millen, A.E.; Ficek, T.L.; Hankinson, S.E. The body of evidence to support a protective role for lutein and zeaxanthin in delaying chronic disease. Overview. *J. Nutr.* **2002**, *132*, 518S–524S.
7. Sajilata, M.G.; Singhal, R.S.; Kamat, M.Y. The carotenoid pigment zeaxanthin—A review. *Compr. Rev. Food Sci. Food Saf.* **2008**, *7*, 29–49.
8. Landrum, J.T.; Bone, R.A. Lutein, zeaxanthin and the macular pigment. *Arch. Biochem. Biophys.* **2001**, *385*, 28-40.
9. Sabour-Pickett, S.; Nolan, J.M.; Loughman, J.; Beatty, S. A review of the evidence germane to the putative protective role of the macular carotenoids for the age-related macular degeneration. *Mol. Nutr. Food Res.* **2012**, *56*, 270–286.
10. Hammond, B.R.; Fletcher, L.M. Influence of the dietary carotenoids lutein and zeaxanthin on visual performance: Application to baseball. *Am. J. Clin. Nutr.* **2012**, *96*, 1207S–1213S.
11. Thomson, L.R.; Toyoda, Y.; Langner, A.; Delori, F.C.; Garnett, K.M.; Craft, N.E.; Nichols, C.R.; Cheng, K.M.; Dorey, C.K. Elevated retinal zeaxanthin and prevention of light-induced photoreceptor cell death in quail. *Investig. Ophthalmol. Vis. Sci.* **2002**, *43*, 3538–3549.
12. Thomson, L.R.; Toyoda, Y.; Delori, F.C.; Garnett, K.M.; Wong, Z.Y.; Nichols, C.R.; Cheng, K.M.; Craft, N.E.; Dorey, C.K. Long term dietary supplementation with zeaxanthin reduces photoreceptor death in light-damaged Japanese quail. *Exp. Eye Res.* **2002**, *75*, 529–542.
13. Tanaka, T.; Shnimizu, M.; Mirowaki, H. Cancer chemoprevention by carotenoids. *Molecules* **2012**, *17*, 3202–3242.
14. Chew, B.P.; Brown, C.M.; Park, J.S.; Mixter, P.F. Dietary lutein inhibits mouse mammary tumor growth by regulating angiogenesis and apoptosis. *Anticancer Res.* **2003**, *23*, 3333–3339.
15. Sumatran, V.N.; Zhang, R.; Lee, D.S.; Wicha, M.S. Differential regulation of apoptosis in normal *versus* transformed mammary epithelium by lutein and retinoic acid. *Cancer Epidemiol. Biomakers Prev.* **2000**, *9*, 257–263.
16. Müller, K.; Carpenter, K.L.H.; Challis, I.R.; Skepper, J.N.; Arends, M.J. Carotenoids induce apoptosis in the T-lymphoblast cell line Jurkat E6.1. *Free Radic. Res.* **2002**, *36*, 791–802.
17. Maccarrone, M.; Bari, M.; Gasperi, V.; Demmig-Adams, B. The photoreceptor protector zeaxanthin induces cell death in neuroblastoma cells. *Anticancer Res.* **2005**, *25*, 3871–3876.
18. Borel, P. Genetic variations involved in interindividual variability in carotenoid status. *Mol. Nutr. Food Res.* **2012**, *56*, 228–240.
19. Hammond, B.R.; Fuld, K.; Snodderly, D.M. Iris color and macular pigment optical density. *Exp. Eye Res.* **1996**, *62*, 293–297.
20. Tran, E.; Demmig-Adams, B. Vitamins and minerals: Powerful medicine or potent toxins? *Nutr. Food Sci.* **2007**, *37*, 50–60.
21. Villanueva, C.; Kross, R.D. Antioxidant-induced stress. *Int. J. Mol. Sci.* **2012**, *13*, 2091–2109.

22. Daicker, B.; Schiedt, K.; Adnet, J.J.; Bermond, P. Canthaxanthin retinophathy-an investigation by light and electron-microscopy and physicochemical analysis. *Graefes Arch. Clin. Exp. Ophthalmol.* **1987**, *225*, 189–197.
23. Weigert, G.; Kaya, S.; Pemp, B.; Sacu, S.; Lasta, M.; Werkmeister, R.M.; Dragostinoff, N.; Simader, C.; Garhofer, G.; Schmidt-Erfurth, U.; *et al.* Effects of lutein supplementation on macular pigment optical density and visual acuity in patients with age-related macular degeneration. *Investig. Ophthalmol. Vis. Sci.* **2011**, *52*, 8174–8178.
24. Ma, L.; Dou, H.L; Huang, Y.M.; Lu, X.R.; Qian, F.; Zou, Z.Y.; Pang, H.L.; Dong, P.C.; Xiao, X.; Wang, X.; *et al.* Improvement of retinal function in early age-related macular degeneration after lutein and zeaxanthin supplementation: A randomized, double-masked, placebo-controlled trial. *Am. J. Ophthalmol.* **2012**, *154*, 625–634.
25. Bartlett, H.E.; Eperjesi, F. Effect of lutein and antioxidant dietary supplementation on contrast sensitivity in age-related macular disease: A randomized controlled trial. *Eur. J. Clin. Nutr.* **2007**, *61*, 1121–1127.
26. Cutler, R.G.; Plummer, J.; Chowdury, K.; Heward, C. Oxidative stress profiling Part II. Theory, technology, and practice. *Ann. N. Y. Acad. Sci.* **2005**, *1055*, 136–158.
27. Gomez-Cabrera, M.-C.; Domenech, E.; Romagnoli, M.; Arduini, A.; Borras, C.; Pallardo, F.V.; Sastre, J.; Viña, J. Oral administration of vitamin C decreases muscle mitochondrial biogenesis and hampers training-induced adaptations in endurance performance. *Am. J. Clin. Nutr.* **2008**, *87*, 142–149.
28. Naviaux, R.K. Oxidative shielding or oxidative stress? *J. Pharmcol. Exp. Ther.* **2012**, *342*, 608–618.
29. De Oliveira, G.P.R.; Rodriguez-Amaya, D.B. Processed and prepared corn products as sources of lutein and zeaxanthin: Compositional variation in the food chain. *J. Food Sci.* **2007**, *72*, S079–S085.
30. Pintea, A.; Dulf, F.V.; Bunea, A.; Matea, C.; Andrei, S. Comparative analysis of lipophilic compounds in eggs of organically raised ISA Brown and Araucana hens. *Chem. Pap.* **2012**, *66*, 955–963.
31. Demmig-Adams, B.; Adams, W.W., III. Photoprotection in an ecological context: The remarkable complexity of thermal dissipation. *New Phytol.* **2006**, *172*, 11–21.
32. Demmig-Adams, B.; Cohu, C.M.; Muller, O.; Adams, W.W., III. Modulation of photosynthetic energy conversion efficiency in nature: From seconds to seasons. *Photosynth. Res.* **2012**, *113*, 75–88.
33. Pogson, B.J.; Nigoyi, K.K.; Björkman, O.; DellaPenna, D. Altered xanthophyll compositions adversely affect chlorophyll accumulation and nonphotochemical quenching in *Arabidopsis* mutants. *Proc. Natl. Acad. Sci. USA* **1998**, *95*, 13324–13329.
34. Havaux, M.; Niyogi, K.K. The violaxanthin cycle protects plants from photooxidative damage by more than one mechanism. *Proc. Natl. Acad. Sci. USA* **1999**, *96*, 8762–8767.
35. Havaux, M.; Dall'Osto, L.; Cuine, S.; Guiliano, G.; Bassi, R. The effect of zeaxanthin as the only xanthophyll on the structure and function of the photosynthetic apparatus in *Arabidopsis thaliana*. *J. Biol. Chem.* **2004**, *279*, 13878–13888.

36. Demmig-Adams, B. Linking the xanthophyll cycle with photoprotective energy dissipation. *Photosynth. Res.* **2003**, *76*, 73–80.
37. Demmig-Adams, B.; Adams, W.W., III. The role of xanthophyll cycle carotenoids in the protection of photosynthesis. *Trends Plant Sci.* **1996**, *1*, 21–26.
38. Davison, P.A.; Hunter, C.N.; Horton, P. Overexpression of beta-carotene hydroxylase enhances stress tolerance in *Arabidopsis*. *Nature* **2002**, *418*, 203–206.
39. Niyogi, K.K. Safety valves for photosynthesis. *Curr. Opin. Plant Biol.* **2000**, *3*, 455–460.
40. Dharmapuri, S.; Rosati, C.; Pallara, P.; Aquilani, R.; Bouvier, F.; Camara, B.; Guiliano, G. Metabolic engineering of xanthophyll content in tomato fruits. *FEBS Lett.* **2002**, *519*, 30–34.
41. Romer, S.; Lubeck, J.; Kauder, F.; Steiger, S.; Adomat, C.; Sandmann, G. Genetic engineering of a zeaxanthin-rich potato by antisense inactivation and cosuppression of carotenoid epoxidation. *Metab. Eng.* **2002**, *4*, 263–272.
42. Albrecht, M.; Misawa, N.; Sandmann, G. Metabolic engineering of the terpenoid biosynthetic pathway of *Escherichia coli* for production of the carotenoids beta-carotene and zeaxanthin. *Biotechnol. Lett.* **1999**, *21*, 791–795.
43. Sin, H.P.Y.; Liu, D.T.L.; Lam, D.S.C. Lifestyle modification, nutritional and vitamin supplements for age-related macular degeneration. *Acta Ophthalmol.* **2013**, *91*, 6–11.
44. Surh, Y.J. Cancer chemoprevention with dietary phytochemicals. *Nat. Rev. Cancer* **2003**, *3*, 768–780.
45. Lapillonne, A.; Clarke, S.D.; Heird, W.C. Polyunsaturated fatty acids and gene expression. *Curr. Opin. Clin. Nutr. Metab. Care* **2004**, *7*, 151–156.
46. Lavrovsky, Y.; Chatterjee, B.; Clark, R.A.; Roy, A.K. Role of redox-regulated transcription factors in inflammation, aging and age-related diseases. *Exp. Gerontol.* **2000**, *35*, 521–532.
47. Seo, T.; Blaner, W.S.; Deckelbaum, R.J. Omega-3 fatty acids: Molecular approaches to optimal biological outcomes. *Curr. Opin. Lipidol.* **2005**, *16*, 11–18.
48. Youdim, K.A.; Spencer, J.P.E.; Schroeter, H.; Rice-Evans, C. Dietary flavonoids as potential neuroprotectants. *Biol. Chem.* **2002**, *383*, 503–519.
49. Maccarrone, M.; Melino, G.; Finazzi-Agrò, A. Lipoxygenases and their involvement in programmed cell death. *Cell Death Differ.* **2001**, *8*, 776–784.
50. Tang, D.G.; La, E.; Kern, J.; Kehrer, J.P. Fatty acid oxidation and signaling in apoptosis. *Biol. Chem.* **2002**, *383*, 425–442.
51. Lebeau, A.; Terro, F.; Rostene, W; Pelaprat, D. Blockade of 12-lipoxygenase expression protects cortical neurons from apoptosis induced by beta-amyloid peptide. *Cell Death Differ.* **2004**, *11*, 875–884.
52. Grichenko, O.E.; Shaposhnikova, V.V.; Kudryavtsev, A.A.; Korystov, Y.N. Apoptosis in p388 leukemia cells induced by specific inhibitors of 5- and 12-lipoxygnease and the product of cyclooxygenase, prostaglandin E-2. *Biol. Bull.* **2004**, *31*, 221–225.
53. Maccarrone, M.; Corasantini, M.T.; Guerrieri, P.; Nistico, G.; Finazzi-Agrò, A. Nitric oxide-donor compounds inhibit lipoxygenase activity. *Biochem. Biophys. Res. Commun.* **1996**, *219*, 128–133.
54. Maccarrone, M.; Lorenzon, T.; Guerrieri, P.; Finazzi-Agrò, A. Resveratrol prevents apoptosis in K562 cells by inhibiting lipoxygenase and cyclooxygenase activity. *Eur. J. Biochem.* **1999**, *265*, 27–34.

55. Chitchumroonchokchai, C.; Bomser, J.A.; Glamm, J.E.; Failla, M.L. Xanthophylls and alpha-tocopherol decrease UVB-induced lipid peroxidation and stress signalling in human lens epithelial cells. *J. Nutr.* **2004**, *134*, 3225–3232.
56. Wrona, M.; Korytowksi, W.; Ròzanowska, M.; Sarna, T.; Truscott, T.G. Cooperation of antioxidants in protection against photosensitized oxidation. *Free Radic. Biol. Med.* **2003**, *35*, 1319–1329.
57. Wrona, M.; Ròzanowska, M.; Sarna, T. Zeaxanthin in combination with ascorbic acid or alpha-tocopherol protects APRE-19 cells against photosensitized peroxidation of lipids. *Free Radic. Biol. Med.* **2004**, *36*, 1094–1101.
58. Bartlett, H.; Eperjesi, F. An ideal ocular nutritional supplement? *Ophthalmic Physiol. Opt.* **2004**, *24*, 339–349.
59. Simopoulos, A.P. Omega-6/omega-3 essential fatty acid ratio and chronic disease. *Food Rev. Int.* **2004**, *20*, 77–90.
60. Haag, M.; Dippenaar, N.G. Dietary fats, fatty acids and insulin resistance: Short review of a multifaceted connection. *Med. Sci. Monit.* **2005**, *11*, RA359–RA367.
61. Blaschke, F.; Takata, Y.; Caglayan, E.; Law, R.E.; Hsueh, W.A. Obesity, peroxisome proliferator-activated receptor and atherosclerosis in type 2 diabetes. *Arterioscler. Thromb. Vasc. Biol.* **2006**, *26*, 28–40.
62. Richardson, A.J.; Ross, M.A. Fatty acid metabolism in neurodevelopmental disorder: A new perspective on associations between attention-deficit/hyperactivity disorder, dyslexia, dyspraxia and the autistic spectrum. *Prostaglandins Leukot. Essent. Fatty Acids* **2000**, *63*, 1–9.
63. Young, G.; Conquer, J. Omega-3 fatty acids and neuropsychiatric disorders. *Reprod. Nutr. Dev.***2004**, *45*, 1–28.
64. Wainwright, P.E. Dietary essential fatty acids and brain function: A developmental perspective on mechanisms. *Proc. Nutr. Soc.* **2002**, *61*, 61–69.
65. Simopoulos, A.P. Omega-3 fatty acids and cancer. *Indoor Built Environ.* **2003**, *12*, 405–412.
66. Simopoulos, A.P. The omega-6/omega-3 fatty acid ratio, genetic variation and cardiovascular disease. *Asia Pac. J. Clin. Nutr.* **2008**, *17*, 131–134.
67. Bazan, N.G.; Molina, M.F.; Gordon, W.C. Docosahexaenoic acid signalolipidomics in nutrition: Significance in aging, neuroinflammation, macular degeneration, Alzheimer's, and other neurodegenerative diseases. *Annu. Rev. Nutr.* **2011**, *31*, 321–351.
68. Roncone, M.; Bartlett, H.; Eperjesi, F. Essential fatty acids for dry eye: A review. *Cont. Lens Anterior Eye* **2010**, *33*, 49–54.
69. Wisniewska-Becker, A.; Nawrocki, G.; Duda, M.; Subczynski, W.K. Structural aspects of the antioxidant activity of lutein in a model of photoreceptor membranes. *Acta Biochim. Pol.* **2012**, *59*, 119–123.
70. Warner, K.; Knowlton, S. Frying quality and oxidative stability of high-oleic corn oils. *J. Am. Oil Chem. Soc.* **1997**, *74*, 1317–1322.
71. Forster, V.A. Genetically modified crop approvals and planted acreages. *Crop Biotechnol.* **2002**, *829*, 17–22.
72. Liu, Q.; Singh, S.P.; Green, A.G. High-stearic and high-oleic cottonseed oils produced by hairpin RNA-mediated posttranscriptional gene silencing. *Plant Physiol.* **2002**, *129*, 1732–1743.

73. Liu, Q.; Singh, S.; Green, A. High-oleic and high-stearic cottonseed oils: Nutritionally improved cooking oils developed using gene silencing. *J. Am. Coll. Nutr.* **2002**, *21*, 205S–211S.
74. Smith, S.A.; King, R.E.; Min, D.B. Oxidative and thermal stabilities of genetically modified high oleic sunflower oil. *Food Chem.* **2007**, *102*, 1208–1213.
75. Herder, R.; Demmig-Adams, B. The power of a balanced diet and lifestyle in preventing cardiovascular disease. *Nutr. Clin. Care* **2004**, *7*, 46–55.
76. Seddon, J.M. Multivitamin-multimineral supplements and eye disease: Age-related macular degeneration and cataract. *Am. J. Clin. Nutr.* **2007**, *85*, 304S–307S.
77. Evans, J.R.; Lawrenson, J.G. Antioxidant vitamin and mineral supplements for slowing the progression of age-related macular degeneration. *Cochrane Database Syst. Rev.* **2012**, *11*, CD000254.
78. Rozanowska, M.; Sarna, T. Light-induced damage to the retina: Role of the rhodopsin chromophore revisited. *Photochem. Photobiol.* **2005**, *81*, 1305–1330.
79. Demmig-Adams, B. University of Colorado, Boulder, CO, USA. Unpublished work, 2013.
80. Hunter, J.J.; Morgan, J.I.W.; Merigan, W.H.; Sliney, D.H.; Sparrow, J.R.; Williams, D.R. The susceptibility of the retina to photochemical damage from visible light. *Prog. Retin. Eye Res.* **2012**, *31*, 28–42.
81. Rozanowska, M. Light-induced damage to the retina: current understanding of the mechanisms and unresolved questions: A symposium-in-print introduction. *Photochem. Photobiol.* **2012**, *88*, 1303–1308.
82. Organisciak, D.T.; Vaughn, D.K. Retinal light damage: Mechanisms and protection. *Prog. Retin. Eye Res.* **2010**, *29*, 113–134.
83. Glaeser, J.; Nuss, A.M.; Berghoff, B.A.; Klug, G. Singlet oxygen stress in microorganisms. *Adv. Microb. Physiol.* **2011**, *58*, 141–173.
84. Kim, S.R.; Nakanishi, K.; Itagaki, Y.; Sparrow, J.R. Photooxidation of A2-PE, a photoreceptor outer segment fluorophore, and protection by lutein and zeaxanthin. *Exp. Eye Res.* **2006**, *82*, 828–839.
85. Loginova, M.Y.; Rostovtseva, Y.V.; Feldman, T.B.; Ostrovsky, M.A. Light damaging action of all-*trans*-retinal and its derivatives on rhodopsin molecules in the photoreceptor membrane. *Biochemistry (Moscow)* **2008**, *73*, 130–138.
86. Bhosale, P.; Serban, B.; Berstein, P.S. Retinal carotenoids can attenuate formation of A2E in the retinal pigment epithelium. *Arch. Biochem. Biophys.* **2009**, *483*, 175–181.
87. Maeda, T.; Golczak, M.; Maeda, A. Retinal photodamage mediated by all-*trans*-retinal. *Photochem. Photobiol.* **2012**, *88*, 1309–1319.
88. Masutomi, K.; Chen, C.H.; Nakatani, K.; Koutalos, Y. All-*trans* retinal mediates light-induced oxidation in single living rod photoreceptors. *Photochem. Photobiol.* **2012**, *88*, 1356–1361.
89. Dall'Osto, L.; Lico, C.; Alric, J.; Giuliano, G.; Havaux, M.; Bassi, R. Lutein is needed for efficient chlorophyll triplet quenching in the major LHCII antenna complex of higher plants and effective photoprotection *in vivo* under strong light. *BMC Plant Biol.* **2006**, *6*, 32.
90. Betterle, N.; Ballottari, M.; Hienerwadel, R.; Dall'Osto, L.; Bassi, R. Dynamics of zeaxanthin binding to the photosystem II monomeric antenna protein Lhcb6 (CP24) and modulation of its photoprotection properties. *Arch. Biochem. Biophys.* **2010**, *504*, 67–77.

91. Demmig-Adams, B.; Cohu, C.M.; Amiard, V.; van Zadelhoff, G.; Veldink, G.A.; Muller, O.; Adams, W.W., III. Emerging trade-offs—Impact of photoprotectants (PsbS, xanthophylls, and vitamin E) on oxylipins as regulators of development and defense. *New Phytol.* **2013**, *197*, 720–729.
92. Li, B.X.; Ahmed, F.; Berstein, P.S. Studies on the singlet oxygen scavenging mechanism of human macular pigment. *Arch. Biochem. Biophys.* **2010**, *504*, 56–60.
93. Jahns, P.; Holzwarth, A.R. The role of the xanthophyll cycle and of lutein in photoprotection of photosystem II. *Biochim. Biophys. Acta* **2012**, *1817*, 182–193.
94. Ruban, A.V.; Johnson, M.P.; Duffy, C.D.P. The photoprotective molecular switch in the photosystem II antenna. *Biochim. Biophys. Acta* **2012**, *1817*, 167–181.
95. Frank, H.A.; Bautista, J.A.; Josue, J.S.; Young, A.J. Mechanism of nonphotochemical quenching in green plants: Energies of the lowest excited singlet states of violaxanthin and zeaxanthin. *Biochemistry* **2000**, *39*, 2831–2837.
96. Holt, N.E.; Zigmantas, D.; Valkunas, L.; Li, X.P.; Niyogi, K.K.; Fleming, G.R. Carotenoid cation formation and the regulation of photosynthetic light harvesting. *Science* **2005**, *307*, 433–436.

9

The Relationship between Lutein and Zeaxanthin Status and Body Fat

Emily R. Bovier [1], **Richard D. Lewis** [2] **and Billy R. Hammond Jr.** [1,*]

[1] Vision Sciences Laboratory, University of Georgia, Athens, GA 30602, USA; E-Mail: erbovier@uga.edu

[2] Foods and Nutrition, University of Georgia, Athens, GA 30602, USA; E-Mail: rlewis@fcs.uga.edu

* Author to whom correspondence should be addressed; E-Mail: bhammond@uga.edu;

Abstract: The objective of this project was to investigate the relationships between total and regional distribution of body fat and tissue lutein (L) and zeaxanthin (Z) status. Healthy men and women ($N = 100$; average age: 22.5 year, average BMI: 23.4 kg/m^2) were evaluated. Total body and regional fat mass were assessed by dual-energy X-ray absorptiometry (Hologic Delphi A). Serum LZ was measured using reverse phase high-performance liquid chromatography, and retinal LZ (referred to as macular pigment optical density; MPOD) was measured using heterochromatic flicker photometry. Body fat percentage (total and regional) was inversely related to MPOD ($p < 0.01$) but no significant relationship was found for serum LZ. Higher body fat percentage, even within relatively healthy limits, is associated with lower tissue LZ status. The results indicate that adiposity may affect the nutritional state of the retina. Such links may be one of the reasons that obesity promotes age-related degenerative conditions of the retina.

Keywords: lutein; zeaxanthin; body fat; adiposity

---

1. Introduction

Lutein and zeaxanthin (LZ), two lipophilic pigments obtained exclusively from the diet, are likely to have a constellation of health effects throughout the body. Higher tissue concentrations of LZ have been associated with a reduced risk of acquired diseases, including cardiovascular disease, various cancers, and age-related eye diseases [1]. LZ status can be quantified by measuring concentrations within the serum and, unlike most nutrients, by noninvasive measurements within tissue. For example, a variety of physical and psychophysical methods are available to directly measure LZ concentrations within the central macular region of the human retina [2]. In the macula, the area that contains the highest carotenoid concentrations within the body, LZ (and a third isomeric intermediary, meso-zeaxanthin) are termed macular pigment (MP). Preliminary evidence has shown that MP correlates with amounts of LZ in adipose tissue, which is a major body store for LZ [3–5].

Although dietary intake is the primary driver of tissue LZ levels, the relation between diet and the ultimate deposition of these pigments within a target tissue is moderated by a number of factors. Hammond *et al.* [6] for instance, found significantly lower MP for women compared to men, despite equivalent plasma concentrations and dietary intakes of LZ. The authors concluded that this relative paucity in women could help explain the higher incidence of age-related eye diseases directly associated with serum LZ and MP, such as age-related macular degeneration and cataracts. Although males and females obviously differ across many biological dimensions, one possible reason for the observed sex differences in MP [5–7] might be the fact that women generally have higher body fat percentages than men. Higher levels of body fat have been shown to be related to lower levels of circulating carotenoids (The reverse is likely also true. Individuals with very low body fat (like anorexics who would then have lower capacity for adipose storage of carotenoids) often have higher circulating carotenoid levels [8]), making these pigments less available to retinal tissue [9]. Consistent with this interpretation, higher body fat levels, especially when approaching obesity, have also been linked to lower levels of MP. Hammond *et al.* [10], for instance, found that both men and women with body fat greater than 27% had 16% lower MP density compared to subjects with lower body fat. One question that was not addressed by Hammond *et al.* is whether the distribution of body fat (also known to differ between men and women [5]) influences serum LZ and/or the ultimate deposition of these pigments within the retina. Chung *et al.* [11] have shown that LZ concentrations in adipose tissue differ according to body site (e.g., levels tend to be higher in the abdomen than in the buttocks).

The primary goal of the present study was to assess the relation between LZ status (measured in serum and retina) to total and regional fat distribution (focusing on the trunk).

2. Methods

2.1. Subjects

Male ($N = 39$) and female ($N = 61$) subjects (average age of 22.5 years; average BMI of 23.4 kg/m^2) were recruited from The University of Georgia and the surrounding Athens area. Subjects were screened for ocular health (e.g., no history of corneal disease, age-related macular degeneration, *etc.*) and corrected visual acuity better than 20/60. All subjects completed informed consent and two measures of MP (an average over the two visits was used in all subsequent analyses) at the Vision Sciences Laboratory. Within two to four weeks, subjects completed assessments of body composition at the UGA Bone Clinic. Serum LZ was determined for 65 subjects. Experimental procedures were approved by the Institutional Review Board of The University of Georgia.

2.2. Assessment of LZ Status: Macular Pigment Optical Density & Serum LZ

Heterochromatic flicker photometry (HFP) was used to measure the optical density of the macular pigments (*i.e.*, macular pigment optical density; MPOD) [12]. This method has been extensively validated [2,13] and is fully described by Wooten *et al.* [12]. Briefly, we used the standardized CAREDs protocol [14], which involves measuring sensitivity to stimuli presented in free-view. A target stimulus alternates in square-wave between a "blue" light maximally absorbed by MP (460 nm) and a "green" light not absorbed by MP (540 nm). Given the differential absorbance of "blue" light compared to "green" light, the discordance in the amount of energy that reaches the photoreceptors is perceived as a flicker. Subjects' thresholds were obtained by having the subjects minimize or eliminate the perception of flicker, a condition known as sensation luminance [15], by adjusting the radiance of the 460 nm light (while the radiance of the 540 nm light was held constant) until the energy of the two lights were perceptually the same. Since flicker sensitivity also differs across subjects, the flicker alternation rates were optimized for each subject using the algorithm described in Stringham *et al.* [13] MPOD was measured at 15′, 30′, 60′, and 105′ retinal eccentricity in the temporal hemi-retina with a macular densitometer, manufactured by Macular Metrics (Rehoboth, MA, USA).

Assessment of serum LZ required collection of blood into 10 mL lithium heparin coated vacutainers (BD) by a licensed phlebotomist. Plasma was separated by centrifugation at 1500× *g* for 20 min at 4 °C and then distributed into light protected Eppendorf vials tubes for storage at −80 °C. The analysis of the blood was done by the analytical laboratories of DSM Nutritional Products Ltd., Kaiseraugst, Switzerland. Serum LZ were quantified with a normal-phase HPLC system after extraction with a *n*-hexane/chlorophorm 20% (v/v) mixture.

2.3. Assessment of Body Composition

Fat mass (g), percentage body fat, and fat-free soft tissue mass (FFST; g) were assessed using dual-energy X-ray absorptiometry (DXA; Delphi A; S/N 70467; Hologic Inc., Bedford, MA, USA). All scans were analyzed by the same technician with the use of Hologic software, version 11.2. Quality assurance for body composition variables was performed by calibration against a 3-step soft tissue wedge (model TBAR; SN 2275) composed of variable thicknesses of aluminum and lucite, calibrated against stearic acid (100% fat) and water (8.6% fat). With respect to test-retest reliability, single intraclass correlation coefficients (ICCs) were calculated from ten females (aged 18 to 30 years) scanned twice within seven days ($R \geq 0.87$).

2.4. Statistical Analyses

Pearson-product moment correlations were conducted to determine associations between LZ status and fat mass, percentage body fat, and FFST. Comparisons between male and female subjects were made with independent samples *t*-tests. Statistical significance was set at $p < 0.05$.

3. Results

The descriptive data for body composition and LZ status stratified by sex are listed in Table 1. The average MPOD at each eccentricity across the retina for the sample was 0.53 at 15′ eccentricity, 0.43 at

30′, 0.29 at 60′, and 0.13 at 105′ eccentricity. Mean serum LZ levels (for the truncated sample, $n = 65$) were 0.26 μmol/L. Women had higher serum LZ than men (0.28 μmol/L compared to 0.21 μmol/L; $t\,(63) = 2.52, p = 0.01$), however, despite the absence of differences in MPOD (see Table 1).

The average body fat percentage was approximately 26%. Women had significantly higher body fat percentage than men (30% compared to 19%; $t\,(98) = 10.52, p < 0.01$). This discrepancy in body fat percentage between men and women was consistent for each region of the body (see Table 1). However, with respect to the amount of fat in the trunk region relative to the rest of the body, men accumulated a higher percentage of total body fat than women (approximately 48% compared to 43%; $t\,(98) = 3.53, p = 0.001$).

Table 1. Means and standard deviations for body composition variables and LZ status.

	Entire Sample ($N = 100$)	**Males ($N = 39$)**	**Females ($N = 61$)**
Body Fat Percentage			
Total Body	25.79 ± 7.60	18.90 ± 4.89	30.19 ± 5.45
Leg	30.05 ± 8.98	20.72 ± 4.86	36.01 ± 5.03
Trunk	23.12 ± 7.95	17.81 ± 6.15	26.51 ± 7.09
Arm	26.15 ± 9.80	16.44 ± 4.47	32.35 ± 6.75
Trunk Fat (Relative) [a]	44.86 ± 6.35	47.52 ± 6.41	43.17 ± 5.76
Body Mass (g)			
Total Body	65,346 ± 13,345	72,423 ± 12,516	60,790 ± 11,853
Fat-Free Soft Tissue	48,796 ± 10,413	58,980 ± 7291	42,284 ± 5891
Total Body Fat	17,062 ± 7090	13,847 ± 6062	19,132 ± 6972
LZ Status			
MPOD 15′	0.53 ± 0.21	0.55 ± 0.20	0.52 ± 0.22
MPOD 30′	0.43 ± 0.18	0.45 ± 0.17	0.42 ± 0.19
MPOD 60′	0.29 ± 0.14	0.29 ± 0.13	0.29 ± 0.14
MPOD 105′	0.13 ± 0.09	0.14 ± 0.09	0.12 ± 0.09
Serum LZ [b]	0.26 ± 0.12	0.21 ± 0.07	0.28 ± 0.14

[a] Refers to the percentage of total body fat in the trunk region; [b] $N = 65$ (39 Females, 26 Males).

Figure 1 illustrates the significant inverse relationship between total body fat percentage and MPOD at 30′ eccentricity ($r = -0.32, p < 0.01$). This relationship was consistent for each region of the body. Furthermore, individuals with higher body fat percentage had lower MPOD at each retinal eccentricity (see Table 2). The relationship between MPOD and the amount of fat in the trunk region relative to the rest of the body was statistically significant ($r = -0.20$, $p = 0.05$). However, when analyses were performed for men and women separately, statistical significance remained for men ($r = -0.32$, $p = 0.02$) but not for women ($r = -0.19, p = 0.07$), as shown in Figure 2. Consistent with its relation to body fat percentage, MPOD at each retinal eccentricity was related to fat mass ($p < 0.05$). Serum LZ was not significantly related to body fat (see Table 2). MPOD and serum LZ were not significantly related to fat-free soft tissue mass (data not reported).

Table 2. Pearson-product moment correlation coefficients for associations between body fat percentage and LZ status.

	Body Fat Percentage				
	Total	Leg	Trunk	Arm	Trunk (Relative) [a]
MPOD 15′	−0.26 *	−0.18	−0.28 **	−0.25 *	−0.10
MPOD 30′	−0.32 **	−0.22 *	−0.37 **	−0.30 **	−0.20 *
MPOD 60′	−0.24 *	−0.14	−0.31 **	−0.21 *	−0.23 *
MPOD 105′	−0.29 **	−0.20 *	−0.32 **	−0.28 **	−0.16
Serum LZ	0.16	0.15	0.16	0.11	−0.02

** $p < 0.01$; * $p < 0.05$; [a] Refers to the percentage of total body fat in the trunk region.

Figure 1. The relationship between MPOD at 30′ eccentricity and total body fat percentage.

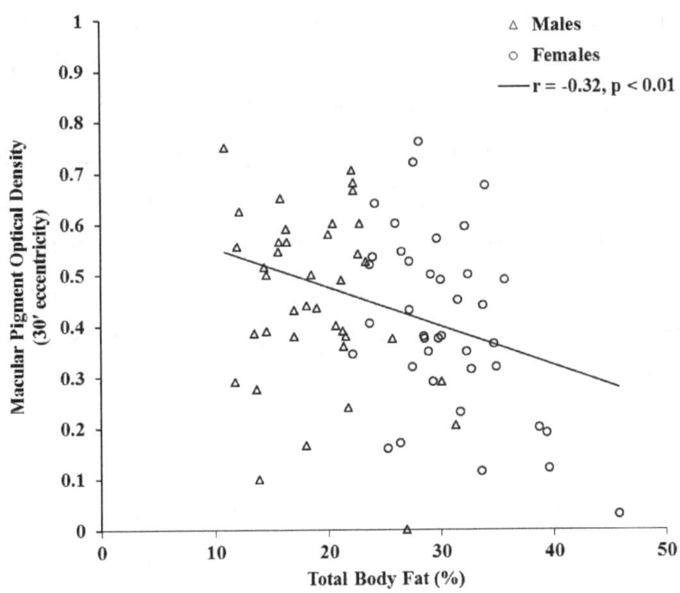

Figure 2. The relationship between MPOD at 30′ eccentricity and the percentage of total body fat that accumulated in the trunk region for male ($N = 39$) and female ($N = 61$) subjects.

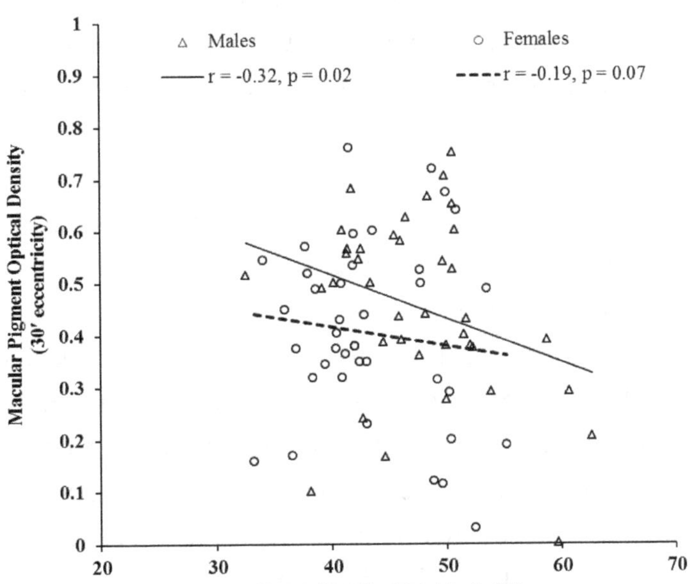

4. Discussion

Consistent with past studies [7,10,16], the primary result of the present study was an inverse relation between MP and body fat across most sites measured. This effect, although statistically significant, and also like past studies of this relation, was only moderate. This may be attributed to the use of young healthy subjects with very limited variability in diet and adiposity: to wit, the group least likely to show effects. Often nutritional relations are driven by the extremes (e.g., those deficient in intake, those showing loss, *etc.*). For example, an inverse relationship between MP and body fat was driven by obese subjects in a study by Hammond *et al.* [10], since the findings were for subjects with over 27% body fat. Limiting our data collection to subjects within a normal range of adiposity, however, was purposeful. Market studies indicate that 85% of Americans take supplements and that these are most often individuals who are already healthy and tend to be affluent and young [17]. We wanted to assess whether normal variation in body fat was related to tissue LZ status within the average range of most Americans, and to determine differences between men and women.

An interaction between adipose and retinal tissue in lutein (L) metabolism was originally proposed by Johnson *et al.* [5] based on findings that changes in adipose L concentration were linked to changes in MP. This relationship, however, was specific to sex: that is, significant negative correlations were found between adipose tissue L concentrations and MP for women, but a significant positive relation was found for men. Broekmans *et al.* [7] reported 13% lower MP in females, despite significantly higher serum and adipose tissue L, and positive associations of adipose L with serum L and MP for male subjects. Nolan *et al.* [16] have argued that their data are consistent with a competition between the retina and body fat for LZ, but only for males. In their sample, MP was inversely related to body fat percentage for men, but no effect was found for women. The results of the current study indicate that higher body percentage, for both men and women, is related to lower MP. This relationship was consistent for each region of the body. However, total fat in the trunk region (relative to the rest of the body) was related to MP in men but not in women. Chung *et al.* [11] reported higher LZ in abdominal adipose tissue compared to buttocks and thighs, and a stronger relationship between LZ in serum and adipose tissue in the abdomen compared to other sites. Our data support the idea that the distribution of body fat, specifically in the abdominal region, influences retinal accumulation of LZ, and that this mechanism may account for differences for men and women in the relationship between adipose and LZ tissue status. This has implications for individual differences in the effectiveness of dietary interventions with LZ.

Dietary supplements containing LZ are being marketed as a way to increase general wellness and protect against conditions linked to oxidative stress. This market trend has been motivated by a large wealth of scientific data showing that a diet deficient in antioxidants is likely to be associated with an elevated risk of degenerative damage. Hammond *et al.* [18] was perhaps the first to note, however, that the same dietary intervention can have significantly different retinal effects across individuals. In that study, some subjects responded vigorously (*i.e.*, tissue LZ increased strongly) to dietary modification with 12 mg of LZ per day (in spinach and corn). Others, however, had no or muted responses.

The nutritional state of the retina has been consistently linked with adiposity. Obesity has also been consistently linked to higher risk of age-related degenerative eye diseases such as macular degeneration [19,20]. Our data suggest that this link can be explained not only by direct stress effects (such as increased inflammatory or oxidative stress) but also by the reduction of some of the natural tissue defenses we evolved to depend upon, such as optimal nutritional status in the form of sufficient LZ concentrations.

Acknowledgments

Funding was provided by DSM Nutritional Products and Kemin Health, LLC.

References

1. Mares-Perlman, J.A.; Millen, A.E.; Ficek, T.L.; Hankinson, S.E. The body of evidence to support a protective role for lutein and zeaxanthin in delaying chronic disease. *J. Nutr.* **2002**, *132*, 518S–524S.
2. Hammond, B.R.; Wooten, B.R.; Smollon, B. Assessment of the validity of *in vivo* methods of measuring human macular pigment optical density. *Optom. Vis. Sci.* **2005**, *82*, 387–404.
3. Parker, R.S. Carotenoids in Human Blood and Tissues. *J. Nutr.* **1989**, *119*, 101–104.
4. Kaplan, L.A.; Lau, J.M.; Stein, E.A. Carotenoid consumption, concentrations, and relationships in various humans organs. *Clin. Physiol. Biochem.* **1990**, *8*, 1–10.
5. Johnson, E.J.; Hammond, B.R.; Yeum, K.; Qin, J.; Wang, X.D.; Castaneda, C.; Snodderly, D.M.; Russell, R.M. Relation among serum and tissue concentrations of lutein and zeaxanthin and macular pigment density. *Am. J. Clin. Nutr.* **2000**, *71*, 1555–1562.
6. Hammond, B.R.; Curran-Celentano, J.; Judd, S.; Fuld, K.; Krinsky, N.I.; Wooten, B.R.; Snodderly, D.M. Sex differences in macular pigment optical density: Relation to plasma carotenoid concentrations and dietary patterns. *Vis. Res.* **1996**, *36*, 2001–2012.
7. Broekmans, W.; Berendschot, T.; Klopping-Ketelaars, I.; de Vries, A.J.; Goldbohm, R.A.; Tijburg L.; Kardinaal, A.F.; van Poppel, G. Macular pigment density in relation to serum and adipose tissue concentrations of lutein and serum concentrations of zeaxanthin. *Am. J. Clin. Nutr.* **2002**, *76*, 595–603.
8. Curran-Celentano, J.; Erdman, J.; Nelson, R.A.; Grater, S.J.E. Alterations in vitamin A, and thyroid hormone status in anorexia nervosa and associated disorders. *Am. J. Clin. Nutr.* **1985**, *42*, 1183–1191.
9. Gruber, M.; Chappell, R.; Millen, A.; LaRowe, T.; Moeller, S.M.; Iannaccone, A. Correlates of serum lutein plus zeaxanthin: Findings from the third national health and nutrition examination survey. *J. Nutr.* **2004**, *134*, 2387–2394.
10. Hammond, B.R.; Ciulla, T.A.; Snodderly, D.M. Macular pigment density is reduced in obese subjects. *Invest. Ophthalmol. Vis. Sci.* **2002**, *43*, 47–50.
11. Chung, H.; Ferreira, A.L.A.; Epstein, S.; Paiva, S.A.R.; Casteneda-Sceppa, C.; Johnson, E.J. Site specific concentrations of carotenoids in adipose tissue: Relations with dietary and serum carotenoids concentrations in healthy adults. *Am. J. Clin. Nutr.* **2009**, *90*, 533–539.
12. Wooten, B.R.; Hammond, B.R.; Land, R.L.; Snodderly, D.M. A practical method for measuring macular pigment optical density. *Invest. Ophthalmol. Vis. Sci.* **1999**, *40*, 2481–2489.

13. Stringham, J.M.; Hammond, B.R.; Nolan, J.M.; Wooten, B.R.; Mammend, A.; Smollen, W.; Snodderly, D.M. The utility of using customized heterochromatic flicker photometry (cHFP) to measure macular pigment in patients with age-related macular degeneration. *Exp. Eye Res.* **2008**, *87*, 445–453.
14. Mares, J.A.; LaRowe, D.; Snodderly, M.; Moeller, S.M.; Gruber, M.J.; Klein, M.L.; Wooten, B.R.; Johnson, E.J.; Chappell, R.J.; CAREDS Macular Pigment Study Group and Investigators. Predictors of optical density of lutein and zeaxanthin in retinas of older women in the Carotenoids in Age-Related Eye Disease Study, an ancillary study of the Women's Health Initiative. *Am. J. Clin. Nutr.* **2006**, *84*, 1107–1122.
15. Kaiser, P.K. Sensation luminance: A new name to distinguish CIE luminance from luminance dependent on an individual's spectral sensitivity. *Vis. Res.* **1988**, *28*, 455–456.
16. Nolan, J.; O'Donovan, O.; Kavanagh, H.; Stack, J.; Harrison, M.; Muldoon, A.; Mellerio, J.; Beatty, S. Macular pigment and percentage of body fat. *Invest. Ophthalmol. Vis. Sci.* **2004**, *45*, 3940–3950.
17. Dietary Supplement Barometer Survey, The Natural Marketing Institute, 2005. Available online: http://www.naturalhealthvillage.com/newsletter/15oct05/264-DSEA_Supplement_Barometer_Survey_Executive%201%20.pdf (accessed on 28 June 2011).
18. Hammond, B.R.; Johnson, E.J.; Russell, R.M.; Krinsky, N.I.; Yeum, K.J.; Edwards, R.B.; Snodderly, D.M. Dietary modification of human macular pigment density. *Invest. Ophthalmol. Vis. Sci.* **1997**, *38*, 1795–1801.
19. Johnson, E.J. Obesity, lutein metabolism, and age-related macular degeneration: A web of connections. *Nutr. Rev.* **2005**, *63*, 9–15.
20. Seddon, J.M.; Cote, J.; Davis, N.; Rosner, B. Progression of age-related macular degeneration: Association with body mass index, waist circumference, and waist-hip ratio. *Arch. Ophthalmol.* **2003**, *121*, 785–792.

10

Retinal Spectral Domain Optical Coherence Tomography in Early Atrophic Age-Related Macular Degeneration (AMD) and a New Metric for Objective Evaluation of the Efficacy of Ocular Nutrition

Stuart Richer [1,2,*], Jane Cho [1,2], William Stiles [1], Marc Levin [1], James S. Wrobel [3], Michael Sinai [4] and Carla Thomas [1]

1 Eye Clinic, James A Lovell Federal Health Care Center, North Chicago, IL 60064, USA; E-Mails: jane.cho@my.rfums.org (J.C.); ilovemabel@aol.com (W.S.); medpat@comcast.net (M.L.); carla.thomas2@va.gov (C.T.)
2 Family & Preventive Medicine, RFUMS Chicago Medical School, North Chicago, IL 60064, USA
3 Internal Medicine, Podiatry Services, University of Michigan, Ann Arbor, MI 48105, USA; E-Mail: jswrobel@med.umich.edu
4 Optovue Inc., Fremont, CA 94538, USA; E-Mail: mike_sinai@optovue.com

* Author to whom correspondence should be addressed; E-Mail: Stuart.Richer1@VA.Gov;

Abstract: Purpose: A challenge in ocular preventive medicine is identification of patients with early pathological retinal damage that might benefit from nutritional intervention. The purpose of this study is to evaluate retinal thinning (RT) in early atrophic age-related macular degeneration (AMD) against visual function data from the Zeaxanthin and Visual Function (ZVF) randomized double masked placebo controlled clinical trial (FDA IND #78973). Methods: Retrospective, observational case series of medical center veterans with minimal visible AMD retinopathy (AREDS Report #18 simplified grading 1.4/4.0 bilateral retinopathy). Foveal and extra-foveal four quadrant SDOCT RT measurements were evaluated in n = 54 clinical and ZVF AMD patients. RT by age was determined and compared to the OptoVue SD OCT normative database. RT by quadrant in a subset of n = 29 ZVF patients was correlated with contrast sensitivity and parafoveal blue cone increment thresholds. Results: Foveal RT in AMD patients and non-AMD patients was preserved with age. Extrafoveal regions, however, showed significant slope differences between AMD patients and non-AMD patients, with the superior and nasal quadrants most vulnerable to retinal thinning (sup quad: −5.5 μm/decade thinning *vs.* Non-AMD: −1.1 μm/decade, $P < 0.02$; nasal quad: −5.0 μm/decade thinning *vs.* Non-AMD: −1.0 μm/decade, $P < 0.04$). Two measures of extrafoveal visual deterioration were correlated: A significant inverse correlation between % RT and contrast sensitivity ($r = -0.33$, $P = 0.01$, 2 Tailed Paired T) and an elevated extrafoveal increment blue cone threshold ($r = +0.34$, $P = 0.01$, 2 Tailed T). Additional SD OCT RT data for the non-AMD oldest age group (ages 82–91) is needed to fully substantiate the model. Conclusion: A simple new SD OCT clinical metric called "% extra-foveal RT" correlates well with functional visual loss in early AMD patients having minimal visible retinopathy. This metric can be used to follow the effect of repleting ocular nutrients, such as zinc, antioxidants, carotenoids, *n*-3 essential fats, resveratrol and vitamin D.

Keywords: atrophic age-related macular degeneration (AMD); spectral domain OCT (SD OCT); contrast sensitivity function (CSF); extrafoveal blue-cone increment thresholds

---

1. Introduction

Age-related macular degeneration (AMD) is the leading cause of vision loss in both developed and developing countries [1–3]. The initial clinical stereoscopic ophthalmoscopic manifestations of the dry form of the disease are drusen formation and RPE hypo/hyper pigmentation. These signs have been used in large scale "ocular nutrient" studies such as AREDS I and II to monitor disease and stratify risk of progression. Yet much pathology is hidden below the surface of the retina. Classic fundus observation and photography even with stereoscopic enhancement by a highly trained physician often reveals merely the gross manifestations of moderate and advanced disease. Emerging sensitive, new technologies include retinal pigment epithelium autofluorescence imaging [4], multi spectral retinal imaging (*i.e.*, Annidis Health Systems, Ottawa, Canada) [5], and high resolution spectral domain OCT imaging for more subtle changes of the retina and choroid [6]. Beyond imaging, lipofuscin is the most consistent and phylogenically constant marker of cellular aging that can be useful for managing AMD [7]. Furthermore, autofluorescence of the A2E fluorophore within the RPE is utilized within AREDS 2 to evaluate geographic atrophic edge expansion [8]. These new technologies, when broadly evaluated in conjunction with preventive medicine/nutritional intervention, may assist eye physicians in preventing the development of moderate and advanced catastrophic AMD.

The Optovue® RTVue (Fremont, CA) was the first commercially available spectral/Fourier domain optical coherence tomography (SD OCT) instrument in the United States. This SD OCT utilizes a low-coherence super luminescent diode light source at a near infrared wavelength of 840 nm (bandwidth 50 nm), and is capable of achieving 5 μm axial tissue resolution. The MM5 scan pattern provides full retinal thickness measurements in the macula as well as nine summary parameters from a 9-zone ETDRS grid.

Clinical observations stimulated the design of this study. We observed that patients with very early, and often subclinical atrophic AMD, display various degrees of parafoveal thinning using the SD OCT

MM5 protocol. For example, Figure 1a depicts the right eye MM5 and contrast sensitivity function (CSF) of four patients with early atrophic AMD, mild and similar lens opacification rating using the LOCS III grading system [9] and 20/20 or better Snellen acuity. The green areas on the thickness maps show regions that have within normal thickness values (compared to the RTVue normative database). The blue areas show regions that have significant thinning ($P < 0.05$). Note that with increasing parafoveal geographic thinning, there is a dramatic declining contrast sensitivity function (CSF) "Area under the curve" (AUC) value. None of these four representative eyes had additional pathology that would decrease the CSF function, *i.e.*, uncorrected refractive error, clinically significant cataract, diabetes, glaucoma or neurodegenerative disease. Figure 1b depicts an image simulation of a high-risk driver-pedestrian traffic scene generated when each of these four CSF functions is analyzed with image processing software (Functional Vision Analyzer®, Stereo Optical, Inc., Chicago, IL). The last driver in particular, with 92% parafoveal + perifoveal thinning preserves his central foveal thickness, has 20/20 Snellen acuity yet profound CSF AUC loss, profound distance visual disability and profound simulated road-scene image degradation. This clinical observation led us to the hypothesis that retinal thinning is quickly measured by SD OCT, may be correlated with subclinical visual disability, and may therefore serve as a new efficient objective clinical metric for diagnosing early atrophic AMD as well as serving as a new adjunct measure of progression.

Figure 1. Retinal thinning, declining contrast sensitivity and simulated impaired driver visibility. (**a**) Spectral Domain OCT MM5 plots of early atrophic AMD phakic retinas from four eyes of four different patients (subject Z22 9% extra-foveal thinning (EFT); Z23 28% EFT; Z18 58% EFT and Z52 92% EFT) in the Zeaxanthin and Vision Function Study (ZVF) FDA IND #78973—see [10]. These subjects all had similar lens opacification by LOCS III analysis and 20/20 or better ETDRS visual acuity. Adjacent CSF plots indicate declining contrast sensitivity with increasing loss of parafoveal retinal thickness. (**b**) Image simulation of a traffic scene of a little girl next to a car computed from each CSF function shown to the left. Images correlate with the monocular CSF of these four patients (clockwise upper left: Z22, Z23, Z18 and Z52), using image processing software (Functional Vision Analyzer®) donated by Stereo Optical, Inc., Chicago, IL.

(a) (b)

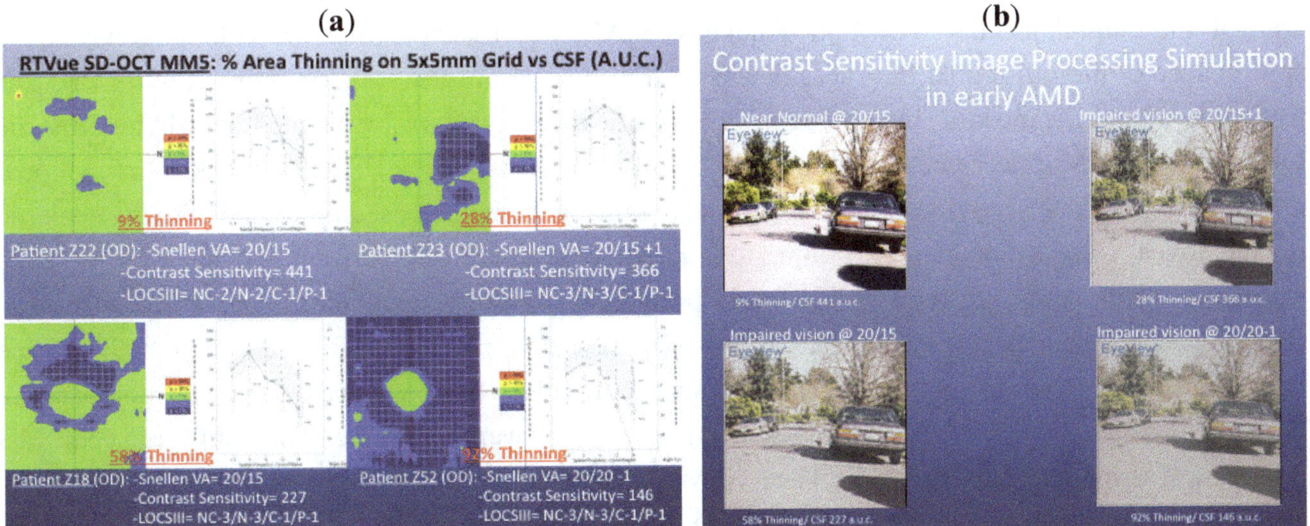

2. Methods

Subjects were included from two data sets: a subset of the Zeaxanthin and Vision Function (ZVF) study data set and an additional de-identified clinical OCT data acquired within the Eye Clinic, DVA Medical Center, North Chicago, IL, during routine clinical care. ZVF is a prospective 12 month n = 119 eye, randomized, placebo controlled (RCT) trial evaluating one degree macular pigment optical density (MPOD) and distribution (MP), visual acuity, CSF, glare recovery, shape discrimination, large field B/Y color vision threshold, and lipofuscin pattern distributions following supplementation with the carotenoids: zeaxanthin at 8 mg, lutein at 9 mg or a combination of both. ZVF was approved by the R&D and Human Subjects Committees of the Department of Veterans' Affairs Medical Center, Hines, IL under the auspices of the FDA (www.ClinicalTrials.Gov IND#78.973; Richer *et al.* [10]). A total of 56 eyes of twenty nine subjects (27 males and 2 females) had completed ZVF with available post-research study SD OCT scans. In the case of the second larger observational SD OCT data set, de-identified clinical data on a random subset of AMD clinic patients was merged with the ZVF 12 month visual function data subset. Thus SD OCT scans of these 29 Clinic subjects, 50 to 88 years (73 ± 10.5 years) of age with mild atrophic AMD cases (but without vision function data) were merged with the ZVF subjects to create a second larger data set consisting of 98 eyes of fifty four subjects (49 males and 5 females) with an age range of 50 to 91 years (74 ± 10.1 years). Only patients with atrophic AMD and typical SD OCT retinal signs were included. For example, RPE/Photoreceptor or photoreceptor integrity line (PIL) disruption, soft drusen, drusenoid RPE detachments, outer nuclear layer reflective (inflammatory) bodies, *etc.* but without evidence of sensory retinal detachment or sub-retinal neovascularization [6]. Subjects with the entity "Age-Related Choroidal Atrophy" manifesting extreme choroidal thinning of less than 125 microns were excluded [11]. Potential retinal thickness and visual function confounders, such as subjects with glaucoma, significant diabetic retinopathy (*i.e.*, macular edema), pre-retinal gliosis and vitreal traction syndrome were excluded. In the ZVF group, four patients had both eyes and three patients had only one eye excluded whereas in the eye clinic AMD patient group, seven patients had both eyes excluded. Subjects were limited to ±6.00 DS refractive error. Informed consent was obtained from ZVF subjects and the Declaration of Helsinki protocols were maintained.

The RTVue provides a detailed sampling of over 19,000 thickness points plotted in a 5 mm × 5 mm area of the central macula. The Full Thickness MM5 Significance Map presentation reveals the significance of the full retinal thickness deviation from normal, of the scanned retina (Figure 1a). The total area of significant loss (blue areas in the Significance Map) was calculated and divided by the total area of the Map to calculate the percent extrafoveal thinning (% EFT), and used for functional correlation. The MM5 provides nine retinal thickness measurements based on the ETDRS, is centered on the fovea with a diameter of 1 mm, four *parafoveal quadrants* surrounding the central fovea extending form 1 mm out to 3 mm, and four perifoveal *quadrants* extending from 3 mm to 5 mm. Extra foveal paramaters refer to the sum of *parafoveal* + *perifoveal* area. Figure 2 depicts these nine regions. An age-matched subset of the RTVue normative database was used for comparison. Normative data from 309 patients (594 retinas) age 50–82 were available. The subfoveal choroidal thickness was measured using the En Face viewing option of the 3D macular presentation. This view presents the sum of all c-scan planes of the same 5 mm macular radius in a top-down fundus view. The choroidal layer was determined to be the distance between Bruch's membrane to a depth at which choroidal vessels can no longer be seen. Two measurements were made for each eye, with an acceptable intra-observer (author JC) coefficient of variation of +0.90. The average choroidal thickness of these two measurements is reported.

Visual psychophysical data, lens opacification and NEI VFQ25 vision questionnaire and retinal grading were available for ZVF patients only. Best refracted distance visual acuity measured with randomly presented ETDRS letters on an M&S Technologies (Chicago, IL) SmartSystem II LCD monitor viewed at 10 feet (SR). The CSF test was performed using best refracted maximum visual acuity and the Functional Vision Anayzer (Stereo Optical, Inc Chicago, IL) as previously described [12,13]. Blue/Yellow Color Vision increment thresholds were ascertained with the ChromaTest® (Bromley, UK) with best corrective lenses according to protocol [10,14,15]. Integrated 6 degree diameter Macular Pigment (MP) area under the curve (AUC) was determined objectively with an ARIS 110 camera (Visual Pathways, Prescott, AZ) by the method of specular reflectance [16].

Figure 2. Full thickness SD OCT MM5 EDTRS significance map schematic. Nine zone ETDRS (Early Treatment of Diabetic Retinopathy) grid provided by the RTVue SDOCT measures an area 5 mm × 5 mm on the retina (MM5 retinal thickness scan pattern). This grid is centered on the fovea and shows the relative location of each of four extra-foveal quadrants defined as the sum of the parafovea + perifovea regions (figure courtesy Optovue Inc., Fremont, CA).

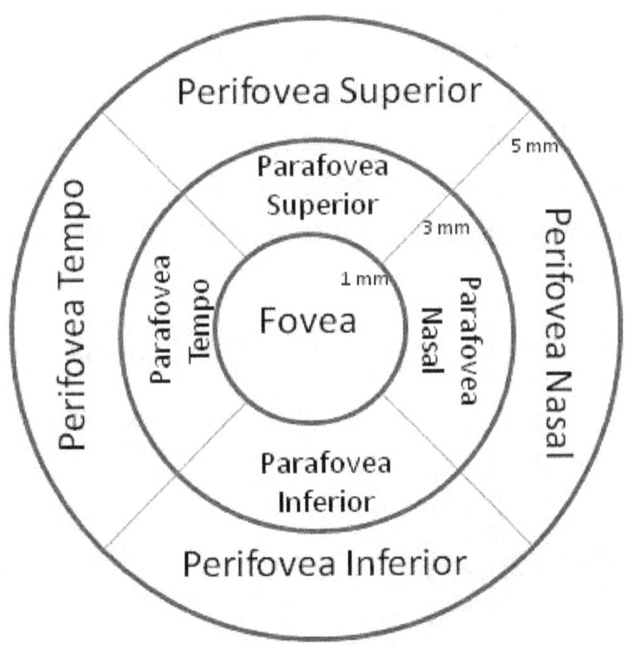

Lens opacification, a confounder of CSF, was qualitatively assessed using a seven increment scaled LOCSIII transparency with multivariate analysis as previously described [9,12,13]. Fifty degree fundus images were taken with a Kowa VX-10 (Tokyo, Japan). Retinal grading of AMD disease state was completed in a double-masked randomized fashion by a retinal specialist (ML) utilizing the AREDS report #18 simplified (0–4) scale for presence of hypo/hyper RPE pigmentation and soft drusen [17]. Overall visual function was assessed with the NEI VFQ25 vision function questionnaire [10].

Statistics: As with ZVF [10], average-eye visual function data from a single subject, and significance, is typically shown for simplicity, in cases in which the analysis did not differ appreciably from evaluating right eyes and left eyes separately. Thus the last three figures in the RESULTS section present data for both eyes. Statistical analysis utilized two sided, student *T*-tests for paired comparison data and $P < 0.05$ was considered significant.

3. Results

The right, left and average eye AMD simplified AREDS grade retinopathy for the ZVF fundus image data set was 0.71 (SD 0.6)/2.0 max score, 0.71 (SD 0.5) 2.0 max score, and 1.43 (SD 0.92)/ 4.0 max bilateral retinal score signifying mild AMD. Average eye ETDRS visual acuity was 20/20-1 (SD 1.2 lines). Figure 3 is a scatter plot of age *vs.* average foveal thickness from n = 594 "Normal" retinas from patients ages 50–82 of various ethnicities. This Optovue normative data suggests a slight foveal thickening with age ($r = 0.09$, $P = 0.02$). AMD patients from the ZVF study ($n = 29$ AMD retinas) and the larger merged clinical/research AMD data set (n = 54 AMD retinas), ages 50+ reveal: (1) slightly thinner foveal thickness compared to these "Normals" and (2) a thickness that does not change with age. Regardless, "Normal" and AMD foveal thickness appears to be highly guarded, conserved, and little changed with age.

Figure 3. Foveal thickness and aging. RTVue SD OCT normative retinal thickness MM5 data from (n = 597) international retinas of an all ethnicities and gender data base between the ages of 50 and 82. The normal fovea thickens approximately 2.5 µm/decade. (Courtesy Optovue, Fremont, CA) Also shown is retinal thickness *vs.* age for post study ZVF AMD subjects (n = 29 retinas) and a combined AMD clinical patient population inclusive of these research (n = 54 retinas) with a greater number of AMD subjects in the 82–91 age group.

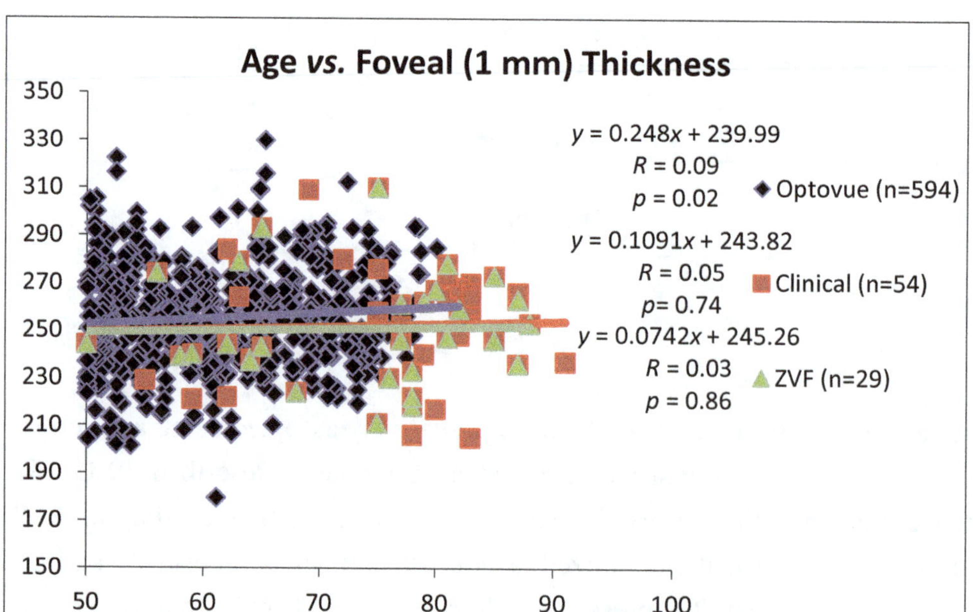

In contradistinction to this slight foveal thickening, Figure 4a–d and Table 1 show parafoveal + perifoveal quadrants slightly *thin* with age in normals, although not significantly: (Superior Quadrant: −1.1 μm/decade; Nasal Quadrant: −1.0 μm/decade; Inferior Quadrant −0.6 μm/decade and Temporal Quadrant −0.3 μm/decade). In both the ZVF AMD study and the larger merged AMD clinical data set, overall macular thickness excluding the fovea show accelerated thinning at a rate of −6.7 μm/decade (P = 0.03) and −4.6 μm/decade (P = 0.04) respectively. Specifically, AMD patients thin by −5.5 μm/decade ($P < 0.02$) superiorly, −5.0 μm ($P < 0.04$) nasally, −4.5 μm ($P < 0.07$ for trend) inferiorly, and −3.3 μm (NS) temporally using data from 54 AMD retinas. Table 1 summarizes this AMD retinal thinning effect. This difference is outside the 5 μm coefficient of variation of the instrument. More specifically, Table 2 depicts accelerated thinning of macular retinal thickness (μm/decade) in the overall 5 mm retinal diameter ETDRS diameter grid *excluding the fovea* and extrafoveal quadrants (but not the fovea) in AMD retinas, compared with the age matched "Optovue normative" population data. A statistically significant AMD retinal thinning effect is particularly evident in the vulnerable superior retinal ETDRS quadrant compared with the temporal quadrant (ns).

Figure 4. Extra-foveal quadrant thickness *vs.* age. (**a**) Superior quadrant; (**b**) Nasal quadrant; (**c**) Inferior quadrant; (**d**) Temporal quadrant. Plots reflect the RTVue SD OCT age matched normative data against the two AMD retina data sets: ZVF and the larger clinical AMD patient data set that includes ZVF study patients. Both AMD data sets display accelerated thinning with age, especially for the superior quadrant ($P < 0.02$). See Table 1.

(a)

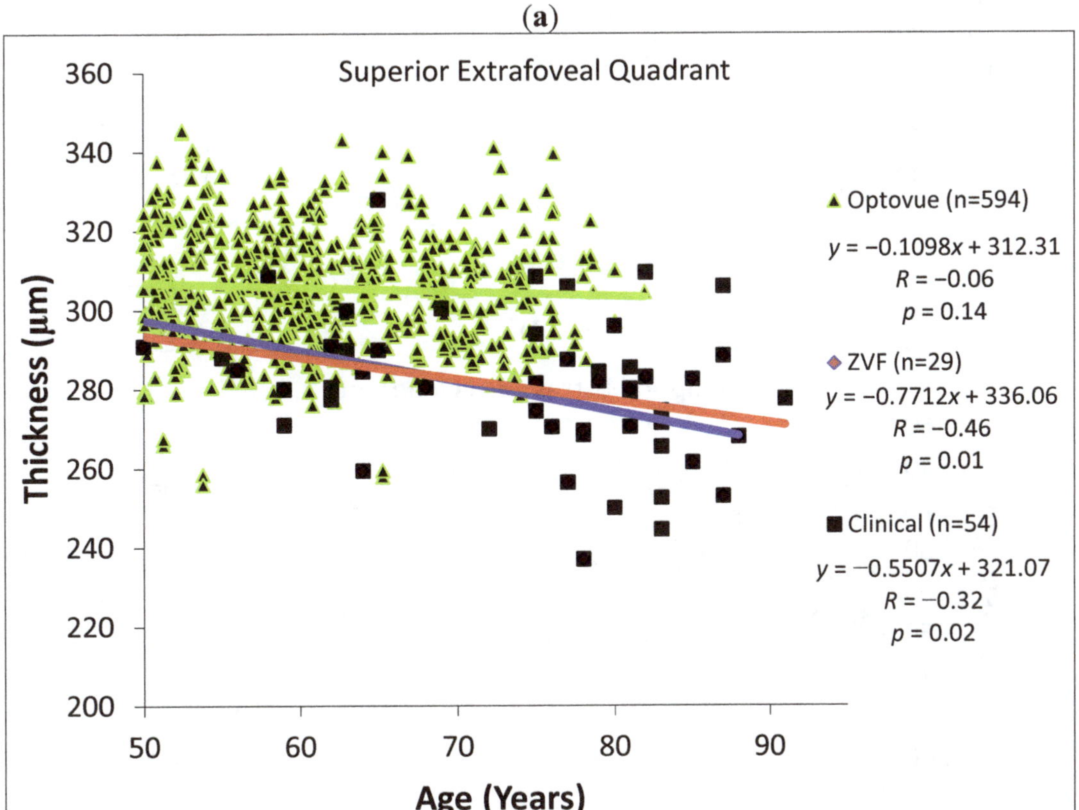

Figure 4. *Cont.*

(b)

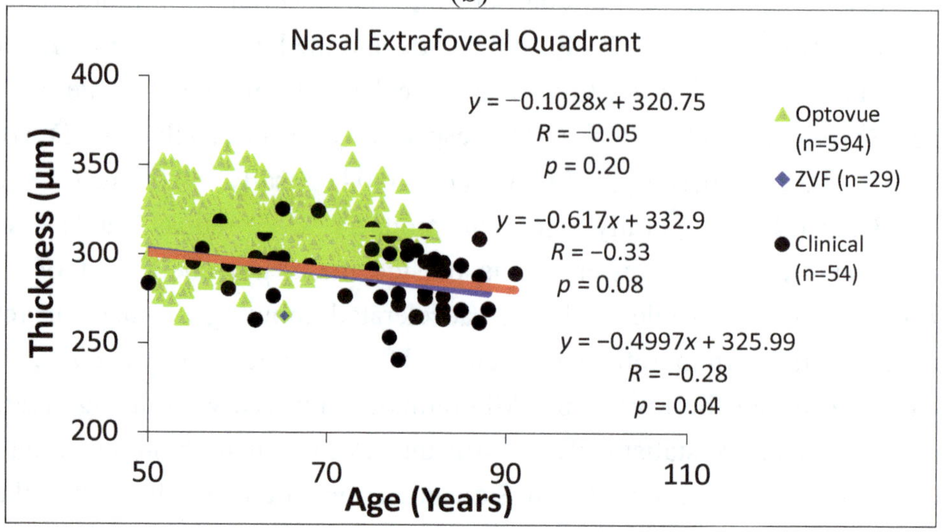

(c)

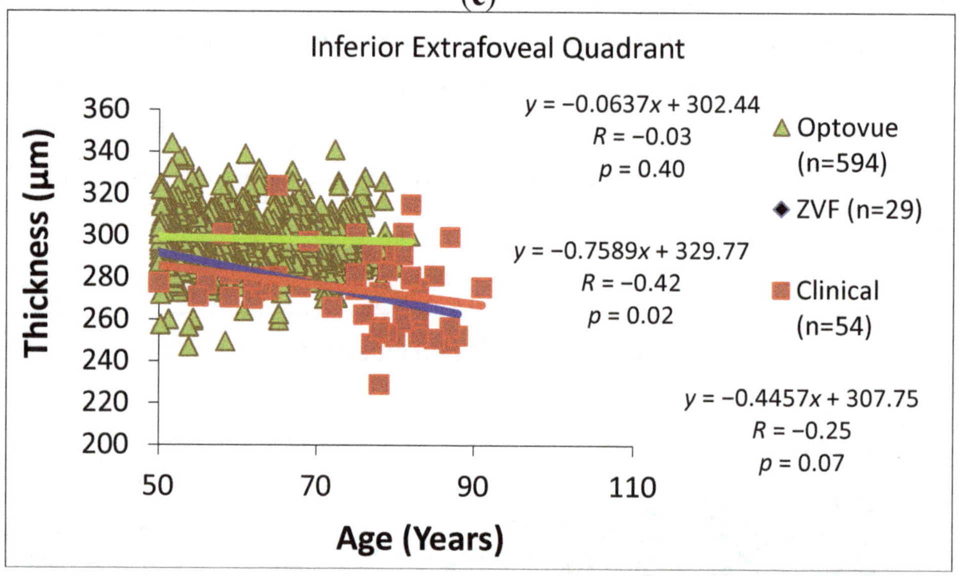

(d)

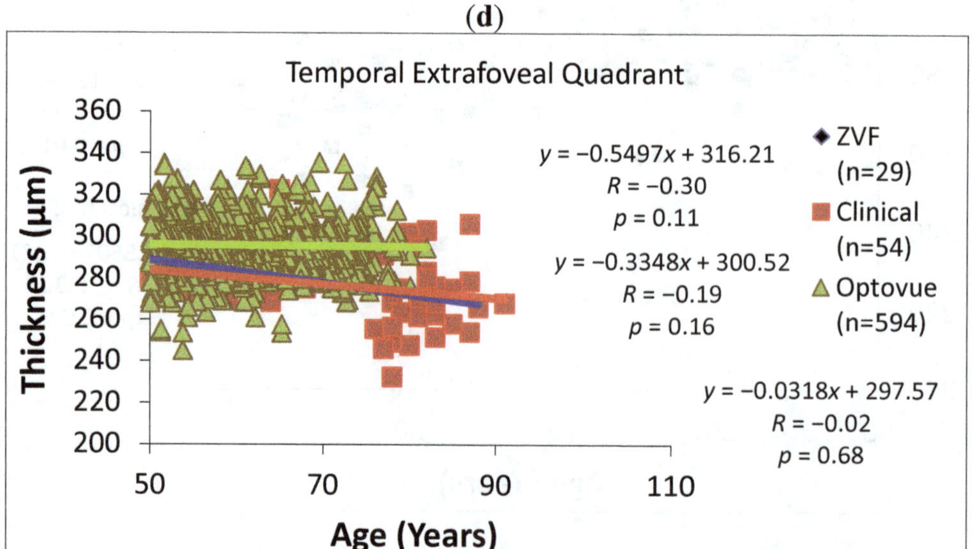

Table 1. The mean (SD) retinal thickness (μm) of patients with AMD is thinner than those from the OptoVue SD OCT "normative" population data base. This difference is outside the 5 μm axial published instrument coefficient of variation.

	Superior	Nasal	Inferior	Temporal
AMD Clinic (n = 54 eyes)	280 ± 17.5 μm	288.7 ± 18	274.5 ± 18	275.5 ± 17.4
AMD ZVF (n = 29 eyes)	279.6 ± 17.7	287.7 ± 19.5	274.2 ± 19.1	276 ± 19.3
Normative (n = 594 eyes)	305.6 ± 14.6	314.4 ± 15.6	298.5 ± 14.8	295.6 ± 14.7

Table 2. Accelerated thinning of macular retinal thickness (μm/decade) in the overall 5 mm retinal diameter ETDRS diameter grid *excluding the fovea and* extrafoveal quadrants (but not the fovea) in ZVF Study and clinical AMD retinas, compared with the age matched "Optovue normative" population data. A statistically significant thinning effect in AMD is particularly evident in the vulnerable superior retinal parafoveal + perifoveal ETDRS quadrant [10], see text.

Region	ZVF AMD Studay (n = 29) μm/decade	Clinical AMD Patients (n = 54) μm/decade	Optovue "Normal" Data [1] (n = 594) μm/decade
Overall (Excluding Fovea)	−6.7 * (P = 0.03)	−4.6 * (P = 0.04)	−0.8 (P = 0.30)
Superior	−7.7 * (P < 0.01)	−5.5 * (P = 0.02)	−1.1 (P = 0.14)
Nasal	−6.2 (P = 0.08)	−5.0 * (P = 0.04)	−1.0 (P = 0.20)
Inferior	−7.6 * (P = 0.02)	−4.5 (P = 0.07)	−0.6 (P = 0.40)
Temporal	−5.5 (P = 0.11)	−3.3 (P = 0.19)	−0.3 (P = 0.68)
Fovea	+0.7 (P = 0.86)	+1.1 (P = 0.74)	+2.5 (P = 0.09)

* Indicates significant data; [1] Optovue, Inc., Fremont, CA, normative database.

Figure 5 depicts loss of CSF with age for the ZVF AMD subjects. Parenthetically, the NEI Vision Function Questionnaire (VFQ 25) total all category summed score (data not shown) was positively correlated with this loss of contrast sensitivity (r = +0.27, P = 0.04) and inversely correlated with % total retinal thinning but not significantly (r = −0.20, P = 0.13). As shown in Figure 6a, CSF is inversely related to % macula thinning (r = −0.33, P = 0.01, 2 Tailed T Paired Comparison) , while Figure 6b depicts the 6.5 degree ChromaTest® B/Y threshold to be heightened and directly related to % macula thinning (r = +0.34, P = 0.01, 2 Tailed T Paired Comparison).

Retinal thickness (excluding the fovea) correlated with choroidal thickness, but not significantly (R = +0.15, P = 0.13). However, Figure 7a shows a significant negative correlation between % thinning and choroidal thickness (r = −0.25, P = 0.01) for all subjects while Figure 7b suggests that parafoveal/perifoveal thinning is associated with declining overall volumetric macular pigment optical density (MPOD), but not significantly (r = −0.21, P = 0.14). Precise three dimensional MPOD data was available only for ZVF subjects.

Figure 5. Contrast sensitivity *vs.* age for ZVF AMD subjects. Loss of CSF with age in n = 56 AMD eyes from the ZVF study. Integrated area under the curve of the contrast sensitivity function (CSF) at four spatial frequencies: 3 cc, 6 cc, 12 cc and 18 cc/degree [10]. (Functional Vision Analyzer®, Stereo Optical, Inc., Chicago, IL).

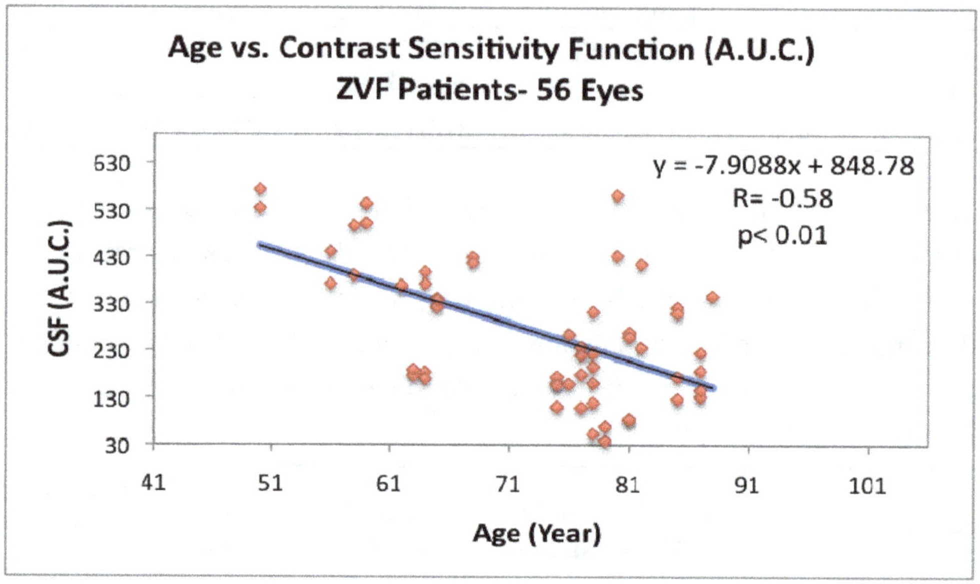

Figure 6. The visual consequences of extra-foveal thinning. (**a**) Contrast sensitivity (area under the curve) is inversely related to % retinal thinning (r = −0.33 P = 0.01, 2 Tailed paired T test). (**b**) 6.5 degree increment blue-threshold is directly related to % retinal thinning (r = +0.34, P = 0.01, 2 Tailed paired T test). Blue/Yellow Color Vision increment thresholds were ascertained with the ChromaTest® (Bromley, UK) with best corrective lenses according to protocol [10,14,15].

(a)

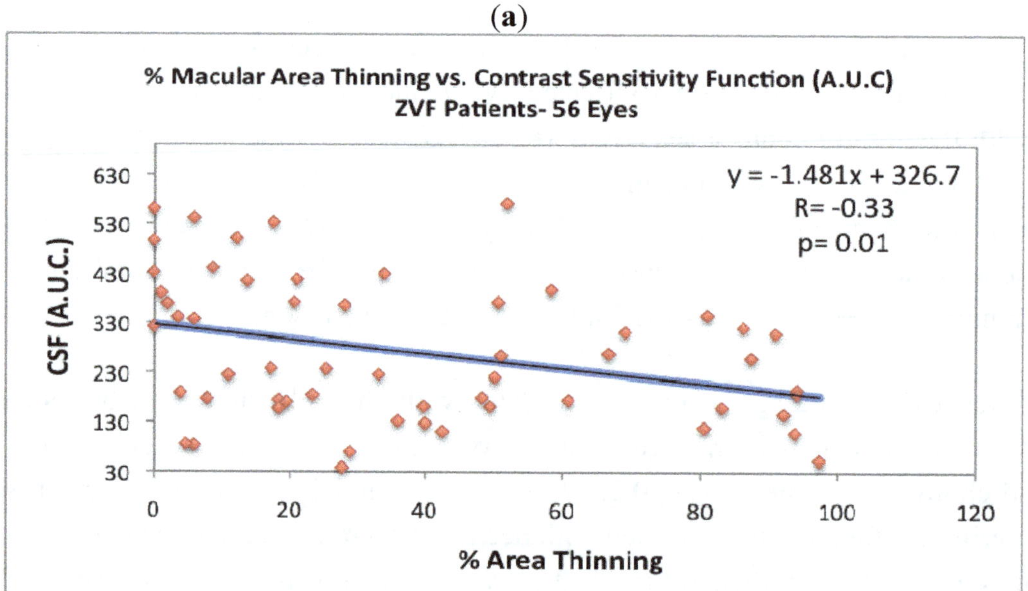

Figure 6. *Cont.*

(b)

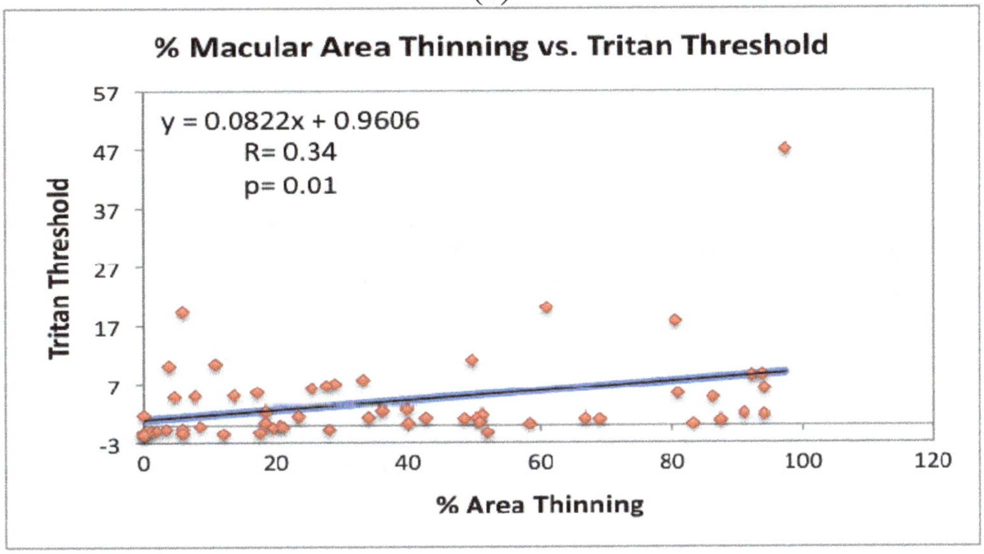

Figure 7. Retinal and choroidal thinning are associated. (**a**) SD OCT measure of choroidal thickness *vs.* % retinal thinning. The coefficient of variation with the manual caliper method, same observer, was $r = 0.90$. Note the significant negative correlation between % retinal thinning and choroidal thickness ($r = -0.25$, $P = 0.01$) for all subjects. (**b**) Three dimensional macula pigment optical density (integrated volume) specular reflectance measurement (ARIS 110 camera, Visual Pathways, Prescott, AZ) *vs.* retinal thinning, reveals % extrafoveal thinning to be associated with declining volumetric macular pigment optic density (MPOD), but not significantly.

(a)

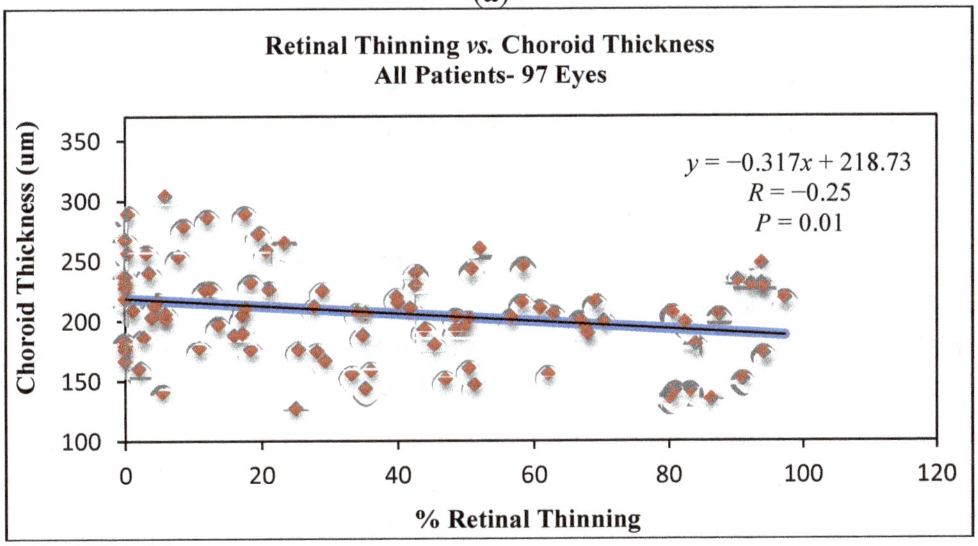

Figure 7. *Cont.*

(**b**)

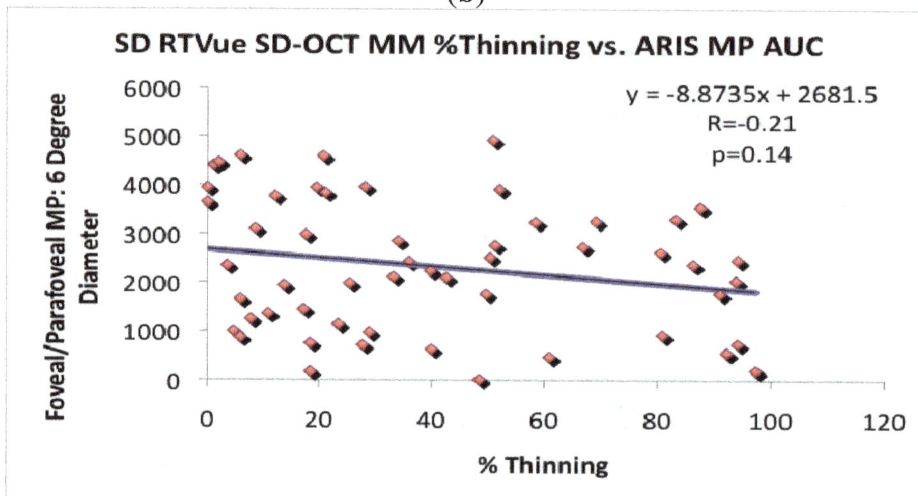

4. Discussion

Foveal thickness appears well protected with age. Even our early AMD patients had no change in central foveal thickness with age. One might expect one or more of the following factors to be associated with age-related retinal thinning: (1) retinal atrophy; (2) choroidal atrophy; or (3) lower foveal macular pigment. We believe the third explanation is germane to this report, as all of the subjects, both post ZVF Study subjects and clinical patients, despite their advancing age had supplemented with approximately 10 mg or more of the oral retinal carotenoids lutein and/or zeaxanthin.

In a manner analogous to neural retinal rim thinning or more recently the concept of pre-glaucomatous ganglionic layer (GCC) cell loss in glaucoma, the atrophic extrafoveal macula appears to thin in AMD at a greater rate than predicted by simple aging. Confounding high myopia was excluded from our database. The order effect with superior most vulnerable and temporal least vulnerable was shown in two data sets—a research data set and a merged research + clinical data set. This pathological patterned loss of tissue was first eloquently revealed by Sarks, Sarks and Killingsworth decades ago using serial fluorescein angiography, white light, and electron microscopy [18]. Our results agree with that historic study.

Our observation that atrophic AMD typically begins in the superior parafovea (at approximately 7 degrees eccentricity) has been confirmed by two other research groups and at the ARVO 2010 meeting (Ft Lauderdale, FL). Significantly, at the Oregon National Primate Research Center, Rhesus monkeys deprived of carotenoids from birth were found to develop atrophic AMD in an extra-foveal superior location [19]. A second group from the Australian National University, using a novel pupillary reaction test, mapped human AMD functional deficits in sector pupillary latency to the superior parafovea [20]. Furthermore, it has been suggested, that the superior half of the retina is vulnerable due to the damaging effects of reflective UV ambient ground reflecting radiation experienced by humans as primates typically walk with a slight head-down gaze (Personal Communication [21]). Ascertaining the health of the superior parafoveal rod rich retina is the basis of the new Maculogix (Atlanta, GA) AMD detection device.

A limitation of this study is the dearth of "normative" patients in the age 82–91 range (Figure 3) combined with the high likelihood of unrecognized subclinical AMD in the "normative" data base especially in old old "normals". However, this lack of patients in the oldest age group combined with the fact that our AMD subjects all had visible retinal pathology creates a counterbalancing bias. This report further supports the conclusion of both the Lutein Antioxidant Supplementation Trial (LAST) and recently published ZVF Study, that subtle signs of photoreceptor—retinal pigment epithelium disturbance characteristic of AMD, such as CSF and increment B/Y color vision thresholds, are impaired long before the appearance of obvious ophthalmoscopic or non-spectral photographic AMD pathological signs appear (*i.e.*, soft drusen or RPE rarefaction). That is, functional visual decline *precedes* photoreceptor—retinal pigment epithelium atrophy [10,12]. The AMD patients in this report had early disease with an AREDS Report #18 five year risk estimate of only 8% for future catastrophic monocular vision loss, near perfect 20/20 ETDRS visual acuity, and no fovea retinal thinning.

In our combined clinical and research experience, patients with even extreme extra-foveal retinal thinning might go undetected in current clinical practice where CSF or even simple, quick near point low contrast Colenbrander visual acuity screening is seldom utilized except perhaps in refractive surgical and contact lens practices [22]. It makes sense that large field (6.5 degree) blue sensitivity suffers earliest in AMD because blue cones are fragile and few in number [14]. By the time the patient is in danger of an acute degenerative change, a flashed 6.5 degree diameter blue/yellow stimulus optotype becomes indistinguishable no matter how intense the color. Once again, subtle color vision disturbances in early AMD are rarely evaluated except in the research laboratory. The decline in visual function in early AMD is far from academic. CSF is related to driving safety and hip fracture risk as well as overall quality of life with mortal implications [23–25]. While a 10-letter (two-line) decrease in best corrected VA is significantly associated with all self-reported measures of visual disability, a mere 2-step decrease in contrast sensitivity is significant [25].

There is increasing recognition that the optical and antioxidant properties of the xanthophyll pigments lutein, zeaxanthin, and lutein's metabolite mesozeaxanthin, play an important role in maintaining the health and function of the human macula [16]. Foveal MPOD has a significant positive, measurement technique independent relationship of approximately $r = +0.30$ with central retinal thickness [26]. Significantly, in that study there was no demonstrable relationship between MPOD at an eccentricity of one or two degrees and central retinal thickness. However in the present AMD study, Figure 7b shows a non-significant trend for extra-foveal thinning to be associated with declining volumetric macular pigment. We also found no significant change in central foveal thickness in agreement with the excellent preservation of visual acuity in both our research and clinical population. Interestingly, several groups have established that MPOD tends to decrease with age [16]. This is conjectured to contribute to the accelerated retinal thinning we observed ostensibly through either direct deposition (*i.e.*, de-pigmentation) or by secondary indirect declining antioxidant tissue protection of the retina and the choriocapillaris/choroidal vascular bed [27]. We also found a significant association between choroidal thinning and retinal thinning. Spaide describes a decrease of 16 μm/decade choroidal thickness in high myopes [11]. Our ZVF AMD patients showed an even greater 22 μm/decade decrease in choroidal thickness with each decade ($r = -0.57$; $P < 0.01$).

5. Conclusion

New technologies and techniques are required to evaluate the effect of nutrient intervention on retinal health in early and moderate AMD. In this report, we present a new objective SD OCT based atrophic AMD metric called "% extra-foveal retinal thinning" or % EFRT. We have shown that % EFRT is associated with loss of contrast sensitivity and extra-foveal blue cones in early AMD. Macular thickness ETDRS SD OCT thickness plots provide eye practitioners with a new clinically useful and objective surrogate measure of early functional visual loss of aging retinas. Indeed, the data and simulations presented in this report explain why practitioners often underestimate the functional impact of a "20/20 AMD diagnosis". Researchers can employ CSF/Low Contrast Screening, SD OCT and MP distribution instrumentation together, to gauge overall and distributional changes in retinal thickness and formally evaluate how prescriptive carotenoid repletion (*i.e.*, lutein/mesozeaxanthin and zeaxanthin along with synergistic *n*-3 fats) impacts % EFRT and visual function. This new metric can be applied to the study of aging, genetic susceptibility and age related choroidal degeneration. The authors believe % EFRT to be superior to the following three currently employed tests: the 150 year old Snellen chart, the 117 year old Amsler Grid and conventional non-spectral fundus cameras. Significantly, % EFRT has potential to meaningfully and efficiently evaluate both nutritional and pharmacologic atrophic AMD intervention(s) in clinical practice as well as retinal research.

Acknowledgements

This material is based on original work supported by the James A Lovell Federal Health Care Center, Eye Clinic (North Chicago, IL) and the Department of Veterans Affairs Research Service/CARES (Hines, IL). Chrysantis/Ball Horticulture (West Chicago, IL) and Kemin Health LC (Des Moines, IA) were the primary granting sponsors of ZVF and LAST respectively. Stereo Optical, Inc. (Chicago, IL) and Optovue (Fremont, CA) provided instrumentation as secondary sponsors of ZVF: FDA IND #78, 973 and our Ocular—Nutrition Laboratory.

References

1. Smith, W.; Assink, J.; Klein, R.; Mitchell, P.; Klaver, C.C.; Klein, B.E.; Hofman, A.; Jensen, S.; Wang, J.J.; de Jong, P.T. Risk factors for age-related macular degeneration: Pooled findings from three continents. *Ophth*almology **2001**, *108*, 697–704.
2. Klein, R.; Peto, T.; Bird, A.; Vannewkirk, M.R. The epidemiology of age-related macular degeneration. *Am. J. Ophthalmol.* **2004**, *137*, 486–495.
3. Harris, G.; Pratt, S.; Richer, S.P. Food and Nutrients in Disease Management. In *Strategies for Medical Doctors, Section I. Conditions of the Ears, Eyes, Nose, and Mouth, Age-Related Macular Degeneration*, 2nd ed.; Kohlstadt, I., Ed.; CRC Press: Philadelphia, PA, USA, 2012; ISBN: 978-1-4200-6720-0.

4. Schmitz-Valkenberg, S.; Fleckenstein, M.; Scholl, H.P.N.; Hlz, F.G. Diagnostic and Surgical Techniques, Fundus Autofluorescense and Progression of Age-Related Macular Degeneration. *Surv. Ophthalmol.* **2009**, *54*, 96–117.
5. Van de Kraats, J.; van Norren, D. Directional and nondirectional spectral reflection from the human fovea. *J. Biomed. Opt.* **2008**, *13*, 024010.
6. Coscas, G. *Optical Coherence Tomography in Age-Related Macular Degeneration*; Springer Medizin Verlag Heidelberg: Heidelberg, Germany, 2009; ISBN: 978-3-642-01468-0.
7. Richer, S.P.; Stiles, W.; Thomas, C. Molecular Medicine in Ophthalmic Care. *Optometry* **2009**, *80*, 695–671.
8. Loane, E.; Kelliher, C.; Beatty, S.; Nolan, J.M. The rationale and evidence base for a protective role of macular pigment in age-related maculopathy. *Br. J. Ophthalmol.* **2008**, *92*, 1163–1168.
9. Chylack, L.T. Function of the lens and methods of quantifying cataract. In *Nutritional and Environmental Influences on the Eye*; Taylor, A., Ed.; CRC Press: Boca Raton, FL, USA, 1999; pp. 25–52.
10. Richer, S.P.; Stiles, W.; Graham-Hoffman, K.; Levin, M.; Ruskin, D.; Wrobel, J.; Park, D.W.; Thomas, C. Randomized, double-blind, placebo-controlled study of zeaxanthin and visual function in patients with atrophic age-related macular degeneration: The Zeaxanthin and Visual Function Study (ZVF) FDA IND #78, 973. *Optometry* **2011**, *82*, 667–680.
11. Spade, R.F. Age-Related Choroidal Atrophy. *Am. J. Ophthalmol.* **2009**, *147*, 801–810.
12. Richer, S.P.; Stiles, W.; Statkute, L.; Pulido, J.; Frankowski, J.; Rudy, D.; Pei, K.; Tsipurski, M.; Nyland, J. Double-masked, placebo-controlled, randomized trial of lutein and antioxidant supplementation in the intervention of atrophic age-related macular degeneration: the Veterans LAST study (Lutein Antioxidant Supplementation Trial). *Optometry* **2004**, *75*, 216–230.
13. Richer, S.P.; Devenport, J.; Lang, J. LAST II: Differential temporal responses of macular pigment optical density (MPOD) in patients with atrophic ARMD to dietary supplementation with xanthophylls. *Optometry* **2007**, *78*, 213–219.
14. Wong, R.; Khan, J.; Adewoyin, T.; Sivaprasad, S.; Arden, G.B.; Chong, V. The ChromaTest, a digital color contrast sensitivity analyzer, for diabetic maculopathy: A pilot study. *BMC Ophthalmol.* **2008**, *8*, 15.
15. Sivagnanavel, V.; Madill, S.A.; Arden, G.B.; Patel, N.; Chong, V.N. Correlation of Colour Contrast Sensitivity With Stage of Age Related Macular Degeneration. *Invest. Ophthalmol. Vis. Sci.* **2005**, *46*, 1398.
16. Bernstein, P.S.; Delori, F.C.; Richer, S.P.; van Kuijk, F.J.; Wenzel, A.J. The value of measurement of macular carotenoid pigment optical densities and distributions in age-related macular degeneration and other retinal disorders. *Vision Res.* **2010**, *50*, 716–728.
17. AREDS Coordinating Center. A Simplified Severity Scale for Age-Related Macular Degeneration. *Arch. Ophthalmol.* **2005**, *123*, 1570–1574.
18. Sarks, J.P.; Sarks, S.H.; Killingsworth, M.C. Evolution of geographic atrophy of the retinal pigment epithelium. *Eye* **1988**, *2*, 552–577.
19. Barker, F.M., II; Snodderly, D.M.; Johnson, E.J.; Schalch, W.; Koepcke, W.; Gerss, J.; Neuringer, M. Nutritional manipulation of primate retinas: Effects of lutein, zeaxanthin, and

n-3 fatty acids on retinal sensitivity to blue-light-induced damage. *Invest. Ophthalmol. Vis. Sci.* **2011**, *52*, 3934–3942.

20. Sabeti, F.; Maddess, T.; James, A. Dichoptic multifocal pupillography identifies retinal dysfunction in early AMD. In *Proceedings of Association for Research in Vision and Ophthalmology Annual Meeting*, Ft Lauderdale, FL, USA, 2–6 May 2010.
21. Sheedy, J. Pacific College of Optometry, Forest Grove, OR, USA. Personal communication, 2010.
22. Colenbrander, A. Assessment of functional vision and its rehabilitation. *Acta Ophthalmol.* **2010**, *88*, 163–173.
23. Owsley, C.; Stalvey, B.T.; Wells, J.; Sloane, M.E.; McGwin, G., Jr. Visual risk factors for crash involvement in older drivers with cataract. *Arch. Ophthalmol.* **2001**, *119*, 881–887.
24. Chew, F.L.; Yong, C.K.; Ayu, S.M.; Tajunisah, I. The association between various visual function tests and low fragility hip fractures among the elderly: A Malaysian experience. *Age Ageing* **2010**, *39*, 239–245.
25. Ivers, R.Q.; Mitchell, P.; Cumming, R.G. Visual function tests, eye disease and symptoms of visual disability: A population-based assessment. *Clin. Exp. Ophthalmol.* **2000**, *28*, 41–47.
26. Liew, S.H.; Gilbert, C.E.; Spector, T.D.; Mellerio, J.; van Kuijk, F.J.; Fitzke, F.; Marshall, J.; Hammond, C.J. Central retinal thickness is positively correlated with macular pigment optical density. *Exp. Eye Res.* **2006**, *82*, 915–920.
27. Nolan, J.M.; Stack, J.O.; Loane, E.; Beatty, S. Risk factors for age related maculopathy are associated with a relative lack of macular pigment. *Exp. Eye Res.* **2007**, *84*, 61–74.

11

The Role of Lutein in Eye-Related Disease

Keyvan Koushan, Raluca Rusovici, Wenhua Li, Lee R. Ferguson and Kakarla V. Chalam *

Department of Ophthalmology, University of Florida, 580 West 8th Street, Tower II, 3rd Fl., Jacksonville, FL 32209, USA; E-Mails: Keyvan.Koushan@jax.ufl.edu (K.K.); Raluca.Rusovici@jax.ufl.edu (R.R.); wenhua_li2003@yahoo.com (W.L.); Lee.Ferguson@jax.ufl.edu (L.R.F.)

* Author to whom correspondence should be addressed; E-Mail: kakarla.chalam@jax.ufl.edu;

Abstract: The lens and retina of the human eye are exposed constantly to light and oxygen. *In situ* phototransduction and oxidative phosphorylation within photoreceptors produces a high level of phototoxic and oxidative related stress. Within the eye, the carotenoids lutein and zeaxanthin are present in high concentrations in contrast to other human tissues. We discuss the role of lutein and zeaxanthin in ameliorating light and oxygen damage, and preventing age-related cellular and tissue deterioration in the eye. Epidemiologic research shows an inverse association between levels of lutein and zeaxanthin in eye tissues and age related degenerative diseases such as macular degeneration (AMD) and cataracts. We examine the role of these carotenoids as blockers of blue-light damage and quenchers of oxygen free radicals. This article provides a review of possible mechanisms of lutein action at a cellular and molecular level. Our review offers insight into current clinical trials and experimental animal studies involving lutein, and possible role of nutritional intervention in common ocular diseases that cause blindness.

Keywords: lutein; age-related macular degeneration; macular pigment; heterochromatic flicker; cataract; macular diseases; uveitis; retinitis pigmentosa

---

1. Introduction

Lutein belongs to the xanthophyll family of carotenoids, which are synthesized within dark green leafy plants, such as spinach and kale [1,2]. On average, Americans consume a daily intake of 1.7 mg lutein [3]. The purified crystalline form of lutein has been generally recognized as being safe for supplementation into foods and beverages [4]. Lutein is absorbed with fat in the gastrointestinal system and transported via lipoproteins. Apolipoprotein E is involved in the transport of lutein in serum [5], with transference being facilitated primarily by High Density Lipoproteins (HDLs) (52%) and Low Density Lipoproteins (LDLs) (22%) [6] In the presence of cholesterol, lutein segregates out from saturated lipid regions (liquid-ordered phase) on cell membranes and accumulate into unsaturated phospholipids in order to form carotenoid-rich domains [7] Tissue specific lutein concentrations are dependent on dietary intake [8,9]. Following dietary ingestion, lutein concentrations of approximately 0.2 μM circulates throughout the body to target tissue sites such as the retina where they are incorporated and serve a functional role in maintenance of tissue homeostasis [3].

In the primate eye lutein, along with zeaxanthin and its isomer meso-zeaxanthin, represent the primary pigment molecule distributed within the macula [6,10]. Lutein and its stereoisomer zeaxanthin are distinguished from other carotenoid compounds based on the chemical composition of hydroxyl group attachments to their structures [11,12]. These macular pigment compounds, which are responsible for the yellow hue of the macula lutea are concentrated in the outer and inner plexiform layers [13,14] as well as in rod outer segment within the macula [15]. Lutein varies in its distribution in the eye. It is found in higher amounts within the peripheral retina, RPE, choroid and ciliary body, while demonstrating small concentrations in the iris and lens [16,17]. Dietary concentrations between 6 and 20 mg per day of lutein have been associated with a reduced risk of ocular disorders such as cataracts and age-related macular degeneration [18,19]. The effects of lutein and other antioxidants in mitigating early onset age related ocular and neurological diseases have been well documented [20–23]. Macular pigments such as lutein have biochemical significance to ocular health by averting disease onset as well as sustaining visual functionality.

2. Structure and Biochemistry of Lutein

2.1. Lutein in the Retina

In terms of tissue concentrations, the presence of lutein and zeaxanthin in the retina represent the highest seen among any other human tissue type. Despite this apparent abundance, the distribution of these carotenoids in the retina is not uniform. In the human fovea, lutein is found in lower quantities relative to zeaxanthin by a ratio of approximate 1:2 [24,25]. In general, the relative amounts of the retinal carotenoids decrease as the point of reference travels farther away from the fovea. This ultimately leads to a ratio amount of 2:1 between lutein and zeaxanthin in the peripheral retina (Figure 1). Moreover, the overall macular pigment optical density for both carotenoids decreases 100 fold in the periphery in comparison to the foveal region [26–30].

Figure 1. Schematic representation of the ratio of lutein to zeaxanthin in central and peripheral retina; L: lutein; Z: zeaxanthin.

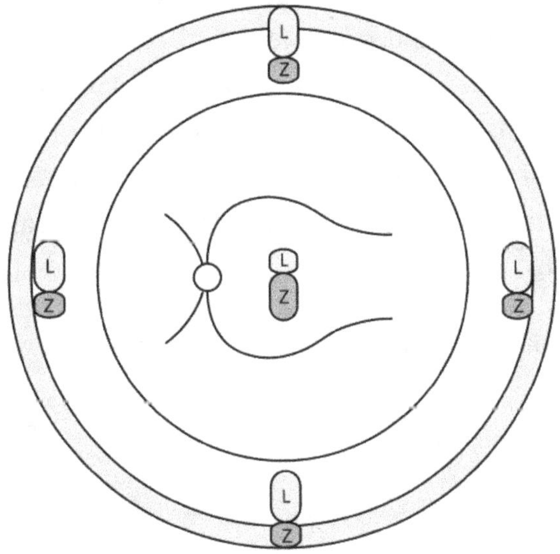

Macular pigment density represents an indirect measure of the amount of lutein present in the body [31–33]. There are several methodologies available that provide some level of quantification of macular pigment density in the retina. Analytical techniques such as heterochromatic flicker [34], fundus reflectometry [35], lipofuscin autofluorescencespectrometry, Resonance Raman Spectroscopy [36], and high performance liquid chromatography (HPLC) [37] provide methods to determine optical density of lutein and other macular pigments. A fairly novel methodology, *in vivo* snapshot hyperspectral imaging with non-negative matrix factorization, analyzes hyperspectral signatures from macular pigments as a means to distinguish biochemical components unique to individual pigment molecules [38].

2.2. Role of Lutein in Prevention of Hypoxia-Induced Cell Damage in the Eye

Free radicals, as defined by the presence of one or more unpaired electrons in an atom or groups of atoms, come in many different forms. The most common type of free radical in biological system is the reactive oxygen species (ROS). ROS such as singlet oxygen species are generated in the retina because of oxygen consumption as well as high energy photon light conversion into electrochemical signaling [39–44]. ROS generated in the retina are believed to be the byproducts of extramitochondrial oxidative phosphorylation in the rod outer segment [44,45]. The accumulation of oxygen radicals and lipid peroxidation, resulting from increased retinal oxygen utilization, has been postulated as a mechanism for photoreceptor apoptosis. Oxidative damage occurring in the rod outer segment causes the release of extra-mitochondrial components like cytochrome c, which initiates apoptosis via caspase 9 activation. One of the major protective roles lutein has in the retina is to serve as an oxygen free radical scavenger during oxidative stress conditions. The ability of lutein to provide effective removal of free radicals, such as singlet oxygen particles, is primarily governed by the chemical structure of two hydroxyl groups acting as strong sinks for reactive oxygen species (Figure 2) [46–48]. Xanthophylls and carotenes are considered the most efficient singlet oxygen scavengers among the carotenoid families [49,50]. The difference in the singlet oxygen extinguishing efficiency primarily relates to the number of double bonds present in the carotenoids. Carotenoids with greater amounts of double bonds are better able to lower their triplet energy state. As a result, molecules such as lycopene, β-carotene, zeaxanthin, cryptoxanthin, and α-carotene can achieve triplet states that facilitate energy transfer with singlet oxygen species. The effective dose (ED50) value of lutein as a free radical scavenger is 0.7 μM. In addition, lutein selectively absorbs blue light, due to its peak absorption spectrum of 446 nm. Blue light produces more light induced damage (100-fold) than orange light, depending on the exposure time. As a consequence of its filtering capabilities, lutein is effective in preventing photoreceptor damage produced by blue light (Figure 3) [51].

Figure 2. Chemical structures of lutein and zeaxanthin.

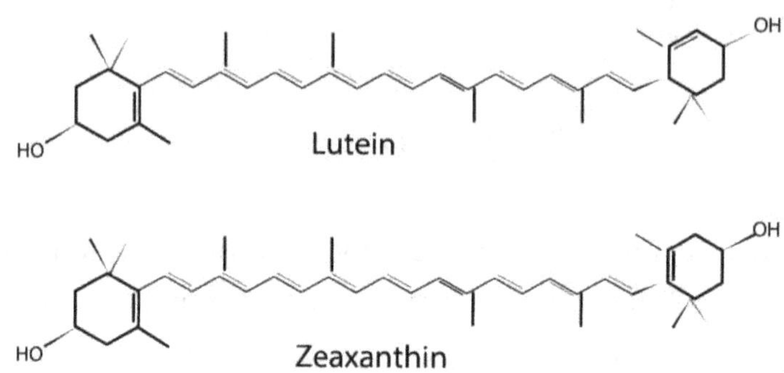

Figure 3. Proposed mechanisms for the protective role of lutein against cellular damage. Lutein reduces the amount of blue light that reaches the photoreceptors. In addition, lutein directly scavenges the reactive oxygen species, thereby preventing them from damaging DNA and protein molecules.

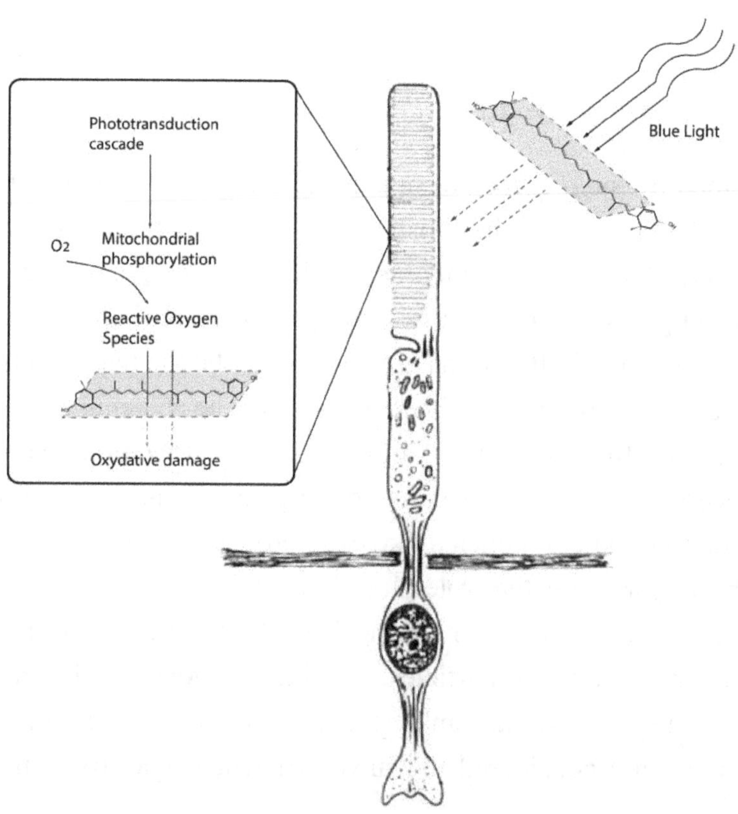

Several *in vivo* and *in vitro* studies have investigated the pharmacokinetic properties of lutein and zeaxanthin as well as the effects xanthophyll supplementation has on prevention of cellular damage due to photochemical and oxidative stress. Snodderly demonstrated that supplementation of cynomolgus and squirrel monkeys with lutein and zeaxanthin resulted in an increase in the plasma concentration of carotenoids [52]. Another study showed serum levels of zeaxanthin in rhesus monkeys can be raised by supplementation with the carotenoids from an extract of Fructus lycii [53]. Some studies have demonstrated reversal of lifelong absence of xanthophylls in primates with lutein supplementation, and subsequent amelioration of acute blue-light photochemical damage [39,54–56]. In retinal pigment epithelial cells, fed native or UV-irradiated photoreceptor outer segments and cultured in 40% oxygen, lutein significantly reduced lipofuscin formation [57,58]. In RGC-5 rat ganglion cell lines, lutein treatment prevented cellular death following oxidative damage via H_2O_2. Similar results were obtained in immortalized Müller cells [59,60].

3. Role of Lutein in Age-Related Macular Degeneration (AMD)

The macula lutea is located in the central and posterior portion of the retina and possesses the highest concentration of photoreceptors, which are responsible for central vision and high-resolution visual acuity. It is a circular area 5–6 mm in diameter that possesses a characteristic yellow pigment that is made up entirely of lutein and zeaxanthin.

Light-induced retinal damage depends largely on the wavelength, exposure time, and intensity of light. For instance, the blue light (440 nm) requires 100 times less intensity to cause damage than orange light (590 nm). The presence of carotenoids in the macula capable of absorbing light of the blue range wavelength would indicate that they serve a protective function. Specifically lutein appears to play a specific role as a photoprotective agent, effectively screening out the damaging blue light from causing excessive damage on the photoreceptors.

AMD is a degenerative process of the macula and is the principle cause of blindness among people age 65 and older in Western countries. AMD can be classified into two categories: non-exudative (or dry) and exudative (or wet) AMD. The former is characterized by accumulation of soft drusen caused by photo-oxidative damage and de-pigmentation of the retinal pigment epithelium. The latter is characterized by neovascularization of the macula, and accumulation of scar tissue.

AMD is a multifactorial disease. Among the important risk factors for AMD are age, genetic susceptibility, sunlight exposure, cigarette smoking, and poor nutritional status.

Combined with the fact that lutein and zeaxanthin are the only carotenoids found in the macula and comprise the macular pigment, this suggests that the observed protective effects of high fruit and vegetable intake may be due primarily to lutein and zeaxanthin intake.

3.1. Experimental Studies

The mechanism by which lutein is transported from blood to RPE and photoreceptors is not well known. It is shown, however, that when lutein and other anti-oxidants (zeaxanthin, lycopene, or α-tocopherol) are added to rabbit and bovine RPE cells under normobaric hyperoxia, formation of lipofuscin is significantly reduced in these cells [61].

A large case-control genetic study on French and North American patients with and without AMD analyzed single nucleotide polymorphism (SNP) rs5888 of the SCARB1 gene, coding for SRBI, which is involved in the lipid and lutein pathways. To investigate whether this SNP polymorphism has an association with AMD, the investigators identified AMD and control subjects who did not carry two known genetic variations associated with AMD (ARMS2 and CHF). They showed that in French and pooled populations (French and North American) without these known mutations, there is a strong association between AMD and SCARB1 gene. Additionally, Subgroup analysis in exudative forms of AMD revealed a pooled OR of 3.6 for individuals heterozygous for rs5888 [62].

Laser-induced choroidal neovascularization (CNV) is widely used in animal models for studying diseases that are associated with CNV, including Age-related Macular Degeneration (AMD). Choroidal vessels invade the subretinal space after photocoagulation in mice. In one study lutein was administered with 0.1% di-methyl sulfoxide (DMSO) as a vehicle daily for 3 days (1, 10, or 100 mg/kg body weight). Lutein significantly inhibited IFK-β-degradation at 4 h in the murine RPE-choroid complex in a dose-dependent fashion. In contrast, lutein administration in mice for 4 days did not affect IFK-β levels in the RPE-choroid. Mice treated with DHMEQ, an inhibitor of NFK-β nuclear translocation, at the dose of 0.5, 1, or 5 mg/kg showed a significant and dose-dependent decrease in the index of CNV volume compared with vehicle-treated mice [63].

3.2. Epidemiological and Clinical Studies

In the late 1980s, a cross-sectional sample from the National Health and Nutritional Examination Survey (NHANES) was used to show that diets high in fruits and vegetables were inversely associated with AMD [64]. Such diets are also high in many carotenoids, including lutein, suggesting that dietary carotenoids may play a role in reducing the risk of AMD [65].

The first epidemiological study to show a direct relationship between lutein intake and AMD risk was reported by Seddon *et al.* in 1994 [18]. Among the specific carotenoids, lutein and zeaxanthin were most strongly associated with decreased AMD risk (57% lower risk for highest quintile of lutein intake). Consistent with this finding was the inverse association between intake of spinach and collard greens, two foods richest in lutein and zeaxanthin, and AMD risk. This was the first study to indicate that individuals deficient in lutein intake may be at higher risk for AMD.

In 1992, the Eye Disease Case-Control Study Group showed that total serum carotenoids (lutein, zeaxanthin, β-carotene, α-carotene, cryptoxanthin and lycopene) were inversely related to AMD risk [66]. Further analysis showed that prevalence of AMD among those in this sample with highest total serum carotenoid concentration was 66% lower than those with the lowest levels. These studies helped provide a basis for the hypothesis that dietary carotenoids may have a protective effect against AMD.

Other observational studies have demonstrated a relationship between lutein and other related outcomes of eye health. A group from the University of New Hampshire examined the relation between serum lutein, lutein intake and macular pigment density (MPD) in a group of 278 healthy volunteers [67]. Their analysis revealed that both serum lutein and dietary lutein significantly correlate with MPD in a positive manner-the higher the level in serum or in the diet, the higher the MPD. These results are consistent with previous observational studies showing a protective effect of serum and dietary lutein against AMD [18,66], and suggest that dietary sources of lutein can influence the amount of lutein deposited in eye tissues.

A revolutionary technique known as Resonance Raman Spectroscopy was used in another observational study to correlate the use of lutein supplements with Macular Pigment Density (MPD) in AMD patients [68]. In a group of age-matched AMD patients and controls, the average MPD was significantly lower in AMD patients compared to controls as long as the subjects were not consuming high-dose lutein supplements. MPD, however, was significantly higher (in the normal range) in AMD patients consuming a lutein supplement (≥4 mg per day) relative to those not receiving the supplement. This study showed that lutein supplementation is associated with increased macular pigmentation and suggests that supplementation may contribute to maintaining eye health.

In another study on enucleated eyes, the investigators obtained donor eyes from AMD patients and control subjects, and measured the actual concentrations of lutein and zeaxanthin in the central regions of the retina (area including and surrounding the macula). Within the inner region (area most closely surrounding the macula), those subjects possessing the highest concentration of lutein were 82% less likely to have AMD relative to those with the lowest concentration [27].

A placebo-controlled, double-masked parallel group study (LISA: Lutein Intervention Study Austria), 126 patients with AMD were randomized into two groups: supplementation with Lutein or placebo for 6 months. Lutein supplementation was found to significantly increase MPOD (Macular Pigment Optical Density), but it showed no effect on macular function (as assessed by microperimetry) or visual acuity [69].

Lutein supplementation has also been shown to improve multifocal electroretingram (mfERG) response in AMD patients. Ma *et al.* have recently randomized 108 AMD patients to receive 10 mg/day lutein ($n = 27$), 20 mg/day lutein ($n = 27$), 10 mg/day lutein plus 10 mg/day zeaxanthin ($n = 27$), or placebo ($n = 27$) for 48 weeks. Their results showed that mfERM responses significantly improved for the 20 mg lutein group and for the lutein and zeaxanthin group. They also showed that macular pigment optical density also improved in all treatment groups [19,21].

Age-Related Eye Disease Study 2 (AREDS2) is a randomized, placebo-controlled, multicenter study designed to determine whether supplementation with 10 mg of lutein and 2 mg of zeaxanthin per day can slow the rate of progression of age-related macular degeneration (AMD) in persons aged 50 to 85 with bilateral intermediate AMD or advanced AMD in 1 eye. All subjects are randomly assigned to placebo ($n = 1012$), Lutein/zeaxanthin (10 mg/2 mg; $n = 1044$), ω-3 long-chain polyunsaturated fatty acids (LCPUFAs; $n = 1069$), or the combination of Lutein/zeaxanthin and ω-3 LCPUFAs ($n = 1078$). All participants are also offered a secondary randomization to 1 of 4 variations of the original AREDS formulations [70]. The results of this study are not published yet. One of the later reports of the original AREDS study, however, has showed that higher dietary intake of lutein/zeaxanthin was independently associated with reduced likelihood of having neovascular AMD, geographic atrophy, and large or extensive intermediate drusen [71].

4. Lutein Role in Diabetic Retinopathy

4.1. Experimental Studies

Diabetic retinopathy in animal models can be induced using streptozocin, a compound that destroys pancreatic insulin-producing β cells. Mice with diabetes show a significant decrease in body weight and a significant increase in blood glucose. As a consequence, retinal ganglion cells and amacrine cells in the inner nuclear layer (INL) undergo apoptosis in this animal model. Results show that lutein prevents reactive oxygen species formation in these diabetic mice and rats. Reactive oxygen species (ROS) in the retina were measured using dihydroethidium and visual function was evaluated by electroretinograms. The decreased amplitude of the oscillatory potentials in the diabetic mice was reversed by administration of lutein [72,73].

4.2. Epidemiological and Clinical Studies

The role of lutein in diabetic retinopathy has not been well studied in human subjects. Only one prospective study on patients with non-proliferative diabetic retinopathy by Hu *et al.* showed that the serum concentration of lutein and zeaxanthin is significantly lower in these patients compared to normal subjects. Their results also suggest that lutein and zeaxanthin supplementation in these patients lead to improvement of visual acuity and decrease in foveal thickness [73]. Their study suggests that lutein and zeaxanthin supplementation may potentially be used as therapeutic agents in treating non-proliferative diabetic retinopathy.

5. Lutein in Retinal Detachment

5.1. Experimental Studies

Retinal detachment was established by subretinal injections of 1.4% sodium hyaluronate in Sprague-Dawley rats. Retinal detachment is traditionally associated with severe photoreceptor cell death. When lutein was given shortly after induction of retinal detachment, it prevented apoptsis of the cells in the outer nuclear layer [74].

5.2. Clinical Studies

Only one study has found high levels of lutein and retinol in the subretinal fluid of a retinal detachment patient. The study found very little β-carotene in subretinal fluid. Lutein was the major carotenoid peak in subretinal fluid (41.4 ± 14.1 ng/mL). The authors suggested that the high proportion of lutein and very low amount of β-carotene in the subretinal fluid support the occurrence of a highly selective transport mechanism of lutein from the blood to the retina [75].

5.3. Lutein in the Lens

Lutein and zeaxanthin are the only carotenoids present in the crystalline lens [76,77]. Cataract is the opacification of the crystalline lens and is caused by precipitation of lens proteins. The development of cataract is facilitated by oxidative damage and often results in impaired vision or blindness.

5.4. Experimental Studies

Lutein reduces fullerol-mediated phototoxic damage of the lens proteins and DNA in human lens epithelial cells in cell culture models. This protective effect is likely due to lutein's antioxidant properties. Other natural antioxidants (*N*-acetyl-L-cysteine nor L-ascorbic acid), however, did not provide any protection for human lens epithelial cells [78].

Animal studies have shown that lutein treatment slows the development and progression of cataracts in diabetic rats (more rats—10 out of 16—presented with clear lenses if treated with lutein *vs.* the non-treated diabetic group). Lipid peroxidation is significantly increased in diabetic lens (up to three-fold) and is reduced by lutein administration in this rat model [3,26,79,80]. In human lens cells, lutein supplementation increases GSH levels which protect against oxidative stress.

5.5. Epidemiological and Clinical Studies

The Carotenoids in Age-Related Eye Disease Study, an ancillary study of the Women's Health Initiative Study showed that women in the highest quintile category of diet or serum levels of lutein and zeaxanthin were 32% less likely to have nuclear cataracts as compared with those in the lowest quintile category [81]. A cross-sectional study of 376 subjects found an inverse relationship between lens optical density (LOD) and MPOD, suggesting that lutein and zeaxanthin may retard aging of the lens [82]. An ancillary study of the Nurses' Health Study cohort on the effect of nutrition on development of age-related cataracts found that the prevalence of nuclear opacification was significantly lower in the highest nutrient intake quintile category relative to the lowest quintile category for vitamin C, vitamin E, riboflavin, folate, beta-carotene, and lutein/zeaxanthin. However, after adjustment for other nutrients, only vitamin C intake remained significantly associated ($p = 0.003$) with the prevalence of nuclear opacities. The prevalence of nuclear cataracts was significantly lower ($p < 0.001$) in the highest vitamin C intake quintile category relative to the lowest quintile category [83].

6. Lutein and the Uvea

Uveitis, a common ophthalmic disorder, is responsible for approximately 10% of blindness in western countries [84,85]. It may be caused by autoimmune disorders, infections or exposure to toxins.

6.1. Experimental Studies

Reactive oxygen species (ROS) play an important role in mediating the inflammatory signals induced by lipopolysaccharides (LPS). It is suggested that natural antioxidants exert protective effects on the LPS-induced uveitis [86].

In an LPS-induced uveitis mice model, oral administration of lutein (125 and 500 mg/kg/day for five days) reduced the nitric oxide level in eye tissues [87]. The same study showed that lutein decreased the malondialdehyde content, increased the oxygen radical absorbance capacity level, glutathione, the vitamin C contents and total superoxide dismutase (SOD) and glutathione peroxidase (GPx) activities and further increased expressions of copper-zinc SOD, manganese SOD and GPx mRNA. Hence the antioxidant properties of lutein contributed to the protection against LPS-induced uveitis, partially through interfering with the inflammatory process.

Multiple animal studies on the neuroprotective effects of lutein against retinal neural damage caused by inflammation in endotoxin-induced uveitis (EIU) [59,88] have shown that the lutein has a dose-dependent anti-inflammatory effect on EIU. The possible mechanism for this effect of lutein may depend on its ability to inhibit the activation of NF-κB and the subsequent inhibition of pro-inflammatory mediators.

6.2. Epidemiological and Clinical Studies

Clinical administration of lutein for prevention or treatment of diseases of the uvea (including uveitis and CNV) has not been reported.

7. Lutein Supplementation

Since lutein is completely insoluble in water, its incorporation into carrier systems has been studied to optimize its nutritional delivery method. Traditionally, lutein is dissolved in an organic solvent and nano-assemblies are obtained by emulsion–solvent evaporation, associating lutein with the amphiphilic cyclodextrin C4:7 at 1:6 molar ratio in aqueous medium. The nano-assemblies allow increased carotenoid solubility in water compared to carotenoid by itself.

It has been suggested that 6 mg of lutein per day, either through diet or using supplements is likely effective in reducing the risk of cataracts and AMD. Although the optimal dose for lutein supplementation has not been established yet, the most common dose in commercial products is 10 mg/day. Lutein is found in many natural products including broccoli, spinach, kale, corn, orange pepper, kiwi fruit, grapes, orange juice, zucchini, and squash. There is 44 mg of lutein per cup of cooked kale, 26 mg/cup of cooked spinach, and 3 mg/cup of broccoli [89]. Toxicity of dietary intake of lutein (supplemental 35 mg per day) has been studied in rats and results show no serious adverse effects [90].

8. Discussion and Conclusions

There are several epidemiological studies that link lutein supplementation with decreased risk of AMD. Lutein supplementation has also been positively linked to increased macular pigment density and improved multifocal electroretingram responses. Building on the findings of the original Age-Related Eye Disease Study, the AREDS2 study is further investigating whether supplementation with lutein and zeaxanthin, in addition to original AREDS formula, would add additional benefit in improving AMD outcomes. Lutein has a significant role in protecting against AMD, most likely through its absorption of the harmful blue light, as well as its inherent antioxidant properties.

The role of lutein in protecting against diabetic retinopathy is not as well established as it is the case for AMD. Serum levels of lutein has been shown to be lower in NPDR patients and lutein supplementation has been shown to improve NPDR [73]. The antioxidant properties of lutein would likely explain its protective function in diabetic retinopathy. Further epidemiologic studies are needed to establish a stronger link between lutein and improvement of diabetic retinopathy.

Several lines of evidence have also suggested a protective role for lutein in the development of nuclear sclerosis cataracts. Considering that oxidative damage of lens proteins plays a major role in development of cataracts, anti-oxidative functions of lutein explain its likely role in slowing the formation of cataracts.

There are weaker lines of evidence to suggest protective roles for lutein against uveitis, and its possible role in the pathogenesis of retinal detachment. Further studies are needed to clarify whether lutein has a role in these ocular diseases.

In conclusion, the antioxidant, anti-inflammatory and blue light-absorptive properties of lutein provide its many protective roles in various ocular diseases especially AMD and cataracts. Lutein has become known as the "eye vitamin" and its dietary intake is important in maintaining its concentration in human lens and retina.

References

1. Snodderly, D.M. Evidence for protection against age-related macular degeneration by carotenoids and antioxidant vitamins. *Am. J. Clin. Nutr.* **1995**, *62*, 1448S–1461S.
2. Subczynski, W.K.; Wisniewska, A.; Widomska, J. Location of macular xanthophylls in the most vulnerable regions of photoreceptor outer-segment membranes. *Arch. Biochem. Biophys.* **2010**, *504*, 61–66.
3. Trumbo, P.R.; Ellwood, K.C. Lutein and zeaxanthin intakes and risk of age-related macular degeneration and cataracts: An evaluation using the Food and Drug Administration's evidence-based review system for health claims. *Am. J. Clin. Nutr.* **2006**, *84*, 971–974.
4. Alves-Rodrigues, A.; Shao, A. The science behind lutein. *Toxicol. Lett.* **2004**, *150*, 57–83.
5. Loane, E.; McKay, G.J.; Nolan, J.M.; Beatty, S. Apolipoprotein E genotype is associated with macular pigment optical density. *Investig. Ophthalmol. Vis. Sci.* **2010**, *51*, 2636–2643.
6. Renzi, L.M.; Hammond, B.R., Jr.; Dengler, M.; Roberts, R. The relation between serum lipids and lutein and zeaxanthin in the serum and retina: Results from cross-sectional, case-control and case study designs. *Lipids Health Dis.* **2012**, *11*, 33; doi:10.1186/1476-511X-11-33.
7. Wisniewska, A.; Draus, J.; Subczynski, W.K. Is a fluid-mosaic model of biological membranes fully relevant? Studies on lipid organization in model and biological membranes. *Cell. Mol. Biol. Lett.* **2003**, *8*, 147–159.
8. Nolan, J.; O'Donovan, O.; Kavanagh, H.; Stack, J.; Harrison, M.; Muldoon, A.; Mellerio, J.; Beatty, S. Macular pigment and percentage of body fat. *Investig. Ophthalmol. Vis. Sci.* **2004**, *45*, 3940–3950.
9. Riso, P.; Porrini, M. Determination of carotenoids in vegetable foods and plasma. *Int. J. Vitam. Nutr. Res.* **1997**, *67*, 47–54.
10. Bhosale, P.; Bernstein, P.S. Vertebrate and invertebrate carotenoid-binding proteins. *Arch. Biochem. Biophys.* **2007**, *458*, 121–127.
11. Lee, B.L.; New, A.L.; Ong, C.N. Simultaneous determination of tocotrienols, tocopherols, retinol, and major carotenoids in human plasma. *Clin. Chem.* **2003**, *49*, 2056–2066.
12. Jenkins, M.Y.; Mitchell, G.V.; Grundel, E. Natural tocopherols in a dietary supplement of lutein affect tissue distribution of tocopherols in young rats. *Nutr. Cancer* **2000**, *37*, 207–214.

13. Snodderly, D.M.; Auran, J.D.; Delori, F.C. The macular pigment. II. Spatial distribution in primate retinas. *Investig. Ophthalmol. Vis. Sci.* **1984**, *25*, 674–685.

14. Sommerburg, O.G.; Siems, W.G.; Hurst, J.S.; Lewis, J.W.; Kliger, D.S.; van Kuijk, F.J. Lutein and zeaxanthin are associated with photoreceptors in the human retina. *Curr. Eye Res.* **1999**, *19*, 491–495.

15. Rapp, L.M.; Maple, S.S.; Choi, J.H. Lutein and zeaxanthin concentrations in rod outer segment membranes from perifoveal and peripheral human retina. *Investig. Ophthalmol. Vis. Sci.* **2000**, *41*, 1200–1209.

16. Bernstein, P.S.; Khachik, F.; Carvalho, L.S.; Muir, G.J.; Zhao, D.Y.; Katz, N.B. Identification and quantitation of carotenoids and their metabolites in the tissues of the human eye. *Exp. Eye Res.* **2001**, *72*, 215–223.

17. Khachik, F.; de Moura, F.F.; Zhao, D.Y.; Aebischer, C.P.; Bernstein, P.S. Transformations of selected carotenoids in plasma, liver, and ocular tissues of humans and in nonprimate animal models. *Investig. Ophthalmol. Vis. Sci.* **2002**, *43*, 3383–3392.

18. Seddon, J.M.; Ajani, U.A.; Sperduto, R.D.; Hiller, R.; Blair, N.; Burton, T.C.; Farber, M.D.; Gragoudas, E.S.; Haller, J.; *et al.* Dietary carotenoids, vitamins A, C, and E, and advanced age-related macular degeneration. Eye Disease Case-Control Study Group. *JAMA* **1994**, *272*, 1413–1420.

19. Ma, L.; Yan, S.F.; Huang, Y.M.; Lu, X.R.; Qian, F.; Pang, H.L.; Xu, X.R.; Zou, Z.Y.; Dong, P.C.; Xiao, X.; *et al.* Effect of lutein and zeaxanthin on macular pigment and visual function in patients with early age-related macular degeneration. *Ophthalmology* **2012**, *119*, 2290–2297.

20. Loughman, J.; Nolan, J.M.; Howard, A.N.; Connolly, E.; Meagher, K.; Beatty, S. The impact of macular pigment augmentation on visual performance using different carotenoid formulations. *Investig. Ophthalmol. Vis. Sci.* **2012**, *53*, 7871–7880.

21. Ma, L,; Dou, H.L.; Huang, Y.M.; Lu, X.R.; Xu, X.R.; Qian, F.; Zou, Z.Y.; Pang, H.L.; Dong, P.C.; Xiao, X.; *et al.* Improvement of retinal function in early age-related macular degeneration after lutein and zeaxanthin supplementation: A randomized, double-masked, placebo-controlled trial. *Am. J. Ophthalmol.* **2012**, *154*, 625–634.

22. Luchsinger, J.A.; Tang, M.X.; Shea, S.; Mayeux, R. Antioxidant vitamin intake and risk of Alzheimer disease. *Arch. Neurol.* **2003**, *60*, 203–208.

23. Ramassamy, C.; Averill, D.; Beffert, U.; Bastianetto, S.; Theroux, L.; Lussier-Cacan, S.; Cohn, J.S.; Christen, Y.; Davignon, J.; Quirion, R.; *et al.* Oxidative damage and protection by antioxidants in the frontal cortex of Alzheimer's disease is related to the apolipoprotein E genotype. *Free Radic. Biol. Med.* **1999**, *27*, 544–553.

24. Trieschmann, M.; Spital, G.; Lommatzsch, A.; van Kuijk, E.; Fitzke, F.; Bird, A.C.; Pauleikhoff, D. Macular pigment: Quantitative analysis on autofluorescence images. *Graefes Arch. Clin. Exp. Ophthalmol.* **2003**, *241*, 1006–1012.

25. Nolan, J.M.; Kenny, R.; O'Regan, C.; Cronin, H.; Loughman, J.; Connolly, E.E.; Kearney, P.; Loane, E.; Beatty, S. Macular pigment optical density in an ageing Irish population: The Irish Longitudinal Study on Ageing. *Ophthalmic Res.* **2010**, *44*, 131–139.

26. Ciulla, T.A.; Hammond, B.R., Jr. Macular pigment density and aging, assessed in the normal elderly and those with cataracts and age-related macular degeneration. *Am. J. Ophthalmol.* **2004**, *138*, 582–587.
27. Bone, R.A.; Landrum, J.T.; Mayne, S.T.; Gomez, C.M.; Tibor, S.E.; Twaroska, E.E. Macular pigment in donor eyes with and without AMD: A case-control study. *Investig. Ophthalmol. Vis. Sci.* **2001**, *42*, 235–240.
28. Bone, R.A.; Landrum, J.T.; Dixon, Z.; Chen, Y.; Llerena, C.M. Lutein and zeaxanthin in the eyes, serum and diet of human subjects. *Exp. Eye Res.* **2000**, *71*, 239–245.
29. Bone, R.A.; Landrum, J.T.; Cao, Y.; Howard, A.N.; Alvarez-Calderon, F. Macular pigment response to a supplement containing meso-zeaxanthin, lutein and zeaxanthin. *Nutr. Metab. (Lond.)* **2007**, *4*, 12; doi:10.1186/1743-7075-4-12.
30. Bone, R.A.; Landrum, J.T.; Guerra, L.H.; Ruiz, C.A. Lutein and zeaxanthin dietary supplements raise macular pigment density and serum concentrations of these carotenoids in humans. *J. Nutr.* **2003**, *133*, 992–998.
31. Stringham, J.M.; Hammond, B.R.; Nolan, J.M.; Wooten, B.R.; Mammen, A.; Smollon, W.; Snodderly, D.M. The utility of using customized heterochromatic flicker photometry (cHFP) to measure macular pigment in patients with age-related macular degeneration. *Exp. Eye Res.* **2008**, *87*, 445–453.
32. Zhao, L.; Sweet, B.V. Lutein and zeaxanthin for macular degeneration. *Am. J. Health Syst. Pharm.* **2008**, *65*, 1232–1238.
33. Johnson, E.J.; Chung, H.Y.; Caldarella, S.M.; Snodderly, D.M. The influence of supplemental lutein and docosahexaenoic acid on serum, lipoproteins, and macular pigmentation. *Am. J. Clin. Nutr.* **2008**, *87*, 1521–1529.
34. Bone, R.A.; Landrum, J.T.; Cains, A. Optical density spectra of the macular pigment *in vivo* and *in vitro*. *Vis. Res.* **1992**, *32*, 105–110.
35. Brindley, G.S.; Willmer, E.N. The reflexion of light from the macular and peripheral fundus oculi in man. *J. Physiol.* **1952**, *116*, 350–356.
36. Bernstein, P.S.; Yoshida, M.D.; Katz, N.B.; McClane, R.W.; Gellermann, W. Raman detection of macular carotenoid pigments in intact human retina. *Investig. Ophthalmol. Vis. Sci.* **1998**, *39*, 2003–2011.
37. Bui, M.H. Simple determination of retinol, alpha-tocopherol and carotenoids (lutein, all-*trans*-lycopene, α- and β-carotenes) in human plasma by isocratic liquid chromatography. *J. Chromatogr. B* **1994**, *654*, 129–133.
38. Lee, N.; Wielaard, J.; Fawzi, A.A.; Sajda, P.; Laine, A.F.; Martin, G.; Humayun, M.S.; Smith, R.T. *In vivo* snapshot hyperspectral image analysis of age-related macular degeneration. *Conf. Proc. IEEE Eng. Med. Biol. Soc.* **2010**, *2010*, 5363–5366.
39. Leung, I.Y. Macular pigment: New clinical methods of detection and the role of carotenoids in age-related macular degeneration. *Optometry* **2008**, *79*, 266–272.
40. Bhosale, P.; Serban, B.; Zhao, da Y.; Bernstein, P.S. Identification and metabolic transformations of carotenoids in ocular tissues of the Japanese quail *Coturnix japonica*. *Biochemistry* **2007**, *46*, 9050–9057.

41. Bhosale, P.; Bernstein, P.S. Quantitative measurement of 3'-oxolutein from human retina by normal-phase high-performance liquid chromatography coupled to atmospheric pressure chemical ionization mass spectrometry. *Anal. Biochem.* **2005**, *345*, 296–301.
42. Khachik, F.; Carvalho, L.; Bernstein, P.S.; Muir, G.J.; Zhao, D.Y.; Katz, N.B. Chemistry, distribution, and metabolism of tomato carotenoids and their impact on human health. *Exp. Biol. Med. (Maywood)* **2002**, *227*, 845–851.
43. Siems, W.G.; Sommerburg, O.; van Kuijk, F.J. Lycopene and β-carotene decompose more rapidly than lutein and zeaxanthin upon exposure to various pro-oxidants *in vitro*. *Biofactors* **1999**, *10*, 105–113.
44. Panfoli, I.; Calzia, D.; Ravera, S.; Morelli, A.M.; Traverso, C.E. Extra-mitochondrial aerobic metabolism in retinal rod outer segments: New perspectives in retinopathies. *Med. Hypotheses* **2012**, *78*, 423–427.
45. Panfoli, I.; Calzia, D.; Ravera, S.; Bruschi, M.; Tacchetti, C.; Candiani, S.; Morelli, A.; Candiano, G. Extramitochondrial tricarboxylic acid cycle in retinal rod outer segments. *Biochimie* **2011**, *93*, 1565–1575.
46. Bone, R.A.; Landrum, J.T. Macular pigment in Henle fiber membranes: A model for Haidinger's brushes. *Vis. Res.* **1984**, *24*, 103–108.
47. Landrum, J.; Bone, R.; Mendez, V.; Valenciaga, A.; Babino, D. Comparison of dietary supplementation with lutein diacetate and lutein: A pilot study of the effects on serum and macular pigment. *Acta Biochim. Pol.* **2012**, *59*, 167–169.
48. Qin, L.; Bartlett, H.; Griffiths, H.R.; Eperjesi, F.; Armstrong, R.A.; Gherghel, D. Macular pigment optical density is related to blood glutathione levels in healthy individuals. *Investig. Ophthalmol. Vis. Sci.* **2011**, *52*, 5029–5033.
49. Conn, P.F.; Schalch, W.; Truscott, T.G. The singlet oxygen and carotenoid interaction. *J. Photochem. Photobiol. B* **1991**, *11*, 41–47.
50. Foote, C.S.; Chang, Y.C.; Denny, R.W. Chemistry of singlet oxygen. X. Carotenoid quenching parallels biological protection. *J. Am. Chem. Soc.* **1970**, *92*, 5216–5218.
51. Nilsson, S.E.; Sundelin, S.P.; Wihlmark, U.; Brunk, U.T. Aging of cultured retinal pigment epithelial cells: oxidative reactions, lipofuscin formation and blue light damage. *Doc. Ophthalmol.* **2003**, *106*, 13–16.
52. Snodderly, D.M.; Russett, M.D.; Land, R.I.; Krinsky, N.I. Plasma carotenoids of monkeys (Macaca fascicularis and Saimiri sciureus) fed a nonpurified diet. *J. Nutr.* **1990**, *120*, 1663–1671.
53. Neuringer, M.; Sandstrom, M.M.; Johnson, E.J.; Snodderly, D.M. Nutritional manipulation of primate retinas, I: Effects of lutein or zeaxanthin supplements on serum and macular pigment in xanthophyll-free rhesus monkeys. *Investig. Ophthalmol. Vis. Sci.* **2004**, *45*, 3234–3243.
54. Huang, L.L.; Coleman, H.R.; Kim, J.; de Monasterio, F.; Wong, W.T.; Schleicher, R.L.; Ferris, F.L., III; Chew, E.Y. Oral supplementation of lutein/zeaxanthin and omega-3 long chain polyunsaturated fatty acids in persons aged 60 years or older, with or without AMD. *Investig. Ophthalmol. Vis. Sci.* **2008**, *49*, 3864–3869.
55. Loane, E.; Nolan, J.M.; O'Donovan, O.; Bhosale, P.; Bernstein, P.S.; Beatty, S. Transport and retinal capture of lutein and zeaxanthin with reference to age-related macular degeneration. *Surv. Ophthalmol.* **2008**, *53*, 68–81.

56. Rehak, M.; Fric, E.; Wiedemann, P. Lutein and antioxidants in the prevention of age-related macular degeneration. *Ophthalmologe* **2008**, *105*, 37–38, 40–45.
57. Lornejad-Schafer, M.R.; Lambert, C.; Breithaupt, D.E.; Biesalski, H.K.; Frank, J. Solubility, uptake and biocompatibility of lutein and zeaxanthin delivered to cultured human retinal pigment epithelial cells in tween40 micelles. *Eur. J. Nutr.* **2007**, *46*, 79–86.
58. Kalariya, N.M.; Ramana, K.V.; Srivastava, S.K.; van Kuijk, F.J. Genotoxic effects of carotenoid breakdown products in human retinal pigment epithelial cells. *Curr. Eye Res.* **2009**, *34*, 737–747.
59. Sasaki, M.; Ozawa, Y.; Kurihara, T.; Noda, K.; Imamura, Y.; Kobayashi, S.; Ishida, S.; Tsubota, K. Neuroprotective effect of an antioxidant, lutein, during retinal inflammation. *Investig. Ophthalmol. Vis. Sci.* **2009**, *50*, 1433–1439.
60. Li, S.Y.; Lo, A.C. Lutein protects RGC-5 cells against hypoxia and oxidative stress. *Int. J. Mol. Sci.* **2010**, *11*, 2109–2117.
61. Sundelin, S.P.; Nilsson, S.E.G. Lipofuscin-formation in retinal pigment epithelial cells is reduced by antioxidants. *Free Radic. Biol. Med.* **2001**, *31*, 217–225.
62. Zerbib, J.; Seddon, J.M.; Richard, F.; Reynolds, R.; Leveziel, N.; Benlian, P.; Borel, P.; Feingold, J.; Munnich, A.; Soubrane, G.; *et al.* rs5888 variant of SCARB1 gene is a possible susceptibility factor for age-related macular degeneration. *PLoS One* **2009**, *4*, e7341; doi:10.1371/journal.pone.0007341.
63. Izumi-Nagai, K.; Nagai, N.; Ohgami, K.; Satofuka, S.; Ozawa, Y.; Tsubota, K.; Umezawa, K.; Ohno, S.; Oike, Y.; Ishida, S. Macular pigment lutein is antiinflammatory in preventing choroidal neovascularization. *Arterioscler. Thromb. Vasc. Biol.* **2007**, *27*, 2555–2562.
64. Goldberg, J.; Flowerdew, G.; Smith, E.; Brody, J.A.; Tso, M.O. Factors associated with age-related macular degeneration. An analysis of data from the first National Health and Nutrition Examination Survey. *Am. J. Epidemiol.* **1988**, *128*, 700–710.
65. Sommerburg, O.; Keunen, J.E.; Bird, A.C.; van Kuijk, F.J. Fruits and vegetables that are sources for lutein and zeaxanthin: The macular pigment in human eyes. *Br. J. Ophthalmol.* **1998**, *82*, 907–910.
66. Risk factors for neovascular age-related macular degeneration. The Eye Disease Case-Control Study Group. *Arch. Ophthalmol.* **1992**, *110*, 1701–1708.
67. Curran-Celentano, J.; Hammond, B.R., Jr.; Ciulla, T.A.; Cooper, D.A.; Pratt, L.M.; Danis, R.B. Relation between dietary intake, serum concentrations, and retinal concentrations of lutein and zeaxanthin in adults in a Midwest population. *Am. J. Clin. Nutr.* **2001**, *74*, 796–802.
68. Bernstein, P.S.; Zhao, D.Y.; Wintch, S.W.; Ermakov, I.V.; McClane, R.W.; Gellermann, W. Resonance Raman measurement of macular carotenoids in normal subjects and in age-related macular degeneration patients. *Ophthalmology* **2002**, *109*, 1780–1787.
69. Weigert, G.; Kaya, S.; Pemp, B.; Sacu, S.; Lasta, M.; Werkmeister, R.M.; Dragostinoff, N.; Simader, C.; Garhofer, G.; Schmidt-Erfurth, U.; *et al.* Effects of lutein supplementation on macular pigment optical density and visual acuity in patients with age-related macular degeneration. *InvestIG. Ophthalmol. Vis. Sci.* **2011**, *52*, 8174–8178.
70. Group, A.R.; Chew, E.Y.; Clemons, T.; Sangiovanni, J.P.; Danis, R.; Domalpally, A.; McBee, W.; Sperduto, R.; Ferris, F.L. The Age-Related Eye Disease Study 2 (AREDS2): Study

design and baseline characteristics (AREDS2 report number 1). *Ophthalmology* **2012**, *119*, 2282–2289.

71. Age-Related Eye Disease Study Research Group; SanGiovanni, J.P.; Chew, E.Y.; Clemons, T.E.; Ferris, F.L., III; Gensler, G.; Lindblad, A.S.; Milton, R.C.; Seddon, J.M.; Sperduto, R.D. The relationship of dietary carotenoid and vitamin A, E, and C intake with age-related macular degeneration in a case-control study: AREDS Report No. 22. *Arch. Ophthalmol.* **2007**, *125*, 1225–1232.
72. Tang, L.; Zhang, Y.; Jiang, Y.; Willard, L.; Ortiz, E.; Wark, L.; Medeiros, D.; Lin, D. Dietary wolfberry ameliorates retinal structure abnormalities in db/db mice at the early stage of diabetes. *Exp. Biol. Med. (Maywood)* **2011**, *236*, 1051–1063.
73. Hu, B.J.; Hu, Y.N.; Lin, S.; Ma, W.J.; Li, X.R. Application of Lutein and Zeaxanthin in nonproliferative diabetic retinopathy. *Int. J. Ophthalmol.* **2011**, *4*, 303–306.
74. Woo, T.T.; Li, S.Y.; Lai, W.W.; Wong, D.; Lo, A.C. Neuroprotective effects of lutein in a rat model of retinal detachment. *Graefes Arch. Clin. Exp. Ophthalmol.* **2013**, *251*, 41–51.
75. Chan, C.; Leung, I.; Lam, K.W.; Tso, M.O. The occurrence of retinol and carotenoids in human subretinal fluid. *Curr. Eye Res.* **1998**, *17*, 890–895.
76. Gao, S.; Qin, T.; Liu, Z.; Caceres, M.A.; Ronchi, C.F.; Chen, C.Y.; Yeum, K.J.; Taylor, A.; Blumberg, J.B.; Liu, Y.; *et al.* Lutein and zeaxanthin supplementation reduces H_2O_2-induced oxidative damage in human lens epithelial cells. *Mol. Vis.* **2011**, *17*, 3180–3190.
77. Zhao, B.; He, Y.Y.; Chignell, C.F.; Yin, J.J.; Andley, U.; Roberts, J.E. Difference in phototoxicity of cyclodextrin complexed fullerene [(gamma-CyD)2/C60] and its aggregated derivatives toward human lens epithelial cells. *Chem. Res. Toxicol.* **2009**, *22*, 660–667.
78. Roberts, J.E.; Wielgus, A.R.; Boyes, W.K.; Andley, U.; Chignell, C.F. Phototoxicity and cytotoxicity of fullerol in human lens epithelial cells. *Toxicol. Appl. Pharmacol.* **2008**, *228*, 49–58.
79. Nolan, J.M.; O'Reilly, P.; Loughman, J.; Stack, J.; Loane, E.; Connolly, E.; Beatty, S. Augmentation of macular pigment following implantation of blue light-filtering intraocular lenses at the time of cataract surgery. *Investig. Ophthalmol. Vis. Sci.* **2009**, *50*, 4777–4785.
80. Barker, F.M., II. Dietary supplementation: Effects on visual performance and occurrence of AMD and cataracts. *Curr. Med. Res. Opin.* **2010**, *26*,2011–2023.
81. Moeller, S.M.; Voland, R.; Tinker, L.; Blodi, B.A.; Klein, M.L.; Gehrs, K.M.; Johnson, E.J.; Snodderly, D.M.; Wallace, R.B.; Chappell, R.J.; *et al.* Associations between age-related nuclear cataract and lutein and zeaxanthin in the diet and serum in the Carotenoids in the Age-Related Eye Disease Study, an Ancillary Study of the Women's Health Initiative. *Arch. Ophthalmol.* **2008**, *126*, 354–364.
82. Berendschot, T.T.; Broekmans, W.M.; Klopping-Ketelaars, I.A.; Kardinaal, A.F.; van Poppel, G.; van Norren, D. Lens aging in relation to nutritional determinants and possible risk factors for age-related cataract. *Arch. Ophthalmol.* **2002**, *120*, 1732–1737.
83. Jacques, P.F.; Chylack, L.T., Jr.; Hankinson, S.E.; Khu, P.M.; Rogers, G.; Friend, J.; Tung, W.; Wolfe, J.K.; Padhye, N.; Willett, W.C.; *et al.* Long-term nutrient intake and early age-related nuclear lens opacities. *Arch. Ophthalmol.* **2001**, *119*, 1009–1019.

84. Suhler, E.B.; Lloyd, M.J.; Choi, D.; Rosenbaum, J.T.; Austin, D.F. Incidence and prevalence of uveitis in Veterans Affairs Medical Centers of the Pacific Northwest. *Am. J. Ophthalmol.* **2008**, *146*, 890–896.
85. Gritz, D.C.; Wong, I.G. Incidence and prevalence of uveitis in Northern California; the Northern California Epidemiology of Uveitis Study. *Ophthalmology* **2004**, *111*, 491–500; discussion 500.
86. Yao, N.; Lan, F.; He, R.R.; Kurihara, H. Protective effects of bilberry (*Vaccinium myrtillus* L.) extract against endotoxin-induced uveitis in mice. *J. Agric. Food Chem.* **2010**, *58*, 4731–4736.
87. He, R.R.; Tsoi, B.; Lan, F.; Yao, N.; Yao, X.S.; Kurihara, H. Antioxidant properties of lutein contribute to the protection against lipopolysaccharide-induced uveitis in mice. *Chin. Med.* **2011**, *6*, 38; doi:10.1186/1749-8546-6-38.
88. Jin, X.H.; Ohgami, K.; Shiratori, K.; Suzuki, Y.; Hirano, T.; Koyama, Y.; Yoshida, K.; Ilieva, I.; Iseki, K.; Ohno, S. Inhibitory effects of lutein on endotoxin-induced uveitis in Lewis rats. *Investig. Ophthalmol. Vis. Sci.* **2006**, *47*, 2562–2568.
89. WebMD L: Lutein. Edited by WebMd Editorial Team, 2013. Available online: http://www.webmd.com/vitamins-supplements/ingredientmono-754-lutein.aspx?activeIngredientId=754&activeIngredientName=lutein (accessed on 9 May 2013).
90. Harikumar, K.B.; Nimita, C.V.; Preethi, K.C.; Kuttan, R.; Shankaranarayana, M.L.; Deshpande, J. Toxicity profile of lutein and lutein ester isolated from marigold flowers (*Tagetes erecta*). *Int. J. Toxicol.* **2008**, *27*, 1–9.

12

Macular Pigment and its Contribution to Vision

Ekaterina Loskutova [1,*], John Nolan [1,2], Alan Howard [3] and Stephen Beatty [1,2]

[1] Macular Pigment Research Group, Department of Chemical and Life Sciences, Waterford Institute of Technology, Waterford, Ireland; E-Mails: jmnolan@wit.ie (J.N.); sbeatty@wit.ie (S.B.)

[2] Institute of Vision Research, Whitfield Clinic, Waterford, Ireland

[3] Howard Foundation, Downing College, Cambridge University, Cambridge, CB22 5LA, UK; E-Mail: alan.howard@howard-foundation.com

* Author to whom correspondence should be addressed; E-Mail: kate@ivr.ie;

Abstract: Three dietary carotenoids, lutein (L), zeaxanthin (Z) and meso-zeaxanthin (MZ) accumulate at the central retina (macula), where they are collectively referred to as macular pigment (MP). MP's pre-receptoral absorption of blue light and consequential attenuation of the effects of chromatic aberration and light scatter are important for optimal visual function. Furthermore, antioxidant activity of MP's constituent carotenoids and the same blue light-filtering properties underlie the rationale for its putative protective role for age-related macular degeneration (AMD). Supplementation with L, Z and MZ augments MP and enhances visual performance in diseased and non-diseased eyes, and may reduce risk of AMD development and/or progression.

Keywords: lutein; zeaxanthin; meso-zeaxanthin; visual performance; macular pigment

---

1. Introduction

Vision is a process by which images of the external world can be interpreted by the seeing part of the brain. The retina facilitates transformation of light into an electrical signal and is an integral part of the visual system.

The posterior pole of the retina is known as the macula. The central part of the macula, the fovea, is only about 2 mm in diameter, but has the highest concentration of light-sensitive cone photoreceptor cells, and is responsible for detailed central and color vision. The macula houses three carotenoid pigments, lutein (L), zeaxanthin (Z) and meso-zeaxanthin (MZ), which are collectively referred to as macular pigment (MP).

In humans, L and Z are entirely of dietary origin, and are found in eggs and many types of brightly colored fruits and vegetables typical of a western diet [1]. The presence of MZ in foodstuffs is currently under investigation, but MZ is known to be produced in the macula following isomerization of retinal L [2].

Of thc 42 dietary carotenoids, 14 are absorbed and used by the human body, yet only L, Z and MZ are found at the macula [3]. The preferential accumulation of L, Z and MZ at the site of sharpest vision is thought to be the result of an uptake mechanism that has evolved in response to the functional needs of the tissue (macula). MP optimizes visual performance in non-diseased eyes because of its pre-receptoral absorption of blue light and consequential attenuation of chromatic aberration and the adverse impact of light scatter ("veiling luminance"). As a result, and because of the known inter-individual variability of MP levels, optimal visual performance in non-diseased eyes is dependent upon optimal MP levels and a peaked spatial profile of this pigment. Furthermore, MP may also protect against age-related macular degeneration (AMD) because of the same blue light-filtering properties and because of the anti-inflammatory and antioxidant activities of MP's constituent carotenoids [4,5].

2. Measures of Visual Function

Vision is a complex process, which includes resolving power, discernment of objects against a contrasting background (contrast sensitivity, or CS), depth perception, color discrimination, movement recognition, amongst other facilities. No single test reflects all of these parameters of visual function, but there are a number of techniques to assess different aspects of visual performance. The most widely used means of testing vision is known as visual acuity (VA), which measures spatial resolving power of the visual system at a 100% contrast. "Normal" VA is deemed to be the ability to discriminate symbols that are 1 arc minute apart. VA is primarily a function of the cones, a type of retinal photoreceptor cell that is also responsible for color vision, and which reaches peak density at the fovea (the central macula). It is important to note that the resolving power of the eye does not describe the ability to discern the foreground from the background within the field of view.

CS is a measure of the visual system's ability to distinguish objects of dissimilar luminance, and is measured, and varies substantially, for different target sizes. CS relates directly to how well a person can perform tasks of everyday life, such as identifying faces, driving or reading [6]. CS declines with increasing age, and is a more sensitive indicator of visual dysfunction attributable to retinal disease than is VA [7]. In other words, measures of CS are more reflective of overall visual performance than is VA, in non-diseased and in diseased eyes.

3. The Process of Vision

The process of vision involves a metabolic response to a physical stimulus. Before the brain can construct an image, light entering the eye needs to be "bent", or refracted, by the optical system in order to be focused on the retina, where it will be transformed into nerve signals, and transmitted to the visual processing center in the occipital cortex for ultimate perception of the stimulus.

3.1. The Optical System of the Eye

The optical system comprises the cornea, the iris and the lens, and is responsible for filtration, refraction and regulation of light intensity. First, light is incident upon the cornea, which filters out ultraviolet (UV) light, and this structure accounts for most of the eye's refractive power. The amount of light passing through the lens is regulated by the pupil. Visible light is then further refracted by the lens, allowing a clear and sharp image to be formed on the retina in an emmetropic eye (emmetropia is the state of vision where an object at infinity is in sharp focus when the crystalline lens is in a neutral or relaxed state).

3.2. Optical Limitations: Glare, Chromatic Aberration, and Light Scatter

Several optical limitations of the visual system can adversely impact upon the quality of vision in the normal eye. It is likely that the ability to accumulate MP at the macula has evolved in order to attenuate the impact of some of these optical imperfections on image quality [8].

3.2.1. Chromatic Aberration

Visible light is spectrally composed of differing wavelengths, from short (blue) to long (red). These wavelengths are refracted by the optical medias to different degrees, with the blue light being refracted substantially more and, therefore, being defocused at the retina. This phenomenon is known as chromatic aberration (CA), and is visually perceived as a bluish blur at the edge of a viewed object, and can substantially and adversely affect the quality of vision, and is reflected in reduced CS [9].

3.2.2. Light Scatter

Particles suspended in the atmosphere and structures within the eye scatter light incident upon them. The lens and cornea cause 70% and 30% of light scattered by the eye, respectively, with the aqueous and vitreous contributions to light scatter being minimal. Importantly, blue light is scattered more than other wavelengths, and the resulting scattered blue light superimposes a bluish "veil" over the retinal image, referred to as veiling luminance [10]. Veiling luminance reduces image contrast and visibility, thereby impairing vision [11].

3.2.3. Glare

Glare is yet another factor which can impair visual performance. There are two types of glare: discomfort glare and disability glare [11]. Discomfort glare is caused by distracting and/or uncomfortable intense light sources, and results in an instinctive desire to squint or look away from the light source. Disability glare, on the other hand, is caused by light scatter and consequential veiling luminance, and impairs visual performance, but is unassociated with discomfort.

In summary, visible blue light is deleterious to the quality of the optical image formed at the retina, because shorter wavelengths are scattered more than other wavelengths, thereby resulting in glare disability and veiling luminance, and also because these short blue wavelengths are more defocused at the retina than other wavelengths, thereby causing chromatic aberration. Further, there are no blue-sensitive cones in the foveola, and blue visible light is therefore solely deleterious to high frequency spatial vision.

3.3. Visual Benefits of MP

Optically, MP is a blue light filter, with maximum absorption circa 460 nm, and screens out deleterious short-wavelength light. It has been shown that MPOD is positively related to the heterochromatic contrast thresholds (obtained by presenting the target with contrast grating stimulus on a blue, 460 nm, background), likely because MP's preferential absorption of blue surround increases target detectability [12]. Under natural conditions, objects are often presented on short-wavelength background, such as blue sky and green leaves, meaning that the filtering properties of MP may be important for real-life vision.

MP's pre-receptoral filtration of blue light is believed to reduce the adverse impact of glare disability, light scatter and chromatic aberration, thereby optimizing CS [13–15]. It follows, therefore, that augmentation of MP would result in enhanced CS and improved glare disability. Indeed, as shown by clinical trials, this can be achieved by supplementation with a formulation containing the macular carotenoids [16–18]. Of interest, in a study by Loughman *et al.*, best visual outcomes were seen when the formulation contained all three of MP's constituent carotenoids (MZ, L and Z in a (mg) ratio of 10:10:2) [18].

However, the visual benefits of MP are not restricted to the effects of its optical properties, reflected in a growing body of evidence that the macular carotenoids may have a favorable effect on neuronal processing [19,20]. These carotenoids have been shown to improve communication through cell-to-cell channels, modulate the dynamic instability of microtubules (structural units of neurons), and prevent degradation of synaptic vesicle proteins [21–23].

Rubin *et al.* have investigated the effects of supplementation with carotenoids (L, Z, lycopene and β-carotene) on plasma levels of these compounds, incidence of prematurity complications, levels of a biomarker of inflammation (C-reactive protein) and electroretinography (ERG) outcomes in preterm infants compared to human milk-fed term infants [24]. Supplementation with carotenoids increased plasma concentrations of these compounds into the range observed for term infants. Moreover, infants who received supplementation showed a significantly greater sensitivity response in rod photoreceptors than infants in the control group, suggesting that carotenoids have an initiative effect on rod function and, thereby, positively affect retinal development in infancy. As discussed by the authors, the proposed mechanism probably involves the same light-absorbing, antioxidant and anti-inflammatory activities of the macular carotenoids that have already been alluded to. Interestingly, levels of the biomarker of inflammation were lower following supplementation, and approximated those of the term infants. This finding is consistent with other reports on the anti-inflammatory properties of the macular carotenoids [4,5].

Indeed, Hammond *et al.* have shown that MP is positively related to a dynamic measure of visual performance, termed critical fusion frequency (CFF) thresholds, which is believed to also reflect post-receptoral processes [19]. In a further study by Renzi *et al.*, these findings were confirmed and expanded upon by measuring the more complete temporal contrast sensitivity function (TCSF) [20]. In this latter study, MPOD was found to be positively related to CFF thresholds and to TCSF, suggesting that MP may be important for central visual processing.

3.4. Neurophysiology of Vision

The process of phototransduction in the retina is essential for vision. Two types of photoreceptors, known as rods and cones, share responsibility for conversion of light into a neural signal. Phototransduction takes place in photoreceptor outer segment membranes, which are organized in stacks. Photopigments within these membranes consist of a light-absorbing chromophore, retinal, and a protein moiety, opsin. When activated by incident light, retinal undergoes photoisomerisation and converts from the 11-*cis* to the all-*trans* form, thus initiating a signal transduction cascade [25].

The photoreceptors are located in the outer layers of the neurosensory retina, which means that they are facing away from incident light. The explanation for this inverted design is that photoreceptors need to be in close contact with the retinal pigment epithelium (RPE), which plays an essential role in sustaining the visual phototransduction cycle.

The RPE supplies photoreceptors with nutrients, and constantly restores the chromophore from the all-*trans* to 11-*cis* configuration, thereby ensuring regeneration of the visual pigment [26]. RPE also recycles shed photoreceptor outer segments, and other metabolic waste. In fact, the metabolism and resultant photo-oxidative damage in the photoreceptor cells is so high that the outer segments must completely renew themselves every 10 days [27].

Disease of the Retina

With the highest metabolic activity in the mammalian world and associated high oxygen consumption, the retina, a tissue rich in readily oxidizable polyunsaturated fatty acids (PUFAs), is an ideal environment for the production of, and damage by, reactive oxygen intermediates (ROIs) [28]. Exposure to light, especially high energy short-wavelength light, and the presence of photosensitizers (chromophores), further increase production of ROIs in this tissue [29,30]. Oxidative stress resulting from excessive production of ROIs, and consequential inflammation, are important in the pathogenesis of AMD [31].

3.5. Protective Role of MP for AMD

MP's pre-receptoral filtration of blue light at the macula (where photoreceptors reach their peak concentration) is believed to protect the vulnerable central retina from oxidative injury by limiting light-induced generation of ROIs [32]. MP's constituent carotenoids also contribute to the antioxidant defense system through their capacity to quench singlet oxygen and scavenge free radicals [33]. Moreover, these compounds may also attenuate the deleterious effects of chronic inflammation in the macular region [4,5].

Accordingly, it is biologically plausible that MP protects against AMD, and supplementation with the macular carotenoids could represent a strategy of preventing and/or delaying the onset of AMD or retarding progression of this disease [34].

4. Conclusion

There is firm evidence that MP is necessary for optimal visual function. Indeed, supplementation with MP's constituent carotenoids can enhance visual performance in non-diseased and diseased eyes, with best results following supplementation with all three of MP's constituent carotenoids (MZ, L and Z in a (mg) ratio of 10:10:2). Finally, there is a biologically plausible rationale whereby MP's optical and antioxidant properties may reduce risk of AMD development and/or progression (as recently shown by AREDS2) [35].

Acknowledgments

Grant support was provided by The Howard Foundation, Cambridge, CB22 5LA, UK.

References

1. Sommerburg, O.; Keunen, J.E.E.; Bird, A.C.; van Kuijk, F.J.G.M. Fruits and vegetables that are sources for lutein and zeaxanthin: The macular pigment in human eyes. *Br. J. Ophthalmol.* **1998**, *82*, 907–910.
2. Bone, R.A.; Landrum, J.T.; Hime, G.W.; Cains, A.; Zamor, J. Stereochemistry of the Human Macular Carotenoids. *Investig. Ophthalmol. Vis. Sci.* **1993**, *34*, 2033–2040.
3. Khachik, F.; Beecher, G.R.; Goli, M.B. Separation, identification and quantification of carotenoids in fruits, vegetables and human plasma by high performance liquid chromatography. *Pure Appl. Chem.* **1991**, *63*, 71–80.
4. Van Herpen-Broekmans, W.M.; Klopping-Ketelaars, I.A.; Bots, M.L.; Kluft, C.; Princen, H.; Hendriks, H.F.; Tijburg, L.B.; van, P.G.; Kardinaal, A.F. Serum carotenoids and vitamins in relation to markers of endothelial function and inflammation. *Eur. J. Epidemiol.* **2004**, *19*, 915–921.
5. Kijlstra, A.; Tian, Y.; Kelly, E.R.; Berendschot, T.T. Lutein: More than just a filter for blue light. *Prog. Retin. Eye Res.* **2012**, *31*, 303–315.
6. Owsley, C.; Sloane, M.E. Contrast sensitivity, acuity, and the perception of "real-world" targets. *Br. J. Ophthalmol.* **1987**, *71*, 791–796.
7. Marmor, M.F. Contrast sensitivity and retinal disease. *Ann. Ophthalmol.* **1981**, *13*, 1069–1071.
8. Walls, G.L.; Judd, H.D. The intra-ocular colour-filters of vertebrates. *Br. J. Ophthalmol.* **1933**, *17*, 705–725.
9. Charalampidou, S.; Nolan, J.; Loughman, J.; Stack, J.; Higgins, G.; Cassidy, L.; Beatty, S. Psychophysical impact and optical and morphological characteristics of symptomatic non-advanced cataract. *Eye (Lond.)* **2011**, *25*, 1147–1154.
10. Wooten, B.R.; Hammond, B.R. Macular pigment: Influences on visual acuity and visibility. *Prog. Retin. Eye Res.* **2002**, *21*, 225–240.
11. Mainster, M.A.; Turner, P.L. Glare's causes, consequences, and clinical challenges after a century of ophthalmic study. *Am. J. Ophthalmol.* **2012**, *153*, 587–593.

12. Renzi, L.M.; Hammond, B.R. The effect of macular pigment on heterochromatic luminance contrast. *Exp. Eye Res.* **2010**, *91*, 896–900.
13. Stringham, J.M.; Hammond, B.R. Macular pigment and visual performance under glare conditions. *Optom. Vis. Sci.* **2008**, *85*, 82–88.
14. Hammond, B.R., Jr.; Wooten, B.R.; Engles, M.; Wong, J.C. The influence of filtering by the macular carotenoids on contrast sensitivity measured under simulated blue haze conditions. *Vis. Res.* **2012**, 58–62.
15. Bone, R.A.; Landrum, J.T.; Cains, A. Optical-density spectra of the macular pigment *in vivo* and *in vitro*. *Vis. Res.* **1992**, *32*, 105–110.
16. Yao, Y.; Qiu, Q.H.; Wu, X.W.; Cai, Z.Y.; Xu, S.; Liang, X.Q. Lutein supplementation improves visual performance in Chinese drivers: 1-year randomized, double-blind, placebo-controlled study. *Nutrition* **2013**, doi:10.1016/j.nut.2012.10.017.
17. Murray, I.J.; Makridaki, M.; van der Veen, R.L.; Carden, D.; Parry, N.R.; Berendschot, T.T. Lutein supplementation over a one year period in early AMD might have a mild beneficial effect on visual acuity; the CLEAR study. *Invest. Ophthalmol. Vis. Sci.* 2013, in press.
18. Loughman, J.; Nolan, J.M.; Howard, A.N.; Connolly, E.; Meagher, K.; Beatty, S. The impact of macular pigment augmentation on visual performance using different carotenoid formulations. *Invest. Ophthalmol. Vis. Sci.* **2012**, *53*, 7871–7880.
19. Hammond, B.R., Jr.; Wooten, B.R. CFF thresholds: Relation to macular pigment optical density. *Ophthalmic Physiol. Opt.* **2005**, *25*, 315–319.
20. Renzi, L.M.; Hammond, B.R., Jr. The relation between the macular carotenoids, lutein and zeaxanthin, and temporal vision. *Ophthalmic Physiol. Opt.* **2010**, *30*, 351–357.
21. Ozawa, Y.; Sasaki, M.; Takahashi, N.; Kamoshita, M.; Miyake, S.; Tsubota, K. Neuroprotective effects of lutein in the retina. *Curr. Pharm. Des.* **2012**, *18*, 51–56.
22. Stahl, W.; Sies, H. Effects of carotenoids and retinoids on gap junctional communication. *Biofactors* **2001**, *15*, 95–98.
23. Crabtree, D.V.; Ojima, I.; Geng, X.; Adler, A.J. Tubulins in the primate retina: Evidence that xanthophylls may be endogenous ligands for the paclitaxel-binding site. *Bioorg. Med. Chem.* **2001**, *9*, 1967–1976.
24. Rubin, L.P.; Chan, G.M.; Barrett-Reis, B.M.; Fulton, A.B.; Hansen, R.M.; Ashmeade, T.L.; Oliver, J.S.; Mackey, A.D.; Dimmit, R.A.; Hartmann, E.E.; *et al.* Effect of carotenoid supplementation on plasma carotenoids, inflammation and visual development in preterm infants. *J. Perinatol.* **2012**, *32*, 418–424.
25. Saari, J.C. Vitamin A metabolism in rod and cone visual cycles. *Annu. Rev. Nutr.* **2012**, *32*, 125–445.
26. Strauss, O. The retinal pigment epithelium in visual function. *Physiol. Rev.* **2005**, *85*, 845–881.
27. Kwok, M.C.; Holopainen, J.M.; Molday, L.L.; Foster, L.J.; Molday, R.S. Proteomics of photoreceptor outer segments identifies a subset of SNARE and Rab proteins implicated in membrane vesicle trafficking and fusion. *Mol. Cell. Proteomics* **2008**, *7*, 1053–1066.
28. Beatty, S.; Koh, H.H.; Henson, D.; Boulton, M. The role of oxidative stress in the pathogenesis of age-related macular degeneration. *Surv. Ophthalmol.* **2000**, *45*, 115–134.

29. Rozanowska, M.; Jarvis-Evans, J.; Korytowski, W.; Boulton, M.E.; Burke, J.M.; Sarna, T. Blue light-induced reactivity of retinal age pigment. *In vitro* generation of oxygen-reactive species. *J. Biol. Chem.* **1995**, *270*, 18825–18830.
30. Rozanowska, M.; Wessels, J.; Boulton, M.; Burke, J.M.; Rodgers, M.A.; Truscott, T.G.; Sarna, T. Blue light-induced singlet oxygen generation by retinal lipofuscin in non-polar media. *Free Radic. Biol. Med.* **1998**, *24*, 1107–1112.
31. Hollyfield, J.G.; Bonilha, V.L.; Rayborn, M.E.; Yang, X.; Shadrach, K.G.; Lu, L.; Ufret, R.L.; Salomon, R.G.; Perez, V.L. Oxidative damage-induced inflammation initiates age-related macular degeneration. *Nat. Med.* **2008**, *14*, 194–198.
32. Kirschfeld, K. Carotenoid pigments: Their possible role in protecting against photooxidation in eyes and photoreceptor cells. *Proc. R. Soc. Lond. B Biol. Sci.* **1982**, *216*, 71–85.
33. Khachik, F.; Bernstein, P.S.; Garland, D.L. Identification of lutein and zeaxanthin oxidation products in human and monkey retinas. *Investig. Ophthalmol. Vis. Sci.* **1997**, *38*, 1802–1811.
34. Sabour-Pickett, S.; Nolan, J.M.; Loughman, J.; Beatty, S. A review of the evidence germane to the putative protective role of the macular carotenoids for age-related macular degeneration. *Mol. Nutr. Food Res.* **2011**, 270–286.
35. Age-Related Eye Disease Study 2 Research Group. Lutein + zeaxanthin and omega-3 fatty acids for age-related macular degeneration: the Age-Related Eye Disease Study 2 (AREDS2) randomized clinical trial. *JAMA* **2013**, *309*, 2005–2015.

Permissions

All chapters in this book were first published by MDPI; hereby published with permission under the Creative Commons Attribution License or equivalent. Every chapter published in this book has been scrutinized by our experts. Their significance has been extensively debated. The topics covered herein carry significant findings which will fuel the growth of the discipline. They may even be implemented as practical applications or may be referred to as a beginning point for another development.

The contributors of this book come from diverse backgrounds, making this book a truly international effort. This book will bring forth new frontiers with its revolutionizing research information and detailed analysis of the nascent developments around the world.

We would like to thank all the contributing authors for lending their expertise to make the book truly unique. They have played a crucial role in the development of this book. Without their invaluable contributions this book wouldn't have been possible. They have made vital efforts to compile up to date information on the varied aspects of this subject to make this book a valuable addition to the collection of many professionals and students.

This book was conceptualized with the vision of imparting up-to-date information and advanced data in this field. To ensure the same, a matchless editorial board was set up. Every individual on the board went through rigorous rounds of assessment to prove their worth. After which they invested a large part of their time researching and compiling the most relevant data for our readers.

The editorial board has been involved in producing this book since its inception. They have spent rigorous hours researching and exploring the diverse topics which have resulted in the successful publishing of this book. They have passed on their knowledge of decades through this book. To expedite this challenging task, the publisher supported the team at every step. A small team of assistant editors was also appointed to further simplify the editing procedure and attain best results for the readers.

Apart from the editorial board, the designing team has also invested a significant amount of their time in understanding the subject and creating the most relevant covers. They scrutinized every image to scout for the most suitable representation of the subject and create an appropriate cover for the book.

The publishing team has been an ardent support to the editorial, designing and production team. Their endless efforts to recruit the best for this project, has resulted in the accomplishment of this book. They are a veteran in the field of academics and their pool of knowledge is as vast as their experience in printing. Their expertise and guidance has proved useful at every step. Their uncompromising quality standards have made this book an exceptional effort. Their encouragement from time to time has been an inspiration for everyone.

The publisher and the editorial board hope that this book will prove to be a valuable piece of knowledge for researchers, students, practitioners and scholars across the globe.

List of Contributors

Stuart Richer
Eye Clinic 112e, Captain James A Lovell Federal Health Care Center, 3001 Green Bay Rd., North Chicago, IL 60064, USA
University of Illinois Eye and Ear Infirmary, University of Illinois at Chicago, Chicago, IL 60612, USA
Chicago Medical School, Rosalind Franklin University of Medicine and Science, 3333 Green Bay Rd., North Chicago, IL 60064, USA

Shana Patel, Shivani Sockanathan and Luke Miller
Chicago Medical School, Rosalind Franklin University of Medicine and Science, 3333 Green Bay Rd., North Chicago, IL 60064, USA

Lawrence J. Ulanski II
Eye Clinic 112e, Captain James A Lovell Federal Health Care Center, 3001 Green Bay Rd., North Chicago, IL 60064, USA
University of Illinois Eye and Ear Infirmary, University of Illinois at Chicago, Chicago, IL 60612, USA

Stuart Richer, William Stiles, Lawrence Ulanski, Donn Carroll and Carla Podella
Eye Clinic 112e, Captain James A Lovell Federal Health Care Center, 3001 Green Bay Rd., North Chicago, IL 60064, USA

Ming Zhong, Riki Kawaguchi, Miki Kassai and Hui Sun
Department of Physiology, Jules Stein Eye Institute, and Howard Hughes Medical Institute, David Geffen School of Medicine, University of California, Los Angeles, CA 90095, USA

El-Sayed M. Abdel-Aal and Humayoun Akhtar
Guelph Food Research Centre, Agriculture and Agri-Food Canada, Guelph, ON N1G 5C9, Canada

Khalid Zaheer
Consultant, Toronto, ON M3M 2E9, Canada

Rashida Ali
Department of Food Science and Technology, ICCBS, University of Karachi, Karachi 75270, Pakistan
English Biscuit Manufacturers Pvt. Ltd., Korangi Industrial Area, Karachi 74900, Pakistan

Lindsay Perusek and Tadao Maeda
Department of Ophthalmology & Visual Sciences, School of Medicine, Case Western Reserve University, Cleveland, OH 44106-4965, USA

Barbara Demmig-Adams and Robert B. Adams
Department of Ecology & Evolutionary Biology, University of Colorado, Boulder, CO 80309-0334, USA

Emily R. Bovier and Billy R. Hammond Jr.
Vision Sciences Laboratory, University of Georgia, Athens, GA 30602, USA

Richard D. Lewis
Foods and Nutrition, University of Georgia, Athens, GA 30602, USA

Molly Schleicher, Caren Garber and Allen Taylor
Laboratory for Nutrition and Vision Research, JM USDA Human Nutrition Research Center on Aging Tufts University, 711 Washington St, Boston, MA 02111, USA

Karen Weikel
Boston Medical Center, 650 Albany Street, Boston, MA 02118, USA

Alfredo García-Layana, Sergio Recalde, Angel Salinas Alamán and Patricia Fernández Robredo
Ophthalmology Department, Clinica Universidad de Navarra, C/Pio XII 36, 31080, Pamplona, Spain

Stuart Richer and Jane Cho
Eye Clinic, James A Lovell Federal Health Care Center, North Chicago, IL 60064, USA
Family & Preventive Medicine, RFUMS Chicago Medical School, North Chicago, IL 60064, USA

William Stiles, Marc Levin and Carla Thomas
Eye Clinic, James A Lovell Federal Health Care Center, North Chicago, IL 60064, USA

James S. Wrobel
Internal Medicine, Podiatry Services, University of Michigan, Ann Arbor, MI 48105, USA

Michael Sinai
Optovue Inc., Fremont, CA 94538, USA

Keyvan Koushan, Raluca Rusovici, Wenhua Li, Lee R. Ferguson and Kakarla V. Chalam
Department of Ophthalmology, University of Florida, 580 West 8th Street, Tower II, 3rd Fl., Jacksonville, FL 32209, USA

Ekaterina Loskutova
Macular Pigment Research Group, Department of Chemical and Life Sciences, Waterford Institute of Technology, Waterford, Ireland

John Nolan and Stephen Beatty
Macular Pigment Research Group, Department of Chemical and Life Sciences, Waterford Institute of Technology, Waterford, Ireland
Institute of Vision Research, Whitfield Clinic, Waterford, Ireland

Alan Howard
Howard Foundation, Downing College, Cambridge University, Cambridge, CB22 5LA, UK

Index

A

Adiposity, 181, 186

Age-related Blindness, 163, 167

Antioxidants, 4, 47, 53-56, 101, 127, 136-137, 148-151, 154, 162, 165, 168-171, 175, 178, 186, 190, 206, 213, 216, 219

B

Binding Protein, 18, 30, 36, 38, 41-45, 53, 60, 82-87, 94-97

C

Carotenes, 48, 53, 82, 92, 163, 207, 217

Carotenoids, 46-62, 65, 80-83, 92-94, 101, 113, 120, 126-129, 131-132, 136, 146-151, 154, 159-166, 174-175, 177, 179, 182, 187-188, 190, 192, 200, 205-206, 208-210, 212-213, 215-220, 222-223, 225-229

Cataract, 47, 53-56, 61, 133, 147, 150-151, 159, 179, 191, 203-205, 212, 220, 227

Cell Culture, 28, 82, 213

Cell Death, 42, 87, 91, 162-164, 167-170, 175, 177, 212

Cholesterol Intake, 118

Choroidal Blood Flow, 64-65

Chromatic Aberration, 222-225

Chromophore, 18-20, 24-26, 29, 31, 33, 35-39, 44, 80-81, 84-93, 97, 99, 163, 172-173, 179, 226

Chylomicron, 31-32, 82-83, 94-95

Color Vision, 5, 19-20, 26-27, 35-37, 192-193, 198, 201, 223

Cornea, 33-34, 45, 224

D

Diabetes, 3, 5-9, 27, 41, 73, 145, 154, 167, 170, 178, 191, 212, 220

Diabetic Retinopathy, 47, 157, 192-193, 212, 214, 220

Dietary Sources, 46-47, 49, 58, 81, 162-163, 165, 211

Docosahexaenoic Acid, 105, 146, 153-154, 156, 160, 170, 178, 217

E

Enzymatic Processing, 84, 86

Enzymatic Reaction, 80

Esterification, 80, 86, 89

Eye Health, 46-48, 51, 53, 57, 107, 111, 113, 164, 210-211

G

Gene Expression, 2, 16, 28-29, 44, 64, 75, 78, 97, 170, 177

Gene Regulation, 81-82, 162

H

Heterochromatic Flicker, 153, 155, 161, 181, 183, 188, 205, 207, 217

Hyperglycemia, 144

Hypotension, 71, 74

I

Intracellular Protein, 30

Isomerization, 25, 37-38, 54, 80, 84-86, 96, 223

Isorhodopsin, 89-91

L

Leber Congenital Amaurosis, 38, 80-81, 89, 97-98, 100

Light Collection, 162-163, 166

Light Scatter, 222-225

Light Sensors, 18 21, 24-25, 34

Lipid Peroxidation, 162, 166, 168-172, 174, 178, 207, 213

Lutein, 46-62, 65, 94, 111, 120-129, 131, 135-136, 142, 145-149, 153-171, 173-176, 178-181, 186-188, 192, 200-203, 205-223, 227-229

M

Macula, 13, 46, 48-49, 51-53, 57, 60, 69, 78, 102, 120, 128, 154, 158, 164, 182, 190, 192, 197, 199-201, 206, 209, 211, 222-224, 226

Macular Degeneration, 1-2, 16-17, 38-39, 42, 46-47, 56-57, 59-61, 63-65, 76-77, 101, 104, 107, 143-153, 156, 159-161, 163, 167, 174-179, 182, 186, 188-190, 202-203, 205-206, 209-211, 215-220, 222-223, 228-229

Macular Pigment, 1, 6, 8-9, 11-15, 51, 53, 57-59, 61, 66, 111, 147-148, 153-156, 159-161, 175-176, 180-183, 187-188, 192-193, 197, 199-201, 203-207, 209-211, 214-220, 222-223, 227-228

Membrane Receptors, 19, 30, 45

Meso-zeaxanthin, 48, 51-53, 127, 154, 158-159, 164, 182, 206, 217, 222-223

Multifocal Electroretingram, 211, 214

N

Neovascularization, 1, 4, 52, 63-64, 66, 74, 76, 102, 111, 150, 192, 209-210, 219

Nutritional Supplement, 1, 16, 63, 74, 76, 153, 157, 178

O

Octogenarians, 4, 16, 63-64, 74, 76

Opsins, 18-21, 24-26, 29, 36, 84

Oxidative Stress, 3-4, 47, 53, 60, 94, 102, 154, 176, 186-187, 207, 209, 213, 219, 226, 228

P

Pathogenesis, 42, 60, 120, 143, 153, 215, 226, 228

Phenolics, 162, 164, 168-171

Phenotype, 33, 38, 43, 45, 86, 89-90, 95

Phospholipids, 51, 206

Photoprotection, 162-163, 166, 170-171, 173-174, 176, 179-180

Photoreceptor, 5, 15, 18-21, 24-26, 28-29, 31, 33-36, 38-39, 42, 44-45, 74-75, 80, 84-88, 90-91, 96-98, 102, 154, 164, 169-170, 175, 178-179, 192, 201, 207-209, 212, 215, 222-223, 226, 228-229

Photoreceptor Cell, 21, 28, 39, 42, 87, 91, 169, 175, 212, 223

Photosensitizer, 172-173

Phototransduction, 85, 87, 91, 96, 205, 226

Physical Inactivity, 171

Pigment Abnormalities, 52, 105, 126, 128-130, 132-133, 137, 139, 141

Polyunsaturated Fat, 114

R

Reactive Oxygen Species, 4, 46, 48, 165, 168-171, 173, 207-208, 212-213

Regenerative Capacity, 63, 75

Resveratrol, 1-3, 16-17, 63-65, 77-78, 177, 190

Retina, 5-7, 10-14, 16, 18-20, 24, 27-29, 34-36, 38, 43, 45-49, 51-53, 57-58, 60, 63-64, 66, 73, 75-76, 78, 80, 82-89, 91-92, 94, 97, 102, 154-155, 159-160, 164, 166, 173-174, 179, 181-183, 186, 190, 192-193, 195, 200-201, 205-207, 209, 211-212, 215-218, 222, 224-226, 228

Retinal Detachment, 192, 212, 215, 220

Retinitis Pigmentosa, 26, 36, 39, 80-81, 98, 205

Retinoic Acid, 19, 27-29, 34, 40-42, 45, 81, 83-85, 93-94, 99, 175

Retinoid, 18-19, 21, 25-30, 34-35, 37-38, 40, 43-44, 81-88, 90-98

Retinoid Storage, 30, 44, 84

Retinoid Toxicity, 28

Retinol, 18-19, 27-32, 40-45, 61, 80-87, 90, 92-98, 131-132, 212, 215, 217, 220

Retinol Binding Protein, 18, 30, 41, 43, 45, 82, 95

Retinyl Ester, 29, 31-32, 44, 82, 85, 89, 94-96

Rhodopsin, 20-22, 24-25, 34-35, 38-39, 84-85, 91, 97-99, 162-163, 171, 173, 179

S

Saturated Fat, 116-117, 120

Small Intestine, 31-32, 82, 93-95

Spectral Domain, 1, 4, 6, 67, 189-191

U

Uveitis, 205, 213-215, 221

V

Vegetable Fat, 119-120

Visual Cycle, 24-27, 37-38, 42-43, 80-81, 84-90, 93, 96-97

Visual Function, 1, 5-6, 9, 12, 15, 64, 67, 71, 74, 76-77, 85, 98, 127, 148, 155, 158, 174, 189, 192-194, 201-204, 212, 216, 222-223, 227-228

Visual Performance, 99, 148, 175, 216, 220, 222-225, 227-228

Visual Pigments, 19-22, 24-25, 27, 30, 34-35, 37, 80, 84-85, 96

X

Xanthophylls, 49-50, 53, 57-58, 60-61, 82, 148, 154, 163-167, 170-174, 178, 180, 203, 207, 209, 215, 228

Z

Zeaxanthin, 46-62, 65, 77, 120-129, 131, 135-136, 142, 145-149, 154-155, 158-171, 173-182, 187-189, 191-192, 200-203, 205-220, 222-223, 227-229

www.ingramcontent.com/pod-product-compliance
Lightning Source LLC
LaVergne TN
LVHW060531210926
848485LV00005B/1184